Public Bioethics

Public Bioethics

Principles and Problems

JAMES F. CHILDRESS

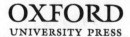

OXFORD
UNIVERSITY PRESS

OXFORD
UNIVERSITY PRESS

Oxford University Press is a department of the University of Oxford. It furthers
the University's objective of excellence in research, scholarship, and education
by publishing worldwide. Oxford is a registered trade mark of Oxford University
Press in the UK and certain other countries.

Published in the United States of America by Oxford University Press
198 Madison Avenue, New York, NY 10016, United States of America.

© Oxford University Press 2020

Library of Congress Cataloging-in-Publication Data
Names: Childress, James F., author.
Title: Public bioethics : principles and problems / James F. Childress.
Description: New York, NY : Oxford University Press, [2020] |
Includes bibliographical references and index.
Identifiers: LCCN 2019038641 (print) | LCCN 2019038642 (ebook) |
ISBN 9780199798483 (hbk) | ISBN 9780197504253 (epub) |
ISBN 9780199798544 (updf) | ISBN 9780197504260 (online)
Subjects: MESH: Bioethical Issues | Public Policy |
Organ Transplantation—ethics | Religion and Medicine
Classification: LCC R724 (print) | LCC R724 (ebook) | NLM WB 60 |
DDC 174.2—dc23
LC record available at https://lccn.loc.gov/2019038641
LC ebook record available at https://lccn.loc.gov/2019038642

1 3 5 7 9 8 6 4 2

Printed by Integrated Books International, United States of America

To my wife Marcia Day Childress

To my grandchildren Ian, Anna, Eric, and Ella Childress

Contents

IV. ETHICS IN PUBLIC HEALTH POLICY

Acknowledgments

I am deeply indebted to numerous individuals and institutions for their substantial contributions to my research and reflections in the chapters that follow. I am particularly grateful for the many illuminating conversations, debates, and deliberations with members of the public bioethics bodies mentioned in the Introduction as well as others not specifically mentioned. Many other individuals have also contributed greatly to this volume, often without knowing that they were doing so. Not surprisingly, I owe a tremendous debt to my long-time collaborator, Tom L. Beauchamp, for a rich, fruitful, enduring, and highly enjoyable partnership through eight editions of *Principles of Biomedical Ethics*, 1979 to the present (the eighth edition is scheduled to appear in late 2019).

Among my numerous valued colleagues at the University of Virginia (UVA)—an institution that has provided a wonderful academic home for me for nearly fifty years—I am particularly grateful to the late John Arras, the late John Fletcher, Larry Bouchard, and Margaret Mohrmann. Ruth Gaare Bernheim has been a most valuable colleague at the Institute for Practical Ethics and Public life at UVA as well as a splendid collaborator on essays and a book in public health ethics. I have also greatly benefited from co-teaching several different courses with her, including courses on public health ethics and law with her and with Richard Bonnie; courses on ethical and legal reasoning in public policy with Bonnie; and seminars on environmental ethics with Jon Cannon. Years earlier I learned much from co-teaching courses on law and bioethics with Patricia King at the Georgetown University Law Center. All these have enriched my reflections on ethics and public policy, and I am grateful to them, as well as to my many colleagues on the UVA Hospital Ethics Committee with whom I have served with pleasure over the last thirty-five years.

Several visiting fellowships provided valuable financial and intellectual support for the preparation of chapters in this book. In 1999–2000, I was a visiting scholar in the Department of Clinical Bioethics at the National Institutes of Health, which provided a remarkably congenial and stimulating environment for bioethical reflection, thanks to Ezekiel Emanuel, the director at the time, and several other colleagues who were generous with their time and ideas. In 2010 (January–May), I held the Carey and Ann Maguire

Chair in American History and Ethics at the Library of Congress, which provided a wonderful opportunity for interactions across various disciplines and allowed for the preparation of the initial drafts of chapters 6 and 13. In May–June 2011 and again for three weeks in 2016, I was a visiting fellow at the Center for Advanced Study in Bioethics at the University of Münster in Münster, Germany. Not only did I work on a number of the chapters in this book on these (and other briefer) visits but also I presented and discussed earlier versions of several of them, particularly chapters 1, 2, 6, 7, 8, and 13, in lectures and seminars and received rigorous and rich feedback that greatly improved the final versions. I cannot adequately thank Bettina Schöne-Seifert, Michael Quante, Thomas Gutmann, and several other colleagues in Münster for their intellectual and social hospitality. Ruth Langer, an administrator at the Center, ensured that my wife and I would have wonderful memories of our time there.

While I was working on these chapters, several graduate students in the Department of Religious Studies at UVA were very helpful, as teaching assistants in my large lecture course Theology, Ethics, and Healthcare, as research assistants, and as conversation partners in and outside seminars. I especially thank Matthew Puffer, Travis Pickell, Mark Storslee, and Laura Alexander, among several others.

Several chapters directly benefited from discussions with different individuals and audiences, and I have attempted to acknowledge these contributions in each chapter.

Finally, most of these chapters, especially when first delivered as lectures or papers, were greatly improved, both substantively and stylistically, by thoughtful criticisms and suggestions offered by my wife, Marcia Day Childress, to whom I owe so much. I dedicate this volume to her and to my grandchildren Ian, Anna, Eric, and Ella Childress.

James F. Childress
Charlottesville, VA
March 15, 2019

Public Bioethics

Introduction

On Doing Public Bioethics

This volume is devoted to "public bioethics."[1] This phrase often refers to doing bioethics with primary attention to public policy, defined as "whatever governments choose to do or not to do."[2] Public bioethics involves analyzing ethical issues in biomedicine, healthcare, and public health in terms of their implications for public policy and proposing public policies to address those issues. The chapters that follow are largely directed at the analysis and assessment of different actual and proposed public policies that implicate bioethical issues, with some attention to public culture and discourse and, at times, to professional culture and practice as well. While analyzing and evaluating public policy is generally considered the primary task in doing public bioethics, reshaping public discourse and public culture is an important goal in and of itself as well as a way to influence public policy.

"Public bioethics" also refers to commissions, councils, task forces, and the like, that are governmentally established, sponsored, or funded for the purpose of deliberating collectively about bioethical issues, again with a primary goal of recommending public policies. This second understanding of public bioethics is also important for this volume. Most chapters grow out of, some reflect on, and all are profoundly shaped by my experiences as a participant in several public bioethics bodies, mainly at the national level in the United States. The processes of publicly deliberating in a group about bioethical issues and appropriate policies and of publicly justifying collective recommendations have been profoundly important for my work.

"Public bioethics body" in this book most commonly refers to a commission or other entity formally established, sponsored, or funded by public authorities to offer guidance about public policies related to ethical concerns in biomedicine, healthcare, and public health. In this conception, a body doing public bioethics is authorized by and responsible, in some way and to some extent, to public authorities.[3] By contrast, other important societal mechanisms to address bioethical issues may be nongovernmental and may be less directed at public policy in a narrow sense. Such groups have a variety of structures, mechanisms, and sponsors.[4] They often focus on institutional, organizational, or professional culture and policy as well as on public culture and discourse. Examples include hospital ethics committees aimed at institutional or organizational policy or ethics committees for professional societies. While such bodies play a subordinate role in the chapters that follow, they have helped to set the context for and to shape my reflections.[5]

In general, contributors to public bioethics, whether as members of or consultants to public bodies or as individual ethicists, analyze bioethical issues, based on careful and thorough interpretations of the factual circumstances, in light of relevant ethical principles and values embedded in the society's history and culture; deliberate about public policies in relation to those principles and values, seeking to resolve any conflicts that may arise; and formulate what they deem to be ethically justifiable public policies in the circumstances. In a non-ideal world, they also pay attention to questions of feasibility.

Public Bioethics: Structures and Personal Experiences

Three main types of structures have been used for public bioethics at the national level, with parallels at state and local levels.[6] Each has distinct advantages and disadvantages. The first is a standing commission, with a broad mandate and rather lengthy term as well as the discretion to identify specific areas for attention. A major advantage of a standing commission is that it has time to mature as a deliberative body, to develop effective practices of collective deliberation, and to build valuable relations of internal trust and cooperation and external credibility. It can also address a range of bioethical issues, often interrelated, over time and be prepared to quickly address new issues when they emerge. For instance, following the announcement of the birth of the cloned sheep "Dolly," President Clinton gave the National Bioethics Advisory Commission (NBAC), which had held its inaugural meeting a few months earlier, ninety days to prepare a report and make recommendations on possible federal policies toward human reproductive cloning. (See the discussion in chapter 5.)

A second type is a commission or committee with a more focused, targeted, and limited mandate to address a particular topic or issue, such as organ transplantation, human fetal tissue transplantation research, or human embryo research. It is usually ad hoc rather than standing. A major advantage of such a focused body is that members can be selected on the basis of their potential contributions to the specific task at hand, which can then be pursued with sufficient expertise and concentrated attention. It may still take some time for such a body to develop effective deliberative capacity and credibility.

A third possibility is the use of nongovernmental committees to produce reports and make recommendations about public policies. The specific studies undertaken by consensus committees under the auspices of the Institute of Medicine (IOM), renamed the National Academy of Medicine (NAM), of the National Academies of Science, Engineering, and Medicine provide one such model.[7] Often set up in response to requests from and with support of federal departments or agencies such as the Food and Drug Administration or the National Institutes of Health, these independent committees prepare consensus reports, usually on specific subjects, such as gene-editing technologies, novel techniques for prevention of maternal transmission of mitochondrial DNA diseases, and organ donor intervention research. Such committees may appear to be more independent and less political than commissions appointed by a governmental body. However, they do have a distinct disadvantage: while they may include public members along with experts, they develop findings, conclusions, and recommendations through processes that are generally less open than those of governmentally established bioethics commissions. Thus, while these committees may appear to be more objective and impartial, they are also less publicly transparent.

I have learned much about public bioethics from serving on all three types of committees.[8] In my judgment, each can contribute significantly to governmental policy-making as well as to shaping public culture and professional practice. This is not the place to do more than note their general advantages and disadvantages. Nor is this the place for a detailed evaluation of the successes and failures of different public bioethics bodies.[9] Which type is best for a particular problem may depend on several factors, including the problem's nature and urgency; its social, cultural, and political context; and the importance of process values such as efficiency, transparency, and public engagement.

Several chapters in this volume were directly influenced by my participation in particular public bioethics bodies—especially NBAC, which was appointed by President Clinton and ably chaired by Harold Shapiro, president of Princeton University—and by presenting oral or written testimony to several predecessor and successor standing national bioethics commissions.[10] In addition, I draw on my experience on other governmentally established bodies that addressed specific bioethical issues. These include standing bodies with specific responsibilities, such as the Recombinant DNA Advisory Committee and the Human Gene Therapy Subcommittee, as well as ad hoc bodies, such as committees for the Office of Technology Assessment, the US Organ Transplantation Task Force (for which I served as vice chair), and the Human Fetal Tissue Transplantation Research Panel.[11] Other public policy bodies also provided important contexts for my reflections, including the United Network for Organ Sharing (UNOS), a private contractor for the Organ Procurement and Transplantation Network (OPTN); I served a term on its board of directors and three terms on its Ethics Committee. I draw too on my experience with the third type of committee noted previously, specifically, committees for the Institute of Medicine, now the National Academy of Medicine, of the National Academies of Sciences, Engineering, and Medicine. I have served on and chaired or cochaired several of these committees, which offer independent advice about public policy.[12]

It is crucial not to overemphasize the role or contribution of academic or professional ethicists for public bioethics bodies. Ethical reflection is not limited to moral, social, or political philosophers or moral theologians, even though that is what these professionals largely emphasize and do. Public bioethics, as I sometimes say, is too important to be left to professional ethicists. In my experience, practical moral insight and wisdom come from a variety of sources—professional ethicists have no corner on that market in collective public deliberation or elsewhere. Hence, it is a mistake to confuse the role of *ethicists* with the role of *ethics* in the formation of public policy.

Nevertheless, ethicists can and often do make significant contributions to the deliberations of public bioethics bodies. First, their familiarity with traditions, methods, and patterns of moral reflection, including a variety of theories that can illuminate ethical controversies, possibilities, and limits, can be helpful in the deliberations of a public bioethics body. Second, they can bring practiced skills in analyzing the logic of moral discourse to particular domains, such as the biological sciences, medicine, healthcare, and public health, all domains examined in bioethics.[13] The processes of bioethics in general and public bioethics in particular are necessarily multidisciplinary and multiprofessional—ideally, interdisciplinary and interprofessional—and the academic or professional ethicist can and should contribute rigorously, creatively, openly, and humbly what he or she can to these processes.

The following chapters reflect the interactions between my experiences as a participant in the work of public bioethics bodies, both contributing to and learning greatly from the processes, and my scholarly ethical analyses and assessments of public policies regarding biomedicine, healthcare, and public health.

Overview of Chapters

Part I, "Principles and Reasoning in Public Bioethics," starts with two chapters that examine selected ethical principles for public policies related to the biological sciences, medicine, and healthcare. Presupposing the framework of *Principles of Biomedical Ethics*,[14] these chapters focus on respect for personal autonomy and on paternalism, based on beneficence/nonmaleficence. Although not developed in Part I, principles of justice and fairness, particularly in the distribution of benefits and burdens, are featured and explicated in subsequent chapters, especially in chapter 9 on organ allocation, chapter 10 on the terrain of public health ethics, and chapter 12 on triage in a public health crisis. Likewise, the principle of utility receives considerable attention later, particularly in those three chapters and in chapter 13 on John Stuart Mill's ethical framework for public health.

Chapter 1, "Respecting Personal Autonomy in Bioethics: Relational Autonomy as a Corrective?," unpacks the dominant, but thin and procedural, conception of the principle of respect for personal autonomy in the context of a medical and legal decision to allow a fourteen-year-old Jehovah's Witness boy to refuse a blood transfusion needed to extend his life. It argues that thicker conceptions of autonomy, closely connected with relational autonomy, can enable us to see more clearly aspects of respect for autonomy too often neglected or downplayed in bioethics. These help us to understand better the interpretive complexity of the principle of respect for autonomy by directing attention beyond a person's immediate decision in the moment to the broader context of relations that in part shape such decisions and to the temporal extensions of the self. It is important not to convert these valuable indicators for respecting autonomous choices and actions into necessary conditions that are too high and too demanding—such a maneuver would deprive ordinary decision-makers of the protection and support needed for their autonomous choices and actions, even to the extent of creating the specter of paternalistic interventions in the name of thicker conceptions of autonomy.

Chapter 2, "Paternalism in Healthcare and Health Policy," seeks to provide conceptual clarity along with a framework for ethically assessing paternalistic actions in both clinical practice and health policy. Not only does paternalism remain common and formidable in both contexts but it has also gained new momentum over the last two decades, for instance, as "neopaternalists" have offered arguments for governmental policies that, at a minimum, seek to protect or benefit individuals through shaping or steering their choices without actually limiting or coercing those choices. This chapter examines the nature of paternalism, particularly by probing its moral foundations and limits and drawing several distinctions that bear on its justification (weak and strong, pure and mixed, hard and soft). It also considers circumstances in which different types of paternalistic interventions may be justified, and, finally, assesses the "new paternalism," based on behavioral economics and psychology, that now figures in many proposals for health-related public policies.

The third chapter in Part I is titled "Narratives versus Norms: A Misplaced Debate in Bioethics?" If properly understood, both narratives, including cases, and norms, including principles and rules, are essential and indispensable to ethics—the difficult questions concern their relations. This chapter attends first to the controversy about cases and case judgments in relation to principles, showing that the debate is largely misplaced. Then, using the well-known case of Donald/Dax Cowart, it stresses the role of narratives in interpreting the requirements of the principle of respect for persons and their autonomous choices. Finally, it examines the value of and tensions between personal and communal narratives as reflected in appeals to personal experience and appeals to principles and rules embedded in societal narratives, particularly shaping public policy.

The chapters in Part II, "Religion, Bioethics, and Public Policy," seek to determine the appropriate place, if any, for religious convictions in the formulation of public policies related to bioethical issues in a pluralistic, democratic society and in the exemptions of conscientious objectors from performing certain procedures or providing certain services.

Chapter 4, "Religion, Bioethics, and Public Policy: Debates about Secularization," begins by analyzing and evaluating two stories about the role of religion in the origin and development of bioethics and about the putative secularization of bioethics. Both stories employ different conceptions of religion, and neglect the range and diversity of bioethics in the United States. Both stories, inaccurate and inadequate in different ways, claim that religion has only a limited place in contemporary bioethics in part as a result of putatively excessive attention to public bioethics and to principles-based reasoning in that context. The chapter then critically examines a prominent and sometimes illuminating but ultimately flawed interpretation of the secularization of public bioethics offered by the sociologist John H. Evans in *Playing God? Human Genetic Engineering and the Rationalization of Public Bioethical Debate*. Much of the controversy featured in this chapter hinges on claims about whether the increasingly prominent role of principles-based reasoning in bioethics, especially in public bioethics, has contributed to and/ or reflected a process of secularization.

Chapter 5, "Religion, Morality, and Public Policy: The Controversy about Human Cloning," explores how religious convictions function in the debate about whether human reproductive cloning should be banned, regulated, or permitted—a debate that erupted in 1997 following the belated announcement of "Dolly's" birth in the previous year. This historical case study examines and assesses the arguments that arose at the time, particularly in the context of NBAC's deliberations and its report, *Cloning Human Beings*. The NBAC hearings included testimony on religious views on human reproductive cloning, and its report examined and assessed those views. The chapter also considers NBAC's deliberations about federal funding of human embryonic stem cell research that further illuminates the place of religious convictions in public bioethics. It concludes that in public bioethics the *process* of reaching a decision—or, in NBAC's case, a recommendation—should attend to the widest possible range of positions and rationales, but that the *outcome* in substance and in public justification needs to involve, as Robert Audi argues, a *sufficient* or *adequate* secular reason.

Chapter 6, "Conscientious Refusals in Healthcare: Protecting Health Professionals' Consciences and Patients' Interests," focuses not on the ethics of individual conscientious refusals but rather on ethically justified responses of institutions, organizations, and governments to such refusals. It asks under what conditions, if any, the state, society, institutions, and professions should exempt conscientiously objecting healthcare professionals from performing procedures or providing services or products that they find objectionable but that are legal and patient-sought. Using several cases and drawing several distinctions (e.g., religious and/or moral objections, and universal and selective objections), this chapter employs the metaphor of constrained balancing to develop a framework for accommodating many conscientious refusals, as distinguished from conscientious obstructions. At a minimum, this balance requires disclosure of information about options in all cases and referral/transfer of patients in certain cases. This chapter also identifies ways to resolve ongoing debates about expansive claims of complicity or unacceptable participation in wrongdoing sometimes invoked by conscientious objectors.[15]

Part III, "Deceased Organ Donation and Allocation," covers interrelated topics that I have long attended to in public bioethics and in my publications. My first article ("Who Shall Live When Not All Can Live?"[16]) grew out of a 1970 interdisciplinary and interprofessional faculty seminar at the University of Virginia that focused on policies regarding artificial and transplantable organs. Subsequent and varied public policy experiences related to organ donation and allocation have further shaped my views and sharpened my arguments.[17]

Chapter 7 is titled "Difficulties of Determining Death: What Should We Do about the 'Dead Donor Rule'?" Widely considered the "ethical linchpin" for the system of voluntary deceased organ donation that depends on public trust, the "Dead Donor Rule" (DDR) and its operation presuppose that the line between life and death can be reliably drawn for purposes of removing vital organs for transplantation. Different but serious conceptual, scientific, and ethical questions surround deceased donation after neurological determination of death and after circulatory determination of death in either controlled or uncontrolled forms. This chapter examines the ethical implications of different approaches to the DDR and asks which public policy should be adopted: (1) abandon the DDR and move to living vital organ donation; (2) retain the DDR but view the determination of death as a legal fiction; (3) retain the DDR but expand individual/familial choices of conceptions of and criteria for determining death; or (4) retain and strengthen the DDR and ethically improve its operation. Attending to both the truthfulness and the probable consequences of different policies, this chapter argues for the fourth option and for improving the process of individual and familial informed consent to deceased organ donation.

In light of the large and persistent gap between the supply of deceased donor organs for transplantation and the number of patients on the waiting list for a transplant, chapter 8, "The Failure to Give: Facilitating First-Person Deceased Organ Donation," first considers different ethical frameworks for evaluating first-person failures to donate organs after death and then assesses selected public policies designed to overcome these failures. Policies to facilitate first-person deceased organ donation often seek to alter the individual's risk/cost-benefit calculations in deciding whether to register as a donor (for instance, by providing financial incentives); these can be ethically justifiable under some circumstances if they encourage donation but do not implicate the sale of organs. Other proposed policies seek to nudge the individual's declaration of organ donation through mandated choice or required response or through opt-out policies, often called "presumed consent," under which not opting out counts as a donative decision. Available evidence suggests that mandated choice, required response, and presumed consent would probably be ineffective and perhaps even counterproductive in the United States at this time, but that some carefully designed combination could possibly be both ethically acceptable and effective.

Chapter 9, "Putting Patients First in Organ Allocation: An Ethical Analysis of Policy Debates in the United States," originated in my testimony before a congressional hearing on organ allocation policy. The ethical issues it addresses remain in play, as evidenced in the 2018–2019 debates about liver allocation policy. This chapter defends the fundamental conviction of the report of the Task Force on Organ Transplantation: Donated organs should be viewed as scarce public resources to be used for the welfare of the community. Organ procurement and transplant teams receive donated organs as "trustees" and "stewards" on behalf of the whole community, that is, the national community (with qualifications). Donated organs should be allocated to patients anywhere in the country according to ethically acceptable standards and logistical constraints, thus reducing the relevance of "accidents of geography" except where these are clearly important for transplantation outcomes. In short, patients, not transplant programs, should be put first. In accord with principles of justice and fairness, it is important to specify and balance, through a public process with public input, several criteria in policies of organ allocation: patient need and probability of successful outcome, along with time on the waiting list. Unless the criteria for patient selection are fair and are perceived to be fair, public distrust may hamper organ donation and perpetuate the scarcity of organs for transplantation.

Part IV is titled "Ethics in Public Health Policy." My public policy involvement in this area has been more on state and local levels, particularly in exploring the allocation of scarce resources in possible pandemics, for instance, of influenza.[18] Chapter 10, which grew out of a Greenwall Foundation–funded working group of a dozen or so ethicists, lawyers, and public health practitioners, provides a rough conceptual map of the terrain of public health ethics. It examines the nature of public health and public health interventions, and it identifies a number of general moral considerations (principles) relevant to public health policy and practice and often, especially as articulated in basic human rights, promotive of public health. Because these moral considerations are general and broad, they require specification and weighting. In cases of conflict, five "justificatory conditions" need to be met: effectiveness, proportionality, necessity, least infringement, and public justification. These conditions help to determine whether protecting or promoting public health warrants overriding individual liberty in particular situations.

Chapter 11, "Public Health and Civil Liberties: Resolving Conflicts," considers public health ethics in a particular context—a liberal, pluralistic, democratic society that embodies explicit commitments to several basic civil liberties: bodily integrity, privacy, freedom of movement, freedom of association, and freedom of religion and conscience. When civil liberties set limits on public health interventions, a presumptivist framework is more defensible and helpful than either an absolutist or a contextualist one for determining appropriate interventions. This framework recognizes several conditions for rebutting the presumption, in certain circumstances, against interventions that infringe civil liberties. Through an exploration of the metaphor of the Intervention Ladder, proposed by the Nuffield Council on Bioethics, this chapter examines several possible ways to secure individuals' cooperation with public health measures, such as vaccinations, directly observed therapy, and quarantine, without infringing their civil liberties. It is often possible to achieve compliance through expressing rather than imposing community.

Chapter 12 examines triage in a public health crisis resulting from a bioterrorist attack. Systems of triage, whether informal or formal, generally have an implicit or explicit utilitarian rationale—they are usually designed to produce the greatest good for the greatest number under conditions of scarcity. In a utilitarian framework, it is important to distinguish *medical utility* from *social utility* and, within the latter, between broad and narrow social utilitarian judgments. Judgments of *broad* social utility recognize the differential social value of people's lives, taken as a whole, while judgments of *narrow* social utility recognize the differential value of specific social functions and roles and assign priority to the individuals discharging certain functions and performing certain roles. Judgments of broad social utility infringe the egalitarian principle of equal regard in a way that judgments of medical utility do not. While it is not justifiable to use broad social utility as a basis for rationing in general or in an emergency, it is possible to justify triage based on medical utility and also on narrow social utility, at least when focused on specific and urgent functions and essential services in a public health crisis. My arguments presuppose a context of public justification: transparency, participation, and cooperation. Public trust will be essential in any public health crisis—hence, the public needs to have confidence in the procedures and standards of triage.

Chapter 13 shows that the controversial legacy of John Stuart Mill's ethical framework for public health is far more complex and interesting than his *On Liberty* suggests, even when that classic work is properly understood. A largely neglected resource in Mill's thought for public health is the ethical framework he actually used, in public testimony and correspondence, to address a heated controversy about the British government's efforts in the Contagious Diseases Acts to reduce the transmission of sexually transmitted diseases. This displays his fuller range of ethical principles for public health, the way he resolved conflicts among those principles, and his somewhat surprising reluctance to endorse what we now call "harm-reduction measures," which many utilitarians, but not Mill, generally find justifiable in public health policy and practice.

Publication History of Chapters

Five chapters were totally or largely written expressly for this volume, while others are republished with modifications as needed. I am grateful to the original publishers for permission to use previously published essays in whole or in part and in unrevised or revised form in this volume.

Chapter 1, "Respecting Personal Autonomy in Bioethics: Relational Autonomy as a Corrective?," has not been previously published. It was originally prepared for and presented at an international conference, "Thick (Concepts of) Autonomy?," University of Münster, Münster, Germany, October 18–20, 2012.

Chapter 2, "Paternalism in Healthcare and Health Policy," originally appeared under this title in *Principles of Health Care Ethics*, 2nd ed., edited by Richard E. Ashcroft, Angus Dawson, Heather Draper, and John McMillan (Chichester, UK: John Wiley & Sons, 2007), pp. 223–231. I thank John Wiley

& Sons for permission to use this chapter, which appears with only minor modifications.

Chapter 3, "Narratives versus Norms: A Misplaced Debate in Bioethics?" appeared under a slightly different title in *Stories and Their Limits*, edited by Hilde Nelson (New York: Routledge, 1997), pp. 252–271. I thank the Taylor and Francis Group for permission to republish this chapter with a few modifications.

Chapter 4, "Religion, Bioethics, and Public Policy: Debates about Secularization," was written specifically for this volume; it incorporates, with permission, much of "An Illuminating and Important but Flawed Analysis: A Critical Response to John Evans' *Playing God*," *Journal of the Society of Christian Ethics* 24 (2004): 195–204.

An earlier version of chapter 5, "Religion, Morality, and Public Policy: The Controversy about Human Cloning," was previously published under the same title in Dena S. Davis and Laurie Zoloth, eds., *Notes from a Narrow Ridge: Religion and Bioethics* (Hagerstown, MD: University Publishing Group, 1999), pp. 65–85. I am grateful to the University Publishing Group for permission to republish much of the earlier version with substantial revisions and additions.

Chapter 6, "Conscientious Refusals in Healthcare: Protecting Health Professionals' Consciences and Patients' Interests," was written for this volume and is published here for the first time.

Chapter 7, "Difficulties of Determining Death: What Should We Do about the 'Dead Donor Rule'?," was first published by *Zentrum für interdisziplinäre Forschung* (ZiF) 1 (2014): 28–39 and is here used by permission with several changes and additions.

Chapter 8, "The Failure to Give: Facilitating First-Person Deceased Organ Donation," was written specifically for this volume. It incorporates several paragraphs, substantially revised, from my earlier article, "The Failure to Give Life: Reducing Barriers to Organ Donation," Hellegers Lecture, Kennedy Institute of Ethics, *Kennedy Institute of Ethics Journal* 11, No. 1 (2001): 1–16.

Chapter 9, "Putting Patients First in Organ Allocation: An Ethical Analysis of Policy Debates in the United States," was published previously in *Cambridge Quarterly of Health Care Ethics* 10, No. 4 (October 2001): 365–376, and, with the journal's permission, is published here with only a few revisions.

Chapter 10, "Public Health Ethics: Mapping the Terrain," authored by James F. Childress, Ruth Faden, Ruth Gaare (Bernheim), et al., was originally published in the *Journal of Law, Medicine, and Ethics* 30, No. 2 (Summer

2002): 170–178. The journal has kindly granted permission to reprint this essay in this volume.

Chapter 11, "Public Health and Civil Liberties: Resolving Conflicts," was previously published in *Routledge Companion to Bioethics*, ed. John Arras, Elizabeth Fenton, and Rebecca Kukla (New York: Routledge, 2015), pp. 325–338. I thank the Taylor and Francis Group for permission to reprint this chapter.

Chapter 12, "Triage in a Public Health Crisis: The Case of a Bioterrorist Attack," appeared under the title "Triage in Response to a Bioterrorist Attack" in *In the Wake of Terror: Medicine and Morality in a Time of Crisis*, ed. Jonathan D. Moreno (Cambridge, MA: MIT Press, 2003), pp. 77–93. I am grateful to The MIT Press for permission to republish this chapter in this volume with modest alterations.

Chapter 13, "John Stuart Mill's Legacy for Public Health Ethics: *On Liberty and Beyond*," was written specifically for this volume.

Notes

1. I have tended to use the phrase "biomedical ethics," rather than "bioethics." See Tom L. Beauchamp and James F. Childress, *Principles of Biomedical Ethics*, 7th edition (New York: Oxford University Press, 2013). However, for economy of expression in this work, I mainly use "bioethics." My late colleague, John C. Fletcher, may have coined the phrase "public bioethics" in his "On Restoring Public Bioethics," *Politics and the Life Sciences* 13 (1994): 84–86. For an attribution of this phrase to Fletcher, see Adam Briggle, *A Rich Bioethics: Public Policy, Biotechnology, and the Kass Council* (Notre Dame, IN: University of Notre Dame Press, 2010), p. 182, fn. 15.
2. Thomas Dye, *Understanding Public Policy*, 15th edition (New York: Pearson, 2016), p. 2. Slightly different statements of this definition appear in different editions.
3. See Alfred Moore, "Public Bioethics and Public Engagement: The Politics of 'Proper Talk,'" *Public Understanding of Science* 99, No. 2 (2010): 197–211. He defines "public bioethics as a complex of institutions, practices and discourses, whose purpose is to connect policy-making with ethical considerations and ethical deliberations, in order to improve political decision-making, and which have a direct or indirect connection to the state, that is, in one way or another initiated, supported, controlled, or commissioned by state actors. Public bioethics can be contrasted with academic, clinical, or corporate bioethics, according to their institutional locations. In a more positive sense we can say that public bioethics refers to the whole range of bodies and procedures, such as national ethics councils, parliamentary ethics commissions, or public consultations on "ethical issues," that are meant to inform and guide political decision-making with respect to ethical considerations."

4. See Ruth Ellen Bulger, Elizabeth Meyer Bobby, and Harvey V. Fineberg, eds., for the Committee on the Social and Ethical Impacts of Developments in Biomedicine, *Society's Choices: Social and Ethical Decision Making in Biomedicine* (Washington, DC: National Academies Press, 1995), pp. 1–2.

5. For instance, the work of the Ethics Committee of the American College of Obstetrics and Gynecology helped to stimulate public and professional debate and federal policy development regarding conscientious refusals by health professionals in reproductive medicine. See chapter 6.

6. Some of the ideas and language in the following four paragraphs are drawn from my "Reflections on the National Bioethics Advisory Commission and Models of Public Bioethics," *Goals and Practice of Pubic Bioethics: Reflections on National Bioethics Commissions*, special report, *Hastings Center Report* 47, no. 3 (May–June 2017): S20–S23, and from "The Bioethical Approach," in the Miller Center's project First Year 2017, presenting a series of essays directed at the US president's first year. It appears at http://www.firstpyear2017.org/essay/the-bioethical-approach.

7. Formerly Institute of Medicine, now the National Academy of Medicine, one of three academies in the National Academies of Sciences, Medicine, and Engineering.

8. Even though I have here focused on the national level, there are, of course, parallel institutional mechanisms at state and local levels too. Most of my interactions with state committees, including the New York Task Force on Life and the Law, have consisted of written and/or oral presentations. Others include testimony to the Virginia State Medicaid Board on funding organ transplants and membership on the State Mandated Health Benefits Panel in Virginia.

9. There are vigorous debates about how successful such bodies are, especially the standing national commissions. I do not go into that debate other than in passing in chapter 5. For an international overview of commissions, see Michael Fuchs, *National Ethics Councils: Their Backgrounds, Functions, and Modes of Operation Compared* (Berlin: Nationaler Ethikrat, 2005). For an examination of possible criteria for evaluating national commissions, see Bulger, Bobby, and Fineberg, eds., *Society's Choices: Social and Ethical Decision Making in Biomedicine*, chaps. 5 and 6; and John Fletcher and Franklin Miller, "The Promise and Perils of Public Bioethics," in *The Ethics of Research Involving Human Subjects: Facing the 21st Century*, ed. Harold Vanderpool (Frederick, MD: University Publishing Group, 1996), pp. 155–184. For selected assessments of particular commissions and directions for future ones, see Elisa Eiseman, *The National Bioethics Advisory Commission: Contributing to Public Policy* (Arlington, VA: RAND Corporation, 2003); Briggle, *A Rich Bioethics: Public Policy, Biotechnology, and the Kass Council*; Jonathan D. Moreno and Sam Berger, eds., *Progress in Bioethics: Science, Policy, and Politics* (Cambridge, MA: MIT Press, 2010); and several valuable contributions to *Goals and Practice of Pubic Bioethics: Reflections on National Bioethics Commissions*, special report, *Hastings Center Report* 47, no. 3 (May–June, 2017): S1–S56.

10. I discuss NBAC in chapters 4 and 5. I also served on the Biomedical Ethics Advisory Committee (BEAC) under the congressional Biomedical Ethics Board—a short-lived body little known even to many in bioethics; for information about the BEAC,

see Bulger, Bobby, and Fineberg, eds., *Society's Choices: Social and Ethical Decision Making in Biomedicine*, pp. 6, 93–94, 436–437.

11. *Report of the Human Fetal Tissue Transplantation Research Panel*, Consultants to the Advisory Committee to the Director, National Institutes of Health, December, 1988, 2 vols. See Childress, "Ethics, Public Policy, and Human Fetal Tissue Transplantation Research," *Kennedy Institute of Ethics Journal* 1 (June 1991): 93–121, which also appears in significantly revised, expanded form in Childress, *Practical Reasoning in Bioethics* (Bloomington: Indiana University Press, 1998), chapter 16. See also Childress, "Consensus in Ethics and Public Policy: The Deliberations of the U.S. Human Fetal Tissue Transplantation Research Panel," in *The Concept of Consensus: The Case of Technology Intervention into Human Reproduction*, ed. Kurt Bayertz, Philosophy and Medicine Vol. 48 (Boston: Kluwer, 1994), pp. 164–188, and Childress, "Deliberations of the Human Fetal Tissue Transplantation Research Panel," a case study in *Biomedical Politics*, ed. Kathi Hanna (Washington, DC: National Academy Press, 1991).

12. In addition to chairing the IOM's Health Sciences Policy Board for three years, I have chaired, cochaired, or served on several consensus committees and workshop planning committees. For some of these, see note 17.

13. Leon Kass, the first chair of President's Council on Bioethics under President George W. Bush, emphasized that this was a "council on bioethics," rather than a "council of bioethicists." Leon Kass, Opening Remarks to the President's Council on Bioethics, Thursday, January 17, 2002, http://www.bioethics.gov/transcripts/jan02/jan17session1.html (accessed September 16, 2007). I generally agree with that orientation, but, to the best of my knowledge, no one has seriously proposed a "council of bioethicists," that is, a council limited to bioethicists. Moreover, that orientation does not—and should not—rule out a possible contribution, however limited it may be, of academic bioethicists or scholars from various fields who concentrate on the ethical issues that arise in the biological sciences, medicine, and healthcare.

14. For a fuller and more extended discussion of the relevant principles, see Beauchamp and Childress, *Principles of Biomedical Ethics*; the 8th edition is scheduled for publication in late 2019.

15. In addition to my long-standing interest in the topic of conscientious objection in several contexts, such as military service, this chapter was stimulated in part by the firestorm occasioned by the release of the report on "The Limits of Conscientious Refusal in Reproductive Medicine" by the American College of Obstetricians and Gynecologists (ACOG). This was Committee Opinion 385 from the ACOG Committee on Ethics. See *Obstetrics and Gynecology* 110 (2007): 1203–1208. I was a member of the ACOG ethics committee at the time of this report and failed to anticipate the controversy that erupted. Chapter 6 in this volume details this controversy at the level of public policy in the Bush, Obama, and Trump administrations. To avoid confusion, I should note that the name of this professional organization has since changed; it is now the American Congress of Obstetricians and Gynecologists rather than the American College of Obstetricians and Gynecologists.

16 PUBLIC BIOETHICS

16. "Who Shall Live When Not All Can Live?" *Soundings: An Interdisciplinary Journal* 53, No. 4 (Winter 1970): 339–355. It was reprinted in *Soundings: An Interdisciplinary Journal* 96, No. 3 (2013): 237–253, along with five response papers. It has also been reprinted in numerous anthologies.

17. In addition to testifying before congressional committees on both organ donation and organ allocation, I served as vice chair of the national Task Force on Organ Transplantation, which produced a report *Organ Transplantation: Issues and Recommendations* (Rockville, MD: US Department of Health and Human Services, Public Health Service, Health Resources and Services Administration, Office of Organ Transplantation, April 1986). Subsequently I served on the United Network for Organ Sharing (UNOS) Board of Directors and its Ethics Committee. I also chaired the Institute of Medicine (IOM) Committee on Increasing the Opportunities for Organ Donation, which produced a consensus report entitled *Organ Donation: Opportunities for Action*, edited by James F. Childress and Catharyn T. Liverman (Washington, DC: National Academies Press, 2006). Most recently, I chaired the Committee on Issues in Organ Donor Intervention Research for the Health and Medicine Division of the Board on Health Sciences Policy of the National Academies of Sciences, Engineering, and Medicine; for this consensus study report, see Childress, Sarah Domnitz, and Catharyn T. Liverman, eds., *Opportunities for Organ Donor Intervention Research: Saving Lives by Improving the Quality and Quantity of Organs for Transplantation* (Washington, DC: National Academies Press, 2017).

18. See Ruth Gaare Bernheim, James F. Childress, Richard J. Bonnie, and Alan L. Melnick, *Essentials of Public Health Ethics* (Burlington, MA: Jones and Bartlett Learning, LLC, 2015).

PART I
PRINCIPLES AND REASONING IN PUBLIC BIOETHICS

1

Respecting Personal Autonomy
in Bioethics

Relational Autonomy as a Corrective?

Crisis of Autonomy and Respect for Autonomy
in Bioethics

From its beginnings in the late 1960s and early 1970s, bioethics has stressed respect for the autonomy of patients and participants in research. This is not surprising—after all, bioethics emerged in part in reaction to centuries of medical paternalism and exploitation in research, and it was infected with a strongly individualistic orientation, particularly in the United States, the site and context of much of the early work in the field.

Now, however, autonomy and respect for autonomy are under attack— at least certain conceptions are under siege. Critics charge that proponents of autonomy—and many policies and practices in contemporary medicine, healthcare, and research that are supposedly based on respect for autonomy—make too much of autonomy, extend autonomy too far, and put too much weight on autonomy over against other ethical principles, such as benefiting the patient or protecting the society.

Critics also contend that much work in bioethics does not adequately characterize and interpret autonomous choices and that it thus distorts the processes of consent and refusal. From this standpoint, many conceptions of autonomous choice and consent/refusal—perhaps the dominant ones—are seen as

- too individualistic, in that they neglect the social context and relational aspects of autonomy;
- too rationalistic, because they ignore the nonrational and emotional aspects of autonomous choices;

- too legalistic, insofar as proponents devote too much attention to laws, regulations, and institutional rules rather than to social practices;
- too formalistic, in view of the excessive attention paid to consent forms over against the process of consent;
- too thin, a common critique of several of these putative deficiencies.

I will examine some key aspects of the standard thin conception of autonomy and respect for autonomy that have come under attack and then explore what one important thicker conception, that of relational autonomy, might add. I will argue that this thicker conception helpfully identifies several aspects of the development and exercise of personal autonomy that further complicate the practice of respect for autonomy. As illuminating and valuable as these insights are, it is important not to convert them into necessary conditions of autonomous choices and actions and of respect for autonomy.

The Principle of Respect for Autonomy

What does it mean to respect persons' autonomous choices and actions? This cumbersome formulation is more accurate and more adequate than the abstract formulation "respect for autonomy," and it's what I mean in this chapter when I use the phrase *respect for autonomy*.

What is involved in respecting autonomy, in the sense of autonomous choices and actions? "Respect" is more than an attitude; it involves actions. Some respectful actions can be stated negatively: *not* interfering with or attempting to interfere with the autonomous choices and actions of others, and *not* subjecting or trying to subject those choices to controlling influences.

Two major types of controlling influence are *manipulation of information* and *coercion*.[1] When persuasion fails, these two types of intervention are sometimes used in efforts to control others' actions. Manipulation of information may occur through nondisclosure or deception, while coercion involves a threat of some kind. These interventions are incompatible with respect for autonomous choices and actions. However, it is not inconsistent to say that we respect another person's autonomous choices and actions by noninterference while, at the same time, we try to persuade that person to act differently. It is not even inconsistent to use modes of influence, such as modest incentives and defaults, which shape action but do not control it.[2]

The first formulation of the principle of respect for autonomy (PRA) is negative. My version slightly modifies one offered by Ruth Faden and Tom Beauchamp: "it is prima facie wrong to subject or attempt to subject the actions (including the choices) of others to controlling influences."[3] The modifications include the addition of "prima facie" and "or attempt to subject" and "including the choices." This negative principle is expressed and specified in various concrete rights or duties—for example, the right to consent to or refuse medical treatments and the right to liberty of action.

Neither the PRA nor the several specified rights and duties can properly be viewed as absolute. They are at most prima facie binding—that is, they are binding, obligatory, other things being equal, and are sometimes justifiably overridden by other principles. An example is protecting public health in an epidemic of serious communicable disease through forcible quarantine against the autonomous choices and actions of recalcitrant citizens.

The PRA is not only negative. It also has clear *positive* implications in several contexts. In research, medicine, and healthcare, for instance—where there are fiduciary relations that involve significant differences in power and knowledge, such as the doctor–patient or researcher–subject relationship—the PRA engenders a positive or affirmative obligation to disclose information and to create the conditions for autonomous choices and actions, for instance, by promoting communication and comprehension. As a result, the PRA is reflected in rules of informed consent and refusal but it is not exhausted by or limited to those rules.

I will explore autonomous choices largely through their expression in consents and refusals. Autonomous choices are often made by autonomous persons, but they may also be made in particular situations by persons who would not be described generally or globally as autonomous persons.

Complexities in Respecting Autonomous Choices:
A Difficult Case

Even if we accept the PRA, it is neither easy nor simple to act on it. Far from being a mechanical task, respecting autonomous choices and actions is a difficult interpretive task, involving, for instance, judgments of competence or capacity, communication (disclosure of information, comprehension, and response), and voluntariness. This interpretive task entails attentive listening, imagination, discernment, and the like, and these are particularly important in determining what the patient or research subject is really saying. The following case provides a useful point of reference as we examine a few of the complexities of respecting persons' autonomous choices:

On November 28, 2007, Dennis Lindberg, age fourteen, died of the effects of acute lymphocytic leukemia and the treatments he was receiving after he refused, on religious grounds (Jehovah's Witness), a blood transfusion that, according to the physicians in this case, could have saved his life and allowed him to live for a few years. His refusal decision was approved by Superior Court Judge John Meyer, who denied a motion filed by the state of Washington to force Dennis to undergo the blood transfusion.

Lindberg was diagnosed with acute lymphocytic leukemia November 8, 2007, and chemotherapy was started but then was stopped because his red blood cell count dropped too low—a common side effect of chemotherapy. Hence the need for the blood transfusion. Medical reports provided to the judge indicated that, with the transfusion and other treatments, Dennis had a 70% chance of surviving the next five years.

This case was complicated by Dennis Lindberg's family circumstances. His biological parents wanted him to receive the transfusion, but they did not have legal custody of their son. The boy's legal guardian at the time of his death was his aunt, Dianna Mincin, with whom he had lived for four years, after his father, now a recovering addict, was jailed for drug possession. (According to some reports, both biological parents had been addicted to methamphetamine.) Ms. Mincin, who is a Jehovah's Witness, supported Dennis's decision to refuse a blood transfusion. Jehovah's Witnesses do not want to die in such cases—therefore, this was not a right-to-die case. Indeed, generally Jehovah's Witnesses accept most medical procedures and treatments, but reject blood transfusions for religious reasons.

Hospital administrators reported this case to the state, which then sought a court order to force the transfusion. Courts in the United States recognize the rights of adults to refuse potentially life-saving blood transfusions and other treatments on religious grounds, but they generally order blood transfusions when medically indicated for children even against parental objections. In reaching his decision, Judge Meyer heard from Dennis's parents, his aunt, social workers, and doctors. Dennis's doctors reportedly supported his decision. Judge Meyer determined that the eighth-grader was a mature minor, who understood that "he's basically giving himself a death sentence." The judge also said, "I don't think Dennis is trying to commit suicide. This isn't something Dennis just came upon, and he believes with the transfusion he would be unclean and unworthy." Finally, according to observers of the court proceedings, the judge indicated that he didn't "believe Dennis's decision is the result of any coercion. He is mature and understands the consequences of his decision."

Some critics of the judge's decision insisted that a fourteen-year-old boy is not competent to make such a life/death decision. According to one critic, adolescents are both more likely to act in ways that seem heroic and very susceptible to influence and pressure. Moreover, they often change their beliefs as they develop. Other critics wondered whether the teenager was experiencing pressure from his immediate caregiver and religious community. In the crisis, his biological parents came from Idaho, where they lived, to indicate their desire for their son to have the transfusion, and to raise questions about whether their son was unduly influenced by his aunt. The father stated, "My sister has done a good job of raising him for the past four years, but her religious beliefs shouldn't be imposed on my son. I want my son to live."

Dr. Benjamin Wilfond, who directs pediatric bioethics at Children's Hospital in Seattle but was not directly involved in this case, focused on several complexities. Dennis would have needed continuing treatments and, with them, repeated transfusions, but it would have been very difficult to force him to cooperate with the treatments over time. As clinicians try to balance protection of children with respect for their autonomous choices, Wilfond observes, "it's not typical to physically restrain children of that age for medical intervention." Dr. Douglas Diekema, another pediatrician and ethicist at Children's Hospital, echoed similar themes—but neither of them could talk specifically about the details of the Lindberg case. Caregivers are "nervous" in such cases because fourteen-year-olds can have an "adultlike" decision-making process, even though they often change their mind as they get older. Diekema too noted the difficulty of "effectively treat[ing] a kid when he's not going to cooperate."

In my mind, if there is a role of the court it would be to test a fourteen-year-old and see just how intense he is about his decision. My approach would be to push it a little further. If he fights you physically, then I'd respect that.

But also, are you willing to tie him down every time he needs a transfusion knowing he'll need treatment for the next three years? You'll have a hard time finding a provider willing to do that.

The natural response, Wilfond noted, is to want to do what is necessary to save the young boy: "But imagine if you heard a story about how this individual was strapped down to be given a transfusion, or tackled as he tried to leave the hospital. At fourteen, if you feel strongly about something, you're going to fight back." In contrast to dealing with very young children, caregivers feel "profoundly conflicted" when adolescents are at the center of such cases.

Dianna Mincin's blog (subsequently deactivated) included this comment a few days before her nephew's death:

> For those reading (about) this journey our family has been on that are not one of Jehovah's Witnesses, we compassionately understand your confusion and, perhaps, even your anger at the decision that Dennis and his family have made. . . . While we empathize with your strong feelings, we ask that you attempt to respect Dennis' fight for what he and his family believe so strongly in.[4]

A first step in respecting persons' autonomous choices is to determine whether they have the capacity to act autonomously. This capacity is often referred to as "competence," and I'll use "competence" and "capacity" interchangeably here, although in the United States "competence" is often used in legal contexts. I am viewing the activity and process of determining capacity/competence in ethical rather than legal terms, but sometimes it will be necessary to obtain a legal determination of competence.

Competence or capacity is task-specific. We ask whether people have the capacity to do X, Y, or Z. They may lack the capacity to do X but have the capacity to do Y—for example, they may have the capacity to drive an automobile but not to make complex transfers of property. In the case of Dennis Lindberg, the judge determined that, even though he was only fourteen years old, he was a "mature minor," that he had the capacity to refuse treatments that could prolong his life for perhaps five years (even though, legally, he lacked the competence to obtain a license to drive an automobile). Commentators note that fourteen-year-olds can have an "adultlike" decision-making process.

Suppose a person lacks competence to give valid consent at a particular time. It is sometimes possible through various interventions to build up or restore a person's capacity for informed consent/refusal. For adults, in contrast to a fourteen-year-old making a life/death decision, we proceed from a presumption of competence and then determine when to disqualify him or her on grounds of limited capacity to make such decisions. Here the fourteen-year-old was presumed to be incompetent, and he had to be evaluated by healthcare professionals and then by a judge to determine whether he was sufficiently competent to refuse treatment. In practice, questions rarely arise about an adult patient's capacity to decide unless he or she *disagrees* with what the clinician proposes. Probing an individual's capacity to decide or his/her understanding and reasons for decisions in routine healthcare would be unnecessary, time-consuming, and very costly, apart from a conviction the decision in question is objectively unreasonable or irrational.[5] By contrast, closer attention to evidence about the adult's level of capacity for autonomous choice is warranted when the diagnostic or therapeutic procedures are more invasive or risky.

For a decision to be autonomous the agent needs an adequate understanding of his or her situation, the available options, the probable consequences of different decisions, and so forth. The judge in the Jehovah's Witness case determined that the teenager understood the implications of his decision to refuse a blood transfusion—that he was "basically giving himself a death sentence" through acting on his beliefs. However, some critics observe that fourteen-year-olds often view themselves as heroic and, furthermore, often change their minds about some of their earlier firm convictions as they mature.

Next it is necessary to determine whether a patient's choice is voluntary or made under undue or controlling influence. In the case of Dennis Lindberg, questions were raised about the voluntariness of his choice because of concerns that he was under undue influence or even coercion. His legal guardian was his aunt, a Jehovah's Witness herself, who in a blog asked for respect for "Dennis's fight for what he and his family believe so strongly in." However, Dennis's biological parents opposed his aunt's imposition of her religious beliefs on their son; the inculcation of those beliefs was probably much more subtle and effective than "imposition" would have been for a teenager, who probably would have resisted "imposition." In any event, the judge did not "believe Dennis' decision [was] the result of any coercion."

Finally, it can be difficult to discern what even clearly competent patients really want. That is, what is the actual content of their choices? Even supposing the Jehovah's Witness teenager was competent, understood his situation and the consequences of his decision, and was acting voluntarily, it still could have been difficult to determine exactly what he wanted in the circumstances as they unfolded. It would have been surprising if he had not been ambivalent. One pediatrician-ethicist recommended pushing the interaction further to test "just how intense he is about his decision," to determine whether he would "fight" it. And this pediatrician-ethicist expressed his hope that the judge had done this sort of probing. It is also important to note that sometimes practitioners of the Jehovah's Witness faith appear to give both healthcare professionals and judges conflicting signals about what they want. I'll return to this later when I discuss cultural beliefs and values.

Relational Autonomy: A Thicker, Richer Conception

Components of Relational Autonomy

Relational autonomy—also called "autonomy in a relational context," "situated autonomy," "contextual autonomy," and so forth—offers an important corrective to some interpretations of the PRA. It directs attention beyond the immediate decision, "the moment of medical decision making,"[6] to the broader context of relations that shape those decisions. Proponents of "relational autonomy," particularly (but not only) feminist thinkers, have helpfully criticized some widespread interpretations and applications of the PRA. I'll focus on relational autonomy rather than on other thick conceptions of autonomy because of limited space, the wide appeal of relational autonomy in bioethics, and its incorporation of elements of some other thick notions. Even so, this is only a brief sketch, hardly representative of the full range of ideas to be found in various conceptions of relational autonomy, and it will concentrate on feminist rather than communitarian conceptions of relational autonomy.[7]

Relational autonomists or relationalists find very problematic the picture of the self that sometimes dominates conceptions of autonomy, understood as self-rule or self-governance: individual, self-made, independent, self-interested, isolated and insulated, and so forth. Of course, not all proponents of thin conceptions of autonomy in bioethics or elsewhere accept all these characteristics—these are at most only tendencies. But relational autonomists offer several criticisms of these tendencies.

Self-rule, self-governance, or self-determination does not mean self-creation. The independence emphasized by the PRA does not or should not deny interdependence and neglect the emergence and expression of the self in relationships. For relationalists, individuals' autonomous choices are not given, individualistically achieved, or fixed. Instead, we need to recognize how supportive social conditions foster autonomous action. In the words of Susan Sherwin, "Relational autonomy redefines autonomy as the social project it is, but it does not deny that autonomy ultimately resides in individuals."[8]

In the first instance, we think of the impact of close, intimate, interpersonal relationships, particularly families, in shaping the self in both positive and negative ways. This was certainly evident in the case of the Jehovah's Witness teenager—(1) the impact of his biological parents' drug problems and his father's imprisonment, and (2) the impact of his relationship with his aunt, who had become his legal guardian and provided him with a home. Broader social, religious, cultural, and political contexts may also be important. In this case, the teenager's affiliation with a particular religious community was very significant, as was his school environment. Even though healthcare professionals are part of the relational context, in this particular case we don't know much about those relations.

In some situations, the self in self-rule or self-determination may actually be an oppressed self. Hence, it is important to examine the conditions of constraint and limitation under which many exercise—or try to exercise—their autonomy. Attention to social injustice is crucially important for relational autonomists. Even culture may be oppressive; for example, some feminists argue that decisions for breast augmentation or even for breast reconstruction following mastectomy for cancer are unduly influenced and perhaps even, in a way, coerced by the dominant culture.

Furthermore, in healthcare, medicine, and research, patients and participants/subjects exercise their choices in relation to and with some dependence on clinicians, researchers, and other professionals. This is one factor that gives rise to the positive obligations of respect for autonomy that I mentioned. Through some of these relations, it may be possible to engender, maintain, or restore autonomous choices.

Several themes featured in relational autonomy now appear in more or less standard accounts of respect for autonomy, in part as a result of the extensive and powerful depictions and defenses of relational autonomy in the literature. In the Jehovah's Witness case, a relational approach would have considered carefully the overall relational context—though perhaps no more carefully than the physicians and judge did. Even under a thin account of autonomy much of what relationalists emphasize would have been incorporated because the case involved a minor, a fourteen-year-old. The same might not have been true for many interactions with adults.

I have already noted the relational context that shaped Dennis's decision-making: parental drug problems; father's imprisonment; home with and legal guardianship under his aunt, a Jehovah's Witness, for four years; religious community and school community; his physicians and other caregivers; and his biological parents, who may have arrived on the scene too late to make a difference in view of how rapidly the crisis developed. The relational context also included the judge who probed the teenager's views. As previously noted, one pediatrician-ethicist indicated that the role of the court should have been to determine the *intensity* of Dennis's beliefs—"to push back a little further" to determine whether he "fights you." Since the treatment over time would have required repeated transfusions, there would have been ongoing fights, and health professionals opposed using physical force in order to provide the rejected blood transfusion.

In sum, valuable insights and helpful correctives to common understandings and misunderstandings of the PRA have emerged from conceptions of "relational autonomy." Some of these correctives were already implicit in or have since been incorporated into the standard approach. No doubt, virtually any thin approach would attend to relational autonomy in the care of minors, but proponents of relational autonomy contend that it should extend to all throughout healthcare. However, not all approaches to or implications and applications of relational autonomy—and there are many different conceptions—are defensible.

Relationally Responsible Choices: A Necessary Condition of Autonomy?

One conception of "relational autonomy" is problematic because it builds a notion of relational, moral responsibility into the conception of autonomy itself. Some interpreters hold that a relationally autonomous choice is one that recognizes its societal repercussions and decides and acts accordingly.[9] Similar issues are raised by "principled autonomy,"[10] which Onora O'Neill and others, following Kant, use to build a notion of responsibility into autonomy (hence, "principled autonomy").[11] From this standpoint, we are not choosing autonomously if we do not attend to the impact of our actions on others.[12]

My approach is quite different, as developed in *Principles of Biomedical Ethics*, coauthored with Tom Beauchamp: people's autonomous choices may be unethical in failing to attend to relational responsibilities and to negative impacts on others; hence, these autonomous choices may sometimes be justifiably overridden. That these choices are unethical does not disqualify them as autonomous; it only means that they are not ethically justifiable, all things considered. And since, like other ethical principles (in the Beauchamp-Childress framework), the PRA is only prima facie binding, it too can be justifiably overridden under some circumstances. Take, for instance, a refusal to follow an order of quarantine in a public health crisis. That refusal could be an autonomous choice but justifiably overridden to protect others.

Respect for an Individual's Social-Cultural Beliefs and Values

Relationalists also stress the larger social-cultural context that shapes individuals' choices, sometimes to the extent of practically constituting their identities, not merely functioning as a causal background. Of course, bioethics needs to attend to various and significant social-cultural contexts of choices. This is crucially important in multicultural societies. How we should do this requires careful thought.

Several empirical studies challenge what they take to be the dominant Western bioethical view of respect for patient autonomy and its implications for determining how much patients should know and decide. All in all, these studies enrich our understanding of the PRA and its applications, but their findings require careful interpretation, both theoretically and practically.

In one study, researchers in California studied the differences in the attitudes of elderly subjects (65 years or older) from four different ethnic backgrounds (Korean American, Mexican American, European American, and African American) toward the roles the individual patient and the family should play in the disclosure of a diagnosis and prognosis of a terminal illness, such as cancer, and in decision-making at the end of life. The study enrolled 800 subjects, 200 from each of the four ethnic groups. Following is the researchers' summary of their main findings:

Korean Americans (47%) and Mexican Americans (65%) were significantly less likely than European Americans (87%) and African Americans (88%) to believe that a patient should be told the diagnosis of metastatic cancer. Korean Americans (35%) and Mexican Americans (48%) were less likely than African Americans (63%) and European Americans (69%) to believe that a patient should be told of a terminal prognosis and less likely to believe that the patient should make decisions about the use of life-supporting technology (28% and 41% vs 60% and 65%). Instead, Korean Americans and Mexican Americans tended to believe that the family should make decisions about the use of life support.[13]

This study determined that the attitudes toward disclosure and toward decision-making primarily correlated with ethnicity and secondarily with respondents' years of education and personal experiences of illness and medical decision-making.

The researchers indicate that their study shows that the "belief in the ideal of patient autonomy is far from universal."[14] They contrast that ideal with a "family-centered model," which emphasizes the individual's web of relationships, and tends to place a higher value on "the harmonious functioning of the family than on the autonomy of its individual members."[15] Hence, there are two divergent models of medical decision-making: a family-centered model and a patient-centered model.[16]

The researchers recommend that physicians "ask their patients if they wish to receive information and make decisions or if they prefer that their families handle such matters."[17] That recommendation is a way both to *recognize* and to *respect* patients' autonomy. Rather than abandoning the ideal of patient autonomy, as the researchers sometimes suppose, this permits individuals to exercise their autonomy by choosing the model they prefer for disclosure of information and decision-making—a patient-centered or a family-centered one. Even a patient's choice of a family-centered model can be an autonomous choice.

In places the authors seem to admit that we don't have to abandon our commitment to individual autonomy or to (the legal doctrine of) informed consent. Instead, they say, what is required is "*broadening* our view of autonomy so that respect for persons includes respect for the cultural values they bring with them to the decision-making process"[18] (italics added). Generally I concur with this conception of broadening the view of respect for autonomy, in contrast to claims of abandonment—perhaps the researchers' earlier statements should be read as an abandonment of excessively *individualistic* notions of autonomy.[19] However, my concurrence includes a strong cautionary note. It is important to avoid reading *individuals'* values off the *cultural* values they generally affirm, or *individuals'* narratives off their *cultural* narratives.

Each year I teach a broad, comparative course, Religion and Medicine, for fourth-year medical students, and I caution the participants as follows: when we learn what a particular religious or cultural tradition affirms, we cannot conclude from this that an individual affiliated with that tradition thinks or believes or acts in a particular way. The individual is not a mere subset of a social-cultural tradition even if that tradition has, in part, shaped the person's identity and the person still identifies with it. We cannot suppose that an observant religious person necessarily holds or acts on a belief or value generally associated with, or even authoritatively promulgated by, his or her particular religion.

This too is important for our central case. It is natural to assume that a self-identified and committed Jehovah's Witness will consistently and adamantly refuse a blood transfusion as contaminating and polluting, based on that tradition's formal statements of beliefs and values. Nevertheless, some Jehovah's Witnesses, perhaps a small minority, actually believe that *consent* to the transfusion, rather than the *transfusion* itself, contaminates the individual—no consent, no contamination! And, according to transcripts of a number of bedside interviews conducted by judges of adult Jehovah's Witnesses who refuse to consent to a blood transfusion recommended by physicians, these patients may appear even to welcome or invite healthcare professionals and courts to help them through this loophole in their beliefs— for some, a court-ordered (but unconsented to) transfusion would not have negative religious repercussions.[20] Healthcare professionals and judges are in a difficult ethical and legal bind when in some circumstances the adult Jehovah's Witness does not want to die but cannot consent to a potentially life-saving blood transfusion without jeopardizing his or her religious standing. Some judges have authorized the transfusions while others have declined to do so.[21]

The suggestion earlier that the Jehovah's Witness teenager's resolve could be tested by seeing whether he would put up a fight should be understood in this connection. As a result of his probing, perhaps the kind required by relational autonomy, the judge understood the teenager to believe that "with the transfusion he would be unclean and unworthy"—even if the court ordered it without his consent or against his refusal. But, as also indicated earlier, we actually don't know what kind of probing the judge used.

In summary, understanding the patient's social-cultural context is very important for clinicians in both disclosing information and interpreting patients' responses. But individuals' appropriations and expressions of their sociocultural traditions and values may be quite idiosyncratic—they may even reject those traditions and values at some key points relevant to the decision at stake. This holds whether these social-cultural traditions and values function causally, as background conditions, or constitutively for those individuals.

Respect for Temporally Extended Selves

Another source of complexity in respecting autonomy stems from the fact that we are "temporally extended selves."[22] We exist in and through time and our choices and actions occur over time. Among the several theorists of relational autonomy who have emphasized this, Susan Sherwin observes, "Under relational theory, selfhood is seen as an ongoing process rather than as something static or fixed."[23] In discharging our obligations under the PRA, we not only have to determine whether a person is choosing autonomously and what he or she chooses, but we also have to put that person's current consents and dissents in a broad temporal context with attention to the past and the future as well as the present. As temporal beings through and through, we frequently express different views and preferences at different times.

Not surprisingly, respecting autonomy in bioethics often focuses on the present moment—for example, do we have the patient's or prospective research subject's informed consent or refusal at this time? However, respecting persons and their autonomous choices becomes very complex when we consider their temporality: Which choices and actions should we respect? In particular, is it ever justifiable to override a patient's present choices and actions in the light of his or her past or (anticipated) future choices and actions? Most dramatically, which person do we respect?

Past or Prior Consent

Past or prior consent/refusal poses no problem if the patient cannot currently autonomously express his or her wishes, perhaps because of mental incapacity. As in the case of advance directives, we respect personal autonomy by acting on that past or prior statement of preference, what is sometimes called precedent autonomy.[24] Matters become more problematic, however, when a person's present choices appear to contradict those prior choices. Sometimes the person may have even made those prior choices to prevent future changes.

For example, in one case, a 28-year-old man decided to terminate chronic renal dialysis because of his poor quality of life and the burdens his condition and its treatment created for his family—his medical conditions included diabetes, legal blindness, and progressive neuropathy that rendered him unable to walk. At his request, his wife and physician finally agreed to this arrangement: when he stopped dialysis, he would receive medication to relieve his pain while he died, and he would not be put back on dialysis even if he requested it. While dying in the hospital, the patient awoke complaining of pain and asked to be put back on dialysis. The patient's wife and physician decided to act on the man's earlier request that he be allowed to die, and he died four hours later.[25]

In my judgment, the spouse and physician should have put the patient back on dialysis in view of his current request and the irreversibility of acting in accord with his earlier, now repudiated, statements. After putting him back on dialysis, they could have determined whether he had autonomously revoked his prior choice. Suppose he said, "Damn it, I told you not to put me back on dialysis whatever I said . . . ." Then they could have proceeded again with greater confidence.

As this case suggests, it is sometimes critically important to determine whether people have autonomously revoked their previous consents/refusals. In such cases, we need to assess a person's level of autonomy over time in order to determine whether the apparent revocation of previous consents or dissents is autonomous. The PRA requires that we attend to both a person's prior consent/refusal and his or her present revocation when there is a conflict, but the present revocation takes priority if it is autonomous.

An important interpretive perspective in respecting autonomous choices is that of narrative unity, integrity and authenticity.[26] One question that often arises is how a patient's current choices fit in with the choices he or she has made over time and in accord with his or her character. Narrative unity and integrity, for example, involve wholeness and constancy over time.

Authenticity, according to one philosopher, means that "an action is consistent with the attitudes, values, dispositions and life plans of the person." Its intuitive idea is "acting in character."[27] Learning whether a person's present choice or action is consistent or inconsistent with that person's life plan and risk budget as embodied over time may help us determine, for example, whether a revocation is genuine. On the one hand, we may wonder whether a person's actions are autonomous if they are out of character (e.g., a person's sudden and unexpected decision to discontinue a needed medical treatment). On the other hand, we are less likely to challenge actions as nonautonomous if they are in character (e.g., a committed Jehovah's Witness's refusal of a blood transfusion).

These ideas of narrative unity, integrity, and authenticity are important, but it would be a mistake to make them criteria for determining whether choices are autonomous. At most, actions apparently out of character and inauthentic raise caution flags that warn others to press for explanations and justifications in order to determine whether those actions are in fact autonomous. However, we cannot rule out in advance the possibility of a change or even a conversion in basic values.

Future or Deferred Consent

Suppose a patient refuses a potentially life-sustaining treatment because of pain, suffering, and apparently limited life prospects. In some such situations clinicians may have good reason to believe that if the patient were kept alive by a particular treatment that she is now refusing, she would eventually ratify the coercive or deceptive treatment on her behalf, perhaps even thanking the professional. Such retrospective ratification does occur in some cases.

But the question is whether *anticipated* future ratification justifies—or helps to justify—acting now against a patient's current express choices in order to respect who that person will become rather than who she currently is. I would argue that predicted future ratification is neither necessary nor sufficient to justify paternalistic interventions against current choices. At most, a patient's probable future ratification may provide supporting (but still inconclusive) evidence that the conditions for justified paternalistic interventions have been met. It is also important to note that the intervention may have changed the person in the process.

Conclusions

I have argued that thicker concepts of autonomy, closely connected with relational autonomy, can enable us—and, indeed, have enabled us—to see more clearly aspects of respect for autonomy that have often been neglected or downplayed in much bioethical theory and practice. In the process, they help us understand better the interpretive complexity of the PRA. This complexity is unavoidable because people—the very people whose autonomy we are to respect—are complex, as indicated by conceptions of relational autonomy.

A danger is that these valuable indicators for respecting autonomous choices might be made into necessary conditions for autonomy, conditions that would then ground respect for autonomy. This would set a standard for autonomous actions that is too high and too demanding and would thus deprive ordinary decision-makers of the protection and support needed for their autonomous choices and actions. It could even create the specter of paternalistic interventions in the name of thicker conceptions of autonomy. The worry is that we will be tempted to override a person's specific minimally but sufficiently autonomous choice because it fails to satisfy the standards of thicker conceptions of autonomy.

Notes

1. Tom L. Beauchamp and James F. Childress, *Principles of Biomedical Ethics*, 7th edition (New York: Oxford University Press, 2013), chap. 4.
2. Richard H. Thaler and Cass R. Sunstein, *Nudge: Improving Decisions about Health, Wealth, and Happiness* (New Haven, CT: Yale University Press, 2008).
3. Tom L. Beauchamp and Ruth R. Faden, *A History and Theory of Informed Consent* (New York: Oxford University Press, 1986).
4. This case was prepared from the following media accounts: Scott Michels, "Judge Allowed 14-Year-Old Jehovah's Witness to Refuse Potentially Lifesaving Care Leukemia Patient Dies after Refusing Blood Transfusion for Religious Reasons," *ABC News Internet Ventures*, with reporting from the Associated Press, November 29, 2007; Cherie Black, "Boy Dies of Leukemia after Refusing Treatment for Religious Reasons," *Seattle Post-Intelligencer*, November 29, 2007; Franny White, "Tragic End to a Troubled Life," *Skagit Valley Herald*, November 29, 2007; Cherie Black, "Jehovah's Witnesses: Boy's Death Ends Battle," *Seattle Post-Intelligencer*, November 29, 2007; Carol M. Ostrom, "Mount Vernon Leukemia Patient, 14, Dies after Rejecting Transfusions," *Seattle Times*, November 29, 2007; "Boy Who Refused Transfusion Dies," *Associated Press*, November 30, 2007.
5. Alasdair Maclean, *Autonomy, Informed Consent and Medical Law: A Relational Challenge* (Cambridge: Cambridge University Press, 2009), p. 248.
6. Susan Sherwin, "A Relational Approach to Autonomy in Health Care," in *The Politics of Women's Health: Exploring Agency and Autonomy*, The Feminist Health Care Ethics

Research Network, coordinator Susan Sherwin (Philadelphia: Temple University Press, 1998), p. 32.

7. See Catriona Mackenzie and Natalie Stoljar, eds., *Relational Autonomy: Feminist Perspectives on Autonomy, Agency, and the Social Self* (New York: Oxford University Press, 2000); Natalie Stoljar, "Feminist Perspectives on Autonomy," in *Stanford Encyclopedia of Philosophy* (Spring 2014 edition), ed. Edward N. Zalta, http://plato. stanford.edu/archives/spr2014/entries/feminism-autonomy/; Diana Tietjens Meyers, ed., *Feminists Rethink the Self* (Boulder, CO: Westview Press, 1997); Marilyn Friedman, "Autonomy and Social Relationships: Rethinking the Feminist Critique," in *Feminists Rethink the Self*, ed. Diana Tietjens Meyers (Boulder, CO: Westview Press, 1997); Anne Donchian, "Understanding Autonomy Relationally: Toward a Reconfiguration of Bioethical Principles," *Journal of Medicine and Philosophy* 26, No. 4 (2001), pp. 365–386; Susan Sherwin, *No Longer Patient: Feminist Ethics and Health Care* (Philadelphia: Temple University Press, 1992).

8. Sherwin, "A Relational Approach to Autonomy in Health Care," p. 39.

9. See the depiction of relational autonomy in Sheila McLean, *Autonomy, Consent and the Law*, Biomedical Law and Ethics Library (London: Routledge-Cavendish, 2010).

10. Onora O'Neill, *Autonomy and Trust in Bioethics* (Cambridge: Cambridge University Press, 2002). See also Onora O'Neill, "Autonomy: The Emperor's New Clothes," *Proceedings of the Aristotelian Society*, sup. Vol. 77 (2003): 1–21.

11. See also Neil C. Manson and Onora O'Neill, *Rethinking Informed Consent in Bioethics* (Cambridge: Cambridge University Press, 2007).

12. It is unclear whether and to what extent the Jehovah's Witness teenager considered the impact of his action on others.

13. Leslie J. Blackhall, Sheila T. Murphy, Gelya Frank, et al., "Ethnicity and Attitudes toward Patient Autonomy," *JAMA: Journal of the American Medical Association* 274 (1995): 820–825, p. 820.

14. Ibid., p. 824.

15. Ibid., p. 825.

16. See also the critique of the individualistic version of respect for autonomy in principlism, from the perspective of Japanese culture, in John Traphagan, *Rethinking Autonomy: A Critique of Principlism in Biomedical Ethics* (Albany: State University of New York Press, 2013).

17. Blackhall et al., "Ethnicity and Attitudes toward Patient Autonomy," p. 820.

18. Ibid., p. 825.

19. See McLean, *Autonomy, Consent and the Law*, for a discussion of both individualistic and relational conceptions of autonomy in English law.

20. James F. Childress, "Jehovah's Witness Refusal of Blood Transfusions: Ethical and Legal Controversies" (2015), unpublished paper.

21. Ibid.

22. Holger Baumann, "Reconsidering Relational Autonomy: Personal Autonomy for Socially Embedded and Temporally Extended Selves," *Analyse & Kritik* 30 (2008): 445–468.

23. Sherwin, "A Relational Approach to Autonomy in Health Care," p. 35.

24. J. K. Davis, "Precedent Autonomy, Advance Directives, and End-of-Life Care," in *The Oxford Handbook of Bioethics*, ed. Bonnie Steinbock (New York: Oxford University Press, 2007), pp. 349–374.
25. Beauchamp and Childress, *Principles of Biomedical Ethics*, p. 113.
26. Bruce Miller, "Autonomy," in *Bioethics* [formerly *The Encyclopedia of Bioethics*], 4th edition, ed. Bruce Jennings (New York: Macmillan Reference, 2014), pp. 302–307.
27. Ibid.

2

Paternalism in Healthcare and Health Policy

When, if ever, may or should a healthcare professional withhold a diagnosis of a serious disease from a patient? Or downplay the seriousness of that disease? Or refrain from mentioning the likelihood of imminent death? Is it justifiable for a healthcare team to continue treating a severely burned young man against his wishes in order to prevent his death, in the belief that he will later be glad to be alive? Under what conditions may and should a clinician seek to have a patient involuntarily hospitalized because of risks of self-harm or suicide? When may or should policy-makers seek to develop laws to control individuals' risky actions even though those actions do not impose risks, costs, or burdens on other individuals or on the society? In short, and more abstractly, when, if ever, are paternalistic actions and policies ethically justified?

Controversies surround the meaning and justification of paternalistic actions in healthcare and of health-related paternalistic public policies. Despite extensive and intensive critiques of paternalism, particularly from the standpoint of respect for personal autonomy, it persists and remains common and important in both contexts. Indeed, it has even gained new appreciation and new momentum over the last fifteen years or so. For instance, in health-related policy, "neopaternalists" have offered arguments for government policies that, at a minimum, seek to protect or benefit individuals through shaping or steering their choices without, in fact, limiting or coercing those choices.[1] Similarly, in healthcare, arguments have emerged that the physician should take a leading role in helping patients select the goals of care, instead of merely presenting in a neutral way "a laundry list of means and insist[ing] that patients choose for themselves."[2]

This chapter will examine the nature of paternalism, particularly by discussing its moral foundations and limits and drawing several distinctions that bear on its interpretation and justification, consider circumstances in which it may be justified, and, finally, explore the new paternalism, based on recent studies in behavioral economics and psychology, that plays a role in a variety of proposals for health-related public policies.

What Is Paternalism?

Paternalistic actions display at least two features: they aim at protecting or promoting the welfare of individuals themselves, and they do so by not acquiescing in the preferences, choices, or actions of those individuals. Paternalism invokes a metaphor of the relationship between father and child, as depicted in the late nineteenth century when the term emerged. Even before the term itself appeared, the metaphor functioned in the language, for instance, of "paternal government" that John Stuart Mill and others used to criticize governmental policies.[3] The metaphor is problematic because it expresses gender roles. However, there are reasons, some feminists argue, for retaining the gendered language of paternalism because it highlights the link between a father's privileges in a patriarchal family and a physician's privileges in a hierarchical medical system.[4] Nevertheless, both "parentalism"[5] and "maternalism—as well as the "nanny state" and various other terms—have been used to cover beneficence-based actions that do not acquiesce in the preferences, choices, and actions of individuals for their own benefit. Each of these terms also has social and cultural baggage. In the final analysis, the term "paternalism" still remains the most appropriate, because of common usage, tradition, and philosophical debates.

Both medical paternalism and governmental paternalism have a moral foundation in the principle of beneficence and/or the virtue of benevolence.[6] In pure paternalistic actions, the intended beneficiary must be an individual whose own good is sought (or, for health-related policies, classes of individuals whose own good is sought). The philosopher Gerald Dworkin has defined paternalism as "the interference of a state or an individual with another person, against their will, and justified by a claim that the person interfered with be better off or protected from harm."[7] (The agent need not be limited to the "state" or an "individual" but can include an institution or a group of individuals in specific roles.)

Gerald Dworkin's definition captures the beneficence/benevolence foundation of paternalism, but there is more debate about how to understand the means employed by paternalists. Specifically, how should we understand "interference" and is it the best term? A broad interpretation of interference is nonacquiescence in the preferences, choices, and actions of others.[8] More limited interpretations focus on interference with liberty. Still others focus on infringement of certain moral rules. And so forth. What is involved in "interference" is important for determining whether and why paternalism is ethically problematic and when, if ever, it can be ethically justified. For instance, efforts to persuade an individual to act in certain ways for his or her own welfare are rarely problematic from an ethical standpoint, while coercion always stands in need of ethical justification. Interferences are most problematic and even prima facie wrong when they infringe the principle of respect for autonomy and/or specific rules such as liberty, privacy, or confidentiality.

Still another distinction may illuminate paternalistic acts in healthcare. Gerald Dworkin's term "interference" captures much *active* paternalism, which occurs, for example, when a clinician intervenes, perhaps by providing information or treatment against a patient's request. But "interference" may be too interventionist and too strong to encompass *passive* paternalism. Consider a healthcare professional's refusal to perform an action requested by a patient, on the grounds that it would not benefit and would even be harmful to that patient. For example, a physician refuses to perform a requested permanent sterilization because of his or her judgment that it would not be in the sexually active, twenty-year-old requester's best interests in the long run. Or a physician declines to participate in assisted suicide in a jurisdiction where it is legal because he or she does not believe it would be in that patient's best interest. Or a physician elects not to provide a futile treatment requested by the patient. In passive paternalism, then, a person refuses to be an agent for the requester, while leaving open the possibility that the requester could find someone else to carry out the request. Other things being equal, it is easier to justify passive paternalism than active paternalism, and the remainder of this chapter will focus largely on active paternalism.

Weak and Strong Paternalism

In the moral analysis and assessment of paternalistic actions or policies, one of the most prevalent and important distinctions is between *weak* and *strong* paternalism, first formulated by Joel Feinberg and subsequently elaborated by many others.[9] In strong paternalism, the intended beneficiary is deemed to be an autonomous or substantially autonomous person whose preferences, choices, and actions appear to damage or threaten to damage his or her best interests. A strong paternalistic action will, at a minimum, infringe the intended beneficiary's autonomous choices and actions and thus infringe an important moral principle of respect for autonomy. It may also infringe other moral principles and rules. The burden of justification for strong paternalism is heavy, though not impossible to meet.

By contrast, in weak paternalism, the intended beneficiary's choices or actions are deemed to be nonautonomous or substantially nonautonomous. As a result, those choices or actions do not carry the same weight as autonomous ones. Indeed, in the absence of patient autonomy, the principle of beneficence encounters no tension with and no resistance from the principle of respect for autonomy. For instance, an incompetent patient—that is, one who lacks the mental capacity to provide informed consent or refusal—may still oppose a particular treatment the clinician believes is necessary. In such a case, the principle of beneficence toward the patient does not conflict with the principle of respect for autonomy because the patient lacks substantial autonomy. Hence, there would be a clear and easy justification for overriding the patient's opposition to the treatment in question, especially if it is necessary to produce a major health benefit. Various means that would otherwise be morally problematic could also be justifiable, such as nondisclosure of information. An example might be nondisclosure of the diagnosis of Alzheimer's disease to a patient who already has advanced symptoms.

Is weak paternalism even a form of paternalism? One important conceptual question is just this: Is weak paternalism even paternalism at all, at least in any morally interesting and significant sense, if the intended beneficiary of a beneficent/benevolent deed lacks substantial autonomy?[10] Answers to this question clearly affect the pattern of justification for nonacquiescence or interference in a patient's preferences, choices, and actions. However, it is helpful to use the term "paternalism" for beneficence-based actions targeting the patient's own best interests when they are in apparent conflict with the patient's preferences, choices, and actions, even if the patient is substantially nonautonomous.

There is a presumption that adult persons can form their own preferences and choose and act with substantial autonomy. In healthcare that presumption provides a starting point from which clinicians address any conflict that emerges. In doing so they may determine that it is justifiable to disqualify the patient as a decision-maker, for example, because of his or her incompetence and hence lack of autonomy. Caution is needed because judgments of incompetence—and of other failures of autonomy—are not merely scientific and technical; they sometimes mask value conflicts. Hence, it is more illuminating and useful to screen actions, including possibly paternalistic actions, in light of the relevant moral principles and the available evidence about the relevant benefits and harms to the patient and about his or her autonomy. Nevertheless, if the patient is not substantially autonomous, beneficence triumphs easily because the principle of respect for autonomy offers no resistance in those circumstances. Weak paternalistic actions are thus easily justified but are not uncontested instances of paternalism.

By contrast, strong paternalistic actions are clearly instances of paternalism, but are not so easily justified, if, indeed, justifiable at all, in part because, as Ronald Dworkin notes, they are disrespectful, demeaning, and insulting to the intended autonomous beneficiary.[11] The most plausible approach, in my judgment, is to keep the door slightly ajar to the justification of some strong paternalistic acts, but to recognize that we should rarely open that door all the way. Beyond the principle of respect for autonomy and related conceptions, John Stuart Mill and others have provided utilitarian reasons for deep suspicion of paternalistic interventions, stressing the odds that the paternalist will be mistaken. According to Mill, "[t]he strongest of all the arguments against the interference of the public with purely personal conduct, is that when it does interfere, the odds are that it interferes wrongly, and in the wrong place."[12] Here Mill offers a more specific utilitarian argument than his broadly utilitarian argument that rules of liberty, where the agent's actions do not put others at risk without their consent, contribute to human fulfillment.[13]

Nevertheless, strong paternalistic actions may sometimes be ethically justifiable. By and large, such actions have a significant moral presumption against them, particularly in a liberal society that emphasizes the principle of respect for autonomy and related principles and rules. Nevertheless, theoretically, both beneficence and respect for autonomy are prima facie binding and their respective weights can only be determined in specific situations. What conditions need to be met in justifying strong paternalistic actions that infringe the principle of respect for autonomy because the intended beneficiary is substantially autonomous? Following are several important conditions for justifying strong paternalistic acts in healthcare; these conditions both modify and expand the conditions presented by Beauchamp and Childress:[14]

1. A patient is at risk of a significant, preventable harm.

2. The paternalistic action will probably prevent the harm.
3. The paternalistic action is necessary to prevent the harm.
4. The projected benefits of the harm prevention to the beneficiary out-weigh its risks to the beneficiary.
5. The paternalistic action involves the alternative that least restricts the beneficiary's autonomy while still securing the benefits for him or her.

These conditions specify for strong paternalistic actions the broader, more general conditions for overriding any prima facie principle in order to maintain another one.[15]

Earlier I suggested that physicians might decline, on grounds of weak paternalism, to disclose a diagnosis of Alzheimer's disease to a patient with *advanced* symptoms. A more difficult ethical question is whether physicians should tell patients in the *early* stages of Alzheimer's disease their diagnosis. Consider the following case: A man in his sixties is brought to the physician by his son, who suspects that his father has Alzheimer's disease because of his apparent problems in interpreting and handling what used to be normal day-to-day activities, in part because of his lapses of memory.[16] The son also asks the physician not to tell the father if she reaches a diagnosis of Alzheimer's disease. After the appropriate tests, the physician has a diagnosis of "probable Alzheimer's disease" and discusses with a nurse and a social worker the son's "impassioned plea" not to tell his father.[17]

The nurse notes that there is now a settled and fairly strong consensus that patients who have cancer should be told their diagnosis—truthful disclosure is required, because beneficence usually does not outweigh respecting the patient's autonomy in these cases. (Of course, beneficence should structure *how* the information is disclosed—a point that is often overlooked.) Nevertheless, the physician wonders just whether and how the principles and precedents regarding the disclosure of cancer illuminate the case of the patient diagnosed with early Alzheimer's disease. After all, there are some important differences between patients diagnosed with cancer and those diagnosed with Alzheimer's disease. First, in contrast to most cancers, the diagnosis of Alzheimer's disease lacks certainty (though over 90% of these diagnoses are confirmed by autopsy). Second, in contrast to many cancers, the course of Alzheimer's disease is unclear for patents. Third, while therapeutic options have greatly increased for patients with many kinds of cancer, the therapeutic options for patients with Alzheimer's disease are still quite limited even though they are improving. Fourth, patients with Alzheimer's

disease face an inevitable erosion of their decision-making capacity, which
may not occur for most patients with cancer.

The physician in this case also has a specifically paternalistic concern.
She worries that telling the patient would harm him, because patients with
Alzheimer's disease tend to have limited coping mechanisms, perhaps because of the neurobiological effects of the disease, and disclosure could lead to
functional decline, depression, agitation, or paranoia—perhaps even suicide.
As the care of patients with Alzheimer's disease has evolved, investigators
have noted the potential positive benefits of disclosure to patients with early
Alzheimer's disease since, for example, they can usually still participate in
important decisions about their present care and in advance about their future care. Although the available evidence indicates that most patients with
cancer want to know their diagnosis, the data are less clear for patients with
Alzheimer's disease, even though the evidence indicates that more and more
patients now want to know their diagnosis particularly in the early stages.

In view of this range of arguments, clinicians (and family members) of
good will may be quite uncertain about the right course of action in these
circumstances—as they affirm beneficence, and nonmaleficence, as well as
respect for autonomy. There is no reason to believe that this patient diagnosed with early Alzheimer's disease is substantially nonautonomous.
Hence, if the physician determines that disclosure would not be in the
patient's best interest, the rationale would be strong paternalism. In view of
the range of arguments just summarized about the disclosure of a diagnosis
of early Alzheimer's disease and the facts of this case, it would be difficult, in
my judgment, to justify nondisclosure as an act of strong paternalism.

Pure and Mixed Paternalism

Suppose the professional's or policy-maker's motives are mixed—suppose he
or she seeks to benefit particular individuals, to protect the public health,
to avoid burdens to third parties, and so forth. How should we characterize
actions that express such a variety of motives? Debates about pure and impure or mixed paternalism surface in deliberations about both clinical
actions and health-related policies. Consider a clinical case in which a cognitively impaired teenager's parents and healthcare professionals are trying
to determine whether it would be appropriate to have her sterilized because
she has become sexually active. They concentrate on the young woman's

best interests but also consider the impact a pregnancy might have on several other parties, including potential offspring, the family, and the society. If they elect sterilization, their primary rationale might be paternalistic (the young woman's best interests), but the other concerns may also be significant in their decision. Hence, their decision might be characterized as impure or mixed rather than pure paternalism.

Rarely are governmental interventions in a liberal society, which professes the value of personal liberty, defended as purely paternalistic. Most often their supporters appeal to the protection of other individuals or of the society, sometimes because of threats to public resources. In contrast to the mid-nineteenth century, when Mill was writing *On Liberty*, a justification based on public resources is now much more plausible. In the context of public expenditures on healthcare and other goods and services, claims arise about the societal impact of individuals' actions that may initially appear to harm only themselves. Hence, relevant third-party effects that justify nonpaternalistic or mixed paternalistic actions include not only traditional public health threats to others through infectious diseases, violence, and so forth, but also excessive burdens on public resources.

A pure paternalistic justification would focus solely on the harms prevented or reduced or on the benefits provided to the affected individuals. For instance, a paternalistic campaign targeting obesity would feature the welfare of potentially or currently obese individuals. However, most campaigns, whether against obesity or cigarette smoking, to take two examples, explicitly invoke both paternalistic and nonpaternalistic justifications, often with an emphasis on the latter because they are more palatable to the public in an individualistic society. It is appropriate to describe such campaigns as impure paternalism or mixed paternalism, because the warrant is directed both at the individuals affected and at the impact their actions have on other individuals or on the society.

In debates about legislation to require motorcycle helmets, some arguments in support of mandatory helmet laws are clearly paternalistic—the legislation is intended, at least in part, to protect the motorcyclists themselves. Other arguments strain to show that nonhelmeted motorcyclists increase the risks of harm to others, for instance, in creating hazards to passing vehicles and in imposing unfair burdens on ambulance drivers, emergency teams, nurses, and neurosurgeons, as well as on the public who, in an interdependent society, may pick up part or all of the costs of the motorcyclist's care. Exempting motorcyclists who internalize the financial costs, perhaps through mandatory health insurance, could reduce some of the externalities. But even so, as in debates about governmental policies to reduce obesity, a contemporary source of major health problems for so many people, the line between what Mill called self-regarding and other-regarding acts and effects may be unclear.[18]

Paternalistic actions often masquerade, at least in part, as protection of others or of the society, rather than the individual himself or herself, again because these justifications can be more easily accommodated within a liberal framework. Hence, it is important to consider, in light of the best available evidence, the respective roles and merits of different arguments focused on protecting individuals' best interests, the public health, and the public treasury. For example, as public health returned to center stage in recent years because of newly emergent infections, the possibility of pandemic influenza, and the threat of bioterrorist attacks, the temptation has been to highjack the language and norms of public health to cover private harms and thus to invoke public health rather than paternalism to justify proposed interventions.

Soft and Hard Paternalism

A similar issue arises with respect to soft and hard paternalistic interventions by the government, what Mill called a "paternal government" or what in Britain has been called "the nanny state, a protective but intrusive matriarch, coddling citizens for their own good."[19] In debates about paternalism, the terms "hard" and "soft" have been used in different but overlapping ways. On one interpretation, soft paternalism appeals to values that the beneficiary actually holds but cannot realize because of problems of limited rationality or limited self-control.[20] The individual's preferences, choices, and actions are unwise even by his or her own standards. By contrast, in hard paternalism, the intended beneficiary does not accept the values that the paternalist uses to define the intended beneficiary's own best interests. While soft paternalism reflects the intended beneficiary's conception of his/her best interests, hard paternalism reflects the benefactor's conception of the beneficiary's unrecognized best interests. According to Glen Whitman, hard paternalists, as representatives of the old paternalism, say: "We know what's best for you, and we'll make you do it," while soft paternalists, as representatives of the new paternalism, say: "*You* know what is best for you, and we'll make you do it."[21]

The relations between two sets of distinctions are complex—hard and soft paternalism, on the one hand, and strong and weak paternalism, on the other hand. The soft paternalist usually claims that limited rationality and/or limited self-control compromise the intended beneficiaries' autonomy and thus prevent them from realizing their own recognized best interests. By contrast, the hard paternalist may hold both weak and strong conceptions of paternalism: the intended beneficiary may be viewed as a substantially autonomous agent who has selected and acts on the wrong values or as a substantially nonautonomous person who suffers from encumbrances in reasoning, willing, or acting.

A related but distinguishable conception of hard and soft paternalism focuses instead on the *means* used to achieve the paternalistic goal. These distinctions are connected because the kinds of means used in soft paternalism generally presuppose greater compatibility with the beneficiary's own beliefs and values, not yet realized or implemented because of inadequate rationality or inadequate self-control. Hard paternalistic interventions generally ban or prescribe or regulate conduct in ways that coerce individuals' actions to secure the desired result. These often involve clear trade-offs, as in "sin taxes" directed at harmful conduct such as smoking cigarettes. By contrast, soft paternalistic means tend to influence, shape, or steer individuals' choices without undermining their freedom to choose—for instance, they often frame information in certain ways while still being truthful and honest. Soft paternalists characterize their means as relatively weak and nonintrusive.[22]

In light of this second version of the distinction between hard and soft paternalism, with particular attention to means, we can now qualify Glen Whitman's striking characterization of soft paternalism. Rather than saying, "*You* know what is best for you, and we'll *make* you do it," the new soft paternalist says, "*You* know what best for you, and we'll *enable* you to do it without curtailing your liberty." Along these lines, some proponents of soft paternalism even label their position "libertarian paternalism" in order to underline the compatibility between liberty and this kind of paternalism. For instance, drawing on literature in psychology and behavioral economics, Sunstein and Thaler write, "The idea of libertarian paternalism might seem to be an oxymoron, but it is both possible and desirable for private and public institutions to influence behavior while also respecting freedom of choice."[23] As soft or as minimal—another term is "minimal paternalism"—as it is, what they propose is still paternalistic because of the "claim that it is legitimate for private and public institutions to attempt to influence people's behavior even when third-party effects are absent."[24]

The new soft paternalists focus on two major limitations on the intended beneficiary's preferences, choices, and actions that may justify interventions to benefit him or her. These two limitations also show the convergence between versions of soft paternalism (in both senses) and weak paternalism. The limitations are what Sunstein and Thaler call "bounded rationality" and "bounded self-control."[25] The conception of bounded rationality focuses on the bounds of rational decisionmaking that lead to departures from the "economic assumption of unbounded rationality."[26] For instance, different default rules on the same action will lead many people to make different choices, or techniques of debiasing may correct biases such as the optimism bias that leads many people to underestimate the risks of some actions for themselves, even if they accurately estimate the risks to the population in general. In the presence of bounded rationality, the state may intervene, softly, in several ways, on paternalistic grounds, that is, to enable individuals to choose and act in accord with their overall best interests over time. As Jolls and Sunstein note, if the available evidence were to establish that smokers discounted the risks of smoking because of an "optimism bias," among other factors, "it is hardly obvious that government would violate their autonomy by giving a more accurate sense of those risks, even if the best way of giving that accurate sense were through concrete accounts of suffering."[27]

If private individuals are limited in their decision-making by bounded rationality, is there any reason to believe that governmental officials are exempt from this limitation? And if they are not exempt, then their policies may be unwise, ineffective, or counterproductive. Recognized flaws in human cognition, Glaeser contends, "should make us more, not less, wary about trusting government decisionmaking," which may even be more flawed than private decision-making.[28]

Some proponents of soft paternalism argue that, in any event, the government cannot avoid using soft paternalism, for instance, in framing the information it presents. After all, any presentation of information involves some standpoint or perspective and hence some framing because pure neutrality is impossible. However, in my judgment, neutrality should remain an important critical (even if ultimately unrealizable) ideal for many, though not all, situations in which the government discloses information about health-related risks. Others contend that soft paternalism is not only unavoidable but also justifiable, at least in some circumstances. Even though it can sometimes be justified, there are good reasons for sounding a cautionary note about the wave of support for soft paternalistic policies.

Several arguments undergird this suspicion,[29] but I will here focus only on a few important points. One apparent advantage of soft paternalism may turn out to be a serious ethical disadvantage from the perspective of social and political philosophy. Recall that this paternalism is soft—that is, it reflects many values that individuals would realize or implement themselves if they did not encounter internal limits of rationality and of control, and the means it employs shape and steer, without thwarting, free choice. As a result, specific paternalistic policies may face little opposition and resistance and provoke few calls for or efforts at monitoring their implementation and effects. Indeed, these policies may even generate their own social and political support. All of this may happen without the transparency and publicity needed for public assessment, in part because some forms of soft paternalistic actions may be incompatible with transparency and publicity—once they are disclosed, explained, and justified, they may be rendered ineffective.

At least, hard paternalistic interventions that involve coercion or serious and explicit trade-offs will be transparent and public, and opponents can mount counterarguments and even resistance. Hence, it is reasonable to suspect that soft paternalistic governmental policies may also be susceptible to abuse in part because of their lack of transparency. Furthermore, government decision-makers may single out some conduct for correction not only or primarily because it involves self-harm over time but also because it displays some moral flaws (e.g., lack of self-control) or is morally distasteful. Not only may such moralistic judgments single out some conduct for correction, among the wide range of acts that involve self-harm, but they may also intensify efforts to censure the conduct and ensure the correction.

Other related ethical concerns also arise. One focuses on stigmatization of conduct that breaches the social norms invoked in soft paternalistic policies. While there is evidence that stigmatization can change behavior, there are also concerns about its psychosocial costs. Proponents of stigmatizing policies usually insist that they target acts, not persons. However, in practice, it is easy to slide from stigmatizing certain conduct to stigmatizing the people who engage in that conduct. For example, this has happened in the United States where, over time, stigmatization has played an increasingly explicit and important role in private and public efforts to curtail smoking: "the anti-tobacco movement has fostered a social transformation that involves the stigmatization of smokers"[30] The slide from stigmatization of acts to stigmatization of the people who engage in those acts can lead, as Glaeser[31] reminds us, to hostility and even hatred for population subgroups. John Stuart Mill cautioned against treating individuals engaged in harmful self-regarding conduct "like an enemy of society."[32] Again, cigarette smoking may be an example, especially as smoking has now become more common among lower socioeconomic groups in the United States. The ethical concerns, as Bayer and Stuber stress, become "all the more pressing as stigmatization falls on the most socially vulnerable—the poor who continue to smoke."[33]

Another possible or even probable slippage provides yet another reason for suspicion of soft paternalism. The acceptance of soft paternalistic interventions, as Glaeser[34] suggests, can prepare the way for and even lead to hard paternalistic interventions. One reason is that soft paternalistic interventions succeed in part by increasing support for the social values and norms that undergird the use of those interventions. The campaign against cigarette smoking again provides an instructive example—the movement from disclosure of information to sharper warnings to hard paternalistic measures such as ever-increasing taxation of cigarettes.[35]

Conclusions

Paternalism is here to stay, in both healthcare and health-related public policies. Yet, that statement is uninformative without a more nuanced analysis of the many different kinds of paternalism this chapter has attempted to identify. Not all paternalistic acts or policies are the same, and they need and receive different justifications and face different limits and constraints. Not all of them, for instance, infringe the principle of respect for personal autonomy. Hence, weak paternalistic acts and policies are more readily justified than strong paternalistic ones. Other distinctions are also important: active and passive paternalism; pure and impure or mixed paternalism; and hard and soft paternalism. While each type of paternalistic act or policy can be justified under some circumstances, the burden of proof is the heaviest for pure, strong, active, and hard paternalism, but other forms, such as soft paternalism, also need close ethical scrutiny for the reasons presented in this chapter.

Notes

1. Cass R. Sunstein and Richard H. Thaler, "Libertarian Paternalism Is Not an Oxymoron," *University of Chicago Law Review* 70 (Fall 2003): 1159–1202; Thaler and Sunstein, "Libertarian Paternalism," *American Economics Review* 93 (2003): 175–179. See also Thaler and Sunstein, *Nudge: Improving Decisions about Health, Wealth, and Happiness* (New Haven, CT: Yale University Press, 2008).
2. Erich H. Loewy, "In Defense of Paternalism," *Theoretical Medicine and Bioethics* 26 (2005): 445–468.
3. John Stuart Mill, *On Liberty*, ed. David Spitz (New York: W.W. Norton & Company, Inc., 1975), p. 94. Mill's critique of "paternal government" receives fuller attention in chapter 13 in this volume.
4. Susan Sherwin, *No Longer Patient: Feminist Ethics and Health Care* (Philadelphia: Temple University Press, 1992).
5. John Kultgen, *Autonomy and Intervention: Parentalism in the Caring Life* (New York: Oxford University Press, 1995).
6. James F. Childress, *Who Should Decide? Paternalism in Health Care* (New York: Oxford University Press, 1982); Tom L. Beauchamp and James F. Childress, *Principles of Biomedical Ethics*, 6th edition (New York: Oxford University Press, 2009).
7. Gerald Dworkin, "Paternalism," in *The Stanford Encyclopedia of Philosophy*, ed. Edward N. Zalta (2006) online http://plato.stanford.edu/entries/paternalism/ (last accessed June 24, 2006).
8. Childress, *Who Should Decide?* and Beauchamp and Childress, *Principles of Biomedical Ethics*, 6th ed.
9. Joel Feinberg, "Legal Paternalism," *Canadian Journal of Philosophy* 1 (1971): 105–124.
10. Tom L. Beauchamp and Laurence B. McCullough, *Medical Ethics: The Moral Responsibilities of Physicians* (Englewood Cliffs, NJ: Prentice-Hall, 1984); see also the discussion in Beauchamp and Childress, *Principles of Biomedical Ethics*, 6th ed., pp. 208–211, where the terms "soft" and "hard" are used as equivalent to and in place of "weak" and "strong." I am using "weak" and "strong" in the conventional sense in this chapter while reserving "soft" and "hard" for another distinction regarding paternalism.
11. Ronald Dworkin, *Taking Rights Seriously* (Cambridge, MA: Harvard University Press, 1977), pp. 262–263.
12. Mill, *On Liberty*, p. 78.
13. Ibid., p. 12.
14. Beauchamp and Childress, *Principles of Biomedical Ethics*, 6th ed., pp. 215–216; this list is slightly revised from the 5th edition (2001).
15. Ibid., p. 23.
16. This fictional case was suggested by the discussion in Margaret A. Drickamer and Mark S. Lachs, "Should Patients with Alzheimer's Disease Be Told Their Diagnosis?" *New England Journal of Medicine* 326 (April 2, 1992): 947–951. The presentation of different pro-con arguments in this section, attributed to different characters, draws heavily on this article. However, the case itself is fictional.

17. Years after this chapter was written, diagnostic tests for Alzheimer's disease are still quite limited. See National Institute of Aging, "Alzheimer's Disease Fact Sheet," at https://www.nia.nih.gov/health/alzheimers-disease-fact-sheet (last accessed May 25, 2019). Even in 2019, the fact sheet notes, "Alzheimer's disease can be definitely diagnosed only after death, by linking clinical measures with an examination of brain tissue in an autopsy." The available diagnostic methods and tools for use with a living patient can determine with a fair degree of accuracy whether a patient with memory problems has "possible Alzheimer's dementia" (i.e., the dementia may have another cause) or "probable Alzheimer's dementia" (i.e., no other cause can be identified).

18. See Mill, *On Liberty*, pp. 10–11, et passim. For example, Mill distinguishes "self-regarding conduct" from conduct that affects others (pp. 76, 78, passim), discusses "self-regarding" virtues, qualities, deficiencies, and faults (pp. 71–73), and notes that "the engines of moral repression have been wielded more strenuously against divergence from the reigning opinion in self-regarding, than even in social matters" (pp. 14–15). See further the discussion of Mill's views in chap. 13 in this volume.

19. "The State Is Looking after You," *The Economist*, April 6, 2006, http://www.economist.com/opinion/displaystory.cfm?story_id=6772346 (last accessed June 23, 2006).

20. Childress, *Who Should Decide?*

21. Glen Whitman, "Against the New Paternalism: Internalities and the Economic of self-Control," *Policy Analysis*, No. 563 (February 22, 2006).

22. Sunstein and Thaler, "Libertarian Paternalism Is Not an Oxymoron."

23. Ibid.

24. Ibid.

25. Ibid.

26. Christine Jolls and Cass R. Sunstein, "Debiasing through Law," *Journal of Legal Studies* 33 (January 2006): 199–237.

27. Ibid.

28. Edward L. Glaeser, "Symposium: Homo Economicus, Homo Myopicus, and the Law and Economics of Consumer Choice: Paternalism and Psychology," *University of Chicago Law Review* 73 (Winter 2006): 133–157.

29. Ibid. Glaeser offers a superb examination of a range of challenges to soft paternalism.

30. Ronald Bayer and Jennifer Stuber, "Tobacco Control, Stigma, and Public Health: Rethinking the Relations," *American Journal of Public Health* 96, No. 1 (January 2006): 47–50.

31. See Glaeser, "Symposium: Homo Economicus, Homo Myopicus, and the Law and Economics of Consumer Choice."

32. Mill, *On Liberty*, p. 74.

33. Bayer and Stuber, "Tobacco Control, Stigma, and Public Health."

34. Glaeser, "Symposium: Homo Economicus, Homo Myopicus, and the Law and Economics of Consumer Choice."

35. W. Kip Viscusi, "The New Cigarette Paternalism," *Regulation* (Winter 2002–2003): 58–64.

3

Narratives versus Norms

A Misplaced Debate in Bioethics?[1]

Introduction

The title of this chapter modifies one used by my teacher, James M. Gustafson, decades ago—"Context versus Principles: A Misplaced Debate in Christian Ethics."[2] In his influential essay, Gustafson argued that the debate over context versus principles is no longer "fruitful": "The umbrella named 'contextualism' has become so large that it now covers persons whose views are as significantly different from each other as they are different from some of the defenders of 'principles.' The defenders of the ethics of principles make their cases on different grounds, and use moral principles in different ways." Gustafson further argued that context and principles represent two of the four major base points in Christian moral discourse (the other two are theology and moral anthropology), and that, whatever a Christian ethicist's starting point, each of the other base points will appear, either implicitly or explicitly.

Even though I borrow from Gustafson's title, our approaches differ in important ways. First, Gustafson concentrated on Christian ethics, while I will focus on ethics broadly conceived—philosophical, religious, and especially practical ethics, including bioethics.

Second, I will often use the broad term "moral norms" of action, rather than the more precise language of moral principles and rules. Moral norms (hereafter "norms" without a modifier) include both principles and rules as "general action guides specifying that some type of action is prohibited, required, or permitted in certain circumstances."[3] I will construe principles as more general norms, which often provide warrants for rules, and rules as more concrete and detailed specifications of the type of prohibited, required, or permitted action. Principles and rules differ in their degree of specificity, but both are norms of actions that are distinguishable from particular judgments in concrete situations.

Third, Gustafson noted that the term "context" marks off no particular position because it covers so many different possibilities, ranging from the Christian community to the actual political situation. Here I deal with narrative(s) as one type of contextual approach to ethics.

However, my topic is not "narrative ethics," at least not in its broadest sense: It is rather "narrative (and norms) *in* ethics." I put matters this way to emphasize that I do not conceive ethics to be exclusively norm-based or always norm-driven. Instead, I will focus on the relations between norms and narratives in ethics. Both, properly understood, are essential and indispensable to ethics—the difficult questions concern their relations.

At the risk of serious oversimplification, I will distinguish the direction I take from some other possibilities by altering the prepositions connecting ethics and narrative as well as the location of the terms "ethics" and "narrative." Possibilities other than "narrative in ethics" include the "ethics *of* narrative," which might refer to the ethics of narration and, equally importantly, the ethics of listening. I will briefly discuss the ethics of narrating and listening in the context of interpreting the norm of respect for persons and their autonomous choices. I will also only mention in passing the "narrative *of* ethics" when I note the importance of tradition, community, and the like, without trying to resolve the larger question of the narrative grounds of ethics.[4]

I won't discuss at all "narrative *for* ethics," by which I mean the use of narrative, mainly but not exclusively fictional narrative, to engender such moral qualities as empathy. In at least some of its versions, such an approach includes "ethics *in* narrative" (with attention to form as well as content) as a way to use "narrative *for* ethics." Still another approach to "narrative *for* ethics" might focus on the "narrative *background of* ethics"—for example, the understanding of the moral self in terms of narrative, an understanding that usually invokes such themes as time, history, community, emotions, and virtues, among others that normist approaches sometimes may appear to neglect.[5]

Such a schematic interpretation of narrative ethics, or narrative and ethics, clearly depends not only on the different prepositions and locations of the key terms (narrative and ethics) but also on the content given to those terms, since narrative includes, for instance, cases, traditions, and fiction, while norms include, at a minimum, principles and rules.

My overall thesis, which echoes Gustafson's charge, is that the debate about narrative(s) versus moral norm(s) in ethics and bioethics is (largely) misplaced because too many different positions fall under each umbrella category, and many of the most vigorous "opponents" in the debate, whether narrativists or normists, actually share more with each other than they recognize and more than they have in common with some who are usually placed in the same camp. Hence, we have to reconsider the broad labels that have probably already outlived any usefulness they ever had.[6] I will focus first on the controversy about cases and case judgments in relation to norms, then I will turn to the role of narratives of different kinds in explicating requirements of the principle of respect for persons, particularly their autonomy, and finally I will examine the tension between personal and communal narratives in the context of appeals to experience and appeals to traditional norms. The last two parts will proceed by reference to two controversial cases.

Cases and Case Judgments in Normative Ethics

I want to start with the largely misplaced debate between casuists, as one type of narrativist, and principlists, as one type of normist, who appear to dispute the relation between the particular and the general, that is, particular case judgments and general moral norms. Each side has contributed to misunderstanding. For instance, normists have contributed to misunderstanding by the way they have discussed theory, applied ethics, and so forth, as well as by formulations and charts that appear to involve only top-down justification.[7] On the other side, casuists such as Albert Jonsen and Steven Toulmin have sometimes overstated their position by unfurling such banners as "the tyranny of principles," when, in fact, they oppose only certain conceptions of principles, that is, principles that are viewed as absolute, invariant, and eternal.[8] Only such principles are tyrannical. In general, principlists who view general norms as prima facie binding, rather than absolute, and who consider "application," as in "applied ethics," an oversimplification, have more in common with many casuists than with many other principlists.

Casuists have greatly illuminated contemporary moral discourse and deliberation by directing our attention to cases, which, after all, are mininarratives. They are narratives because of "the presence of a story and a story teller,"[9] but they are appropriately construed as "mininarratives" in order to distinguish them from much fuller stories. Casuists have further shown that our particular case judgments are often independent of and enter into the formulation of general norms rather than simply being derived from those norms.[10]

However, sometimes casuists who insist on paradigm cases and analogical reasoning are more formalistic and even legalistic than some principlists, especially principlists who recognize only prima facie binding norms. In their effort to categorize cases, casuists sometimes neglect the narrative quality of the cases they examine by forcing those cases into categories or "boxes" labeled as medical indications, patient preferences, quality of life, and external factors.[11]

Richard Miller wonders whether paradigms and stories are compatible and thus whether casuists and narrativists can have a "happy marriage." For him:

> narratives are not clear and uncontroversial, but murky and complicated. It is usually difficult to see through them until the end, and even then the interpretation of the narrative is often up for grabs. Such a device for practical reasoning would seem to make casuistry interminable. Paradigms boost the ability to enable casuists to proceed more efficiently, without interpretative complications. In contrast to narratives, paradigms are more or less self-evident or self-interpreting.[12]

However, cases have an ineliminable narrative structure; this holds even for the fairly thin cases often used in bioethics whether they are considered to be paradigmatic or not.

Miller further argues (against John Arras) that it is a mistake to bring casuistry and narrative close together because casuistry is occasioned, in large measure, by the two experiences of doubt and perplexity, the former involving uncertainty about the meaning or applicability of a moral principle, and the latter stemming from the experience of moral conflict.[13] Miller contends that casuistry's sense of separation or alienation of self, even if momentarily, from the guiding principle(s) is "difficult to reconcile with the dominant strand of narrative ethics, which views narrative as the antidote to doubt and perplexity—indeed, to practical reasoning itself." As presented by Alasdair MacIntyre and Stanley Hauerwas, among others with a strong interest in virtue, narrative is connected with the unity of the self and virtue, rather than with problems, dilemmas, and quandaries: "Narrative is a genre in the service of an undivided, unconflicted character, one which is not anxious about practical decisions or conflicts of duties." However, the

MacIntyre-Hauerwas conception of narrative and ethics is only one, even though it is clearly very influential. No particular approach to narrative and ethics, such as the MacIntyre-Hauerwas approach, should be taken as definitive, for, as my earlier schema suggested, there are so many different approaches to narrative and ethics.

Rather than focusing on the method of casuistry, perhaps we should focus on "particular cases" and "particular case judgments," with attention to the moral judgments made in the context of a particular case narrative. Particular case judgments are not always problematic or dilemmatic. Indeed, quite often—even usually—it is clear what we should do in particular circumstances, for example, to assist someone in need, without any appeal to general moral norms or paradigm cases (that is, same type cases). However, many who focus on particular cases and particular case judgments argue not only for their independence but also for their primacy or priority. What does it mean to affirm, as Jonsen and Toulmin do, the primacy or priority of particular judgments, that is, judgments related to particular cases?[14]

First, it might mean that particular judgments chronologically come first. But then the question is: For whom? Each individual participates in communities, many of which involve traditions of moral reflection. These traditions include both general moral norms and judgments about particular cases. Even if the particular judgments came first historically, we do not encounter the moral traditions of our communities only through their particular judgments; they usually present general norms too. Indeed, it is hard to imagine moral education proceeding without general norms as well as paradigm cases. Hence, the Jonsen-Toulmin view of principles as "top down" holds only if we think in terms of theoretical derivation; it does not fit with a historical, communal interpretation of morality.

Second, the primacy of particular judgments could mean logical priority. However, it is not clear that either general norms or particular case judgments have logical priority. Their relation is better construed as dialectical, with neither fully and completely derived from the other, but with each potentially modifying the other.

Third, assigning primacy to particular judgments could indicate normative priority. Here again the language of dialectic is more appropriate. Where particular judgments appear to conflict with general norms, adjustments are required, but it is not plausible to say that either should always take priority over the other.

We should note further what is implied when we make a judgment that an action is wrong in a particular set of circumstances. R. M. Hare argues that "if we, as a result of reflection on something that has happened, have made a certain moral judgment, we have acquired a precept or principle which has application in all similar cases. We have, in some sense of that word, learnt something."[15] If we learn something useful from reflection on a particular case, Hare claims, the principle we gain must be *somewhat general*; it cannot have unlimited specificity. Since no two real cases are exactly alike, we have results of reflection that can be useful in the future only if we "have isolated certain broad features of the cases we were thinking about—features which may recur in other cases." Hare's argument presupposes the formal principle of universalizability, which he rightly identifies as a condition of moral judgments. Accepting the principle of universalizability does not distinguish principlism from casuistry. Indeed, casuistry, as Jonsen and Toulmin conceive it, also presupposes this formal principle of universalizability—after all, casuistry depends on identifying relevant similarities and differences between cases in analogical reasoning. (The principle of universalizability also appears in the common law doctrine of precedent, which provides one major model for casuistry.)

Once generated, norms still require interpretation, and this interpretive process also involves narratives. A case may not clearly fall under a general norm; a single norm may point in two different directions in the same situation; and norms may come into apparent or real conflict—perhaps even dilemmas as well as interpersonal conflicts. Henry Richardson identifies three models of connection between principles and cases: (1) application, which involves the deductive application of principles and rules, (2) balancing, which depends on intuitive weighing, and (3) specification, which proceeds by "qualitatively tailoring our norms to cases."[16]

Even though Tom Beauchamp and I use the metaphors of both application and balancing, we most often balance principles, especially if application is construed as deduction. A balancing approach is the most consistent with a conception of principles as prima facie binding. However, we have attempted to reduce the reliance on intuition by developing a rough decision procedure of constrained balancing that attends to such matters as the necessity of breaching one principle in order to protect another, the effectiveness of doing so, minimization of the extent of the breach, and so forth.[17]

What Richardson calls "specification" also figures prominently in our work, because, as Hare notes, "any attempt to give content to a principle involves specifying the cases that are to fall under it . . . Any principle, then, which has content *goes some way down the path of specificity*" (italics added).[18] We have always used some form of specification (though the label was added only in the fourth edition) in determining the meaning, range, and scope of principles such as respect for autonomy, and in indicating how principles can take shape in rules, such as rules requiring voluntary informed consent. It also appears in our discussion of lying.[19] Furthermore, as Richardson notes, specification overlaps with casuistical categories—who, when, why, and so on—which themselves involve narratives, such as A is doing X to Y for Z reasons.

Instead of viewing application, balancing, and specification as three alternative models, it is better, I believe, to recognize that all three are important in parts of morality and for different situations or aspects of situations. Sometimes, however infrequently, we apply norms, sometimes we specify norms, but sometimes we can resolve conflicts only by balancing norms.

Perhaps *interpretation* is the most adequate general category, as long as interpretation includes attention to the meaning, scope, and range of different general norms, along with their weight or strength, as well as attention to particular situations (narratives). If determinations of meaning, scope, and weight are not possible in total abstraction from situations (narratives), or at least types of situations, as I would argue, then the putative differences between casuistry and principlism may be less significant than is often supposed. These apparently different approaches may share more than many recognize. Beauchamp and I do not claim that appeals to norms are indispensable for every particular judgment and moral decision, but we do claim that norms play an important role in many moral judgments and decisions, in moral education, and in moral justification in a communal setting (for example, regarding public policy). At the very least, there is an important similarity in spirit between some casuistical approaches and our principlism.

Not all conceptions of norms are equally hospitable to narratives. A conception of norms as prima facie binding and thus subject to balancing rather than subject merely to application or even specification fits more closely with narrative approaches. Sometimes we have to balance general norms in the situation, the case, as appropriately described. While application and specification need to attend more to the narrative structure of cases than their proponents often recognize, balancing clearly requires thoughtful attention to the case narrative.

Many different kinds of cases appear in biomedical ethics—for example, real, hypothetical but realistic, hypothetical but fantastic. Writers in bioethics tend to use real cases drawn from practice and literature in healthcare and public policy and from legal decisions. However, as Hare suggests, the main contrast should be drawn between realistic cases, whether actual or hypothetical, and fantastic ones. Nevertheless, if we take ethical imagination seriously, fantastic cases may also play a significant if only occasional role in stimulating our moral reflection, in testing the consistency of our judgments, and in challenging our formulation of norms and their applicability to certain cases. A superb example is Judith Jarvis Thomson's famous case of the person who is kidnapped and plugged into an unconscious violinist with a fatal kidney ailment to save the latter's life.[20] This case has helped to reshape the way we ethically imagine or conceive the problem of abortion. Abortion does not merely concern agents' obligations not to harm or kill but also their obligations to assist others by providing bodily life support—what is the basis of the latter obligation, how far does it extend, and how much weight does it have? Thomson's fantastic case provided an imaginative reconstrual of the relationship between a pregnant woman and a fetus, which others then extended through analogy with organ donation to explore the basis and limits of moral obligations to provide bodily life support.[21] Much of the debate about fantastic cases concerns their analogical significance for real or realistic cases.

Real and realistic cases are not merely matters of accurate description, they also raise difficult questions of narration.[22] One question is how thick cases must be—narrativists are inclined to make them very thick to create a fuller picture, and this is often quite appropriate but not always necessary or unproblematic. There is also a place for thin cases. Much depends on what we hold about "moral relevance." If, according to the condition of universalizability, we are to treat (relevantly) similar cases in a (relevantly) similar way, then the criteria of relevance obviously become important—and these may stem from the narratives of the community(ies). According to Dena Davis, "we need thick descriptions [as in the case of Donald/Dax Cowart, to be discussed later] to allow cases to remain open to different interpretations over time, and also to enable cases to ground an ethics of care. The thicker the case, the more contextual the response."[23]

Even real cases, whether thick or thin, are not mere reports of objective reality. Tod Chambers and others have forcefully called our attention to unarticulated assumptions in bioethics cases. All narratives are constructed, even the mininarratives of cases, however "true" to objective happenings they may be. These points drive another nail into the coffin of the fact/value distinction or separation that appears in some theories of the deductive application of norms to concrete cases. Application breaks down in part because so much evaluative work goes into the very construction of the case. Even real cases as narrated are, in Gustafson's phrase, "evaluative descriptions."

In moving from actual case to actual case, the ethicist (casuist) may be limited to mininarratives that practitioners and others offer for analysis and assessment as their felt problems or dilemmas. General moral norms may help identify other cases that should be on the moral agenda, and they may direct our attention to real problems and dilemmas, which have not yet been experienced as such. But even general moral norms cannot be applied, specified, or balanced without narrative contexts, a point that I will develop in relation to the principle of respect for personal autonomy and the ongoing debate about the best way to interpret a particular case.

Norms and Narratives: Respect for Personal Autonomy and the Case of Donald/Dax Cowart

The powerful case of Donald Cowart (later known as Dax Cowart), particularly as presented in the videotape *Please Let Me Die*, has long been a focal point for bioethical debates about the respective roles of narratives and norms. Some commentators have sharply contrasted William May's "narrative approach" to this case with my (and Courtney Campbell's) principlist approach.[24] Even though the contrasts may appear to be immediately instructive, they are often overdrawn, and in fact, the narrativist and principlist approaches to this case may be closer than many suppose. Despite their different starting points—narratives and norms respectively—there is considerable convergence between these positions, even though one ethicist claims that they "could not be more different."[25]

This case involves a very athletic man in his twenties who is severely burned in an accident that kills his father, and who over time indicates that he does not want to continue the treatment necessary to save his life.[26] Using a dramatic narrative approach to illuminate the burned person's shattered world, May argues that this case "challenges the conventional analysis of great moral issues in medical ethics," with its customary focus on conflicts between two rival values of life and quality of life and between two rival principles of paternalism and autonomy for selecting the right decision-maker. In his rich and powerful discussion, May contends that conventional frameworks fail in these world-shattering cases, mainly because the catastrophe is so devastating that the terms life/quality of life cannot adequately express what is at stake. The dramatic, narrative language of life/death/rebirth, May suggests, better expresses what is involved. However, May later returns to debates about paternalism and autonomy, observing that the image of rebirth, of the construction of a new identity, does not eliminate—and may even intensify— the problem of paternalism.[27]

By contrast, Campbell and I start with debates about the meaning and weights of the principles of beneficence and respect for autonomy in conflicts about paternalistic interventions; but we then attempt to show how difficult it is to respect persons in their concreteness, because they are temporal creatures (past, present, and future) and because they are social creatures (embedded in different communities). We cannot respect other persons' autonomy without listening to their narratives in order to determine what their wishes, choices, and actions really are. (Even though Campbell and I did not use the language of narrative, it is consistent with and further explicates what we argued.)

So May begins with narratives but moves to norms; we begin with norms but move to narratives. And, substantively, we come to the same conclusion about what ought to have been done (or not done). Campbell and I conclude that "it was imperative to acknowledge Dax's right to decide for himself whether to accept or refuse treatment after enough time had elapsed to determine his prognosis, his competence, and his settled wishes. At some point paternalistic interventions were unjustified." And May concludes: "Whatever the team can do for the victim, it cannot bring him to new life without his consent. It cannot provide him with such parenting. The domestic analogy is wrong." Furthermore, just as May recognizes the dangers of both paternalism and antipaternalism—paternalists are tempted by the sins of the overbearing, and antipaternalists by the sins of the underbearing—so Campbell and I stress both principles of respect for persons and of beneficence in order to avoid such temptations.[28]

The fact that May's rich, narrative discussion also concludes that Cowart should have been allowed to make his own decision about treatment is, according to some commentators, very important—a different conclusion would have called into question his narrative analysis. In short, norms can check narratives, just as narratives can check principles.[29] Here again we can see a dialectical relation between norms and cases.

May reaches his conclusion by arguing that paternalistic interventions are wrong in cases such as Cowart's largely because they are ineffective for the end that is sought. He takes a pro-autonomy position, in the sense of pro-choice as a resolute will to make good on a primary decision. Pro-autonomy is justified in such cases because it is a necessary condition for the constitution or reconstitution of moral identity following such a catastrophic loss. May thus offers a consequentialist justification for allowing Cowart to choose/refuse treatment: "Perhaps . . . leaving the door open to the possibility of his refusing treatment may make it easier for him to accept treatment and to persevere in the consequences of that acceptance and make good" on it. The healthcare team cannot bring Cowart to a new life "without his consent." If he chooses to live, he cannot simply "take up his old life. He must become a new man. Don Cowart becomes Dax. No parentalist can force him down that role." What is required is an "interior transformation . . . the reordering of one's identity from the ground up." While the community can assist this "heroic movement" in various ways, "without consent to transformation the patient cannot move from saying 'please let me die' to 'I am glad to be alive.'"[30]

In contrast to May's consequentialist argument, Campbell and I accept a (nonabsolutist) norm of respect for personal autonomy that justifies Cowart's and others' prima facie right to make decisions in both catastrophic and noncatastrophic cases—it is morally important to respect persons and their own stories. To respond otherwise would insult Cowart and treat him with disrespect. Why our position is more adequate as a baseline than May's, even though it too needs a narrative perspective, emerges more clearly in the light of some problems that May's approach encounters.

May appeals to some broad interpretive categories to locate and illuminate Cowart's experience, his ordeal, as a severely burned patient. Especially important are the categories of life/death/rebirth and Christian conversion as well as the hero in Greek tragedy. Such broad narrative categories can indeed be illuminating for certain purposes but confusing and even dangerous for others. In particular, they are confusing and dangerous when used to illuminate others' particular narratives in order to determine how caregivers ought to respond to their refusal of (or request for) treatment. Archetypal narratives may obscure individual narratives and thus seriously distort what a particular patient is saying—for instance, May's use of religious, often Christian, narrative patterns may be quite inappropriate for a severely burned patient who is atheistic or agnostic. Any interpretive categories must be sufficiently broad and neutral to encompass a wide range of conceptions of a good life and death.[31]

Physicians and other healthcare professionals should attend to the patient's own narrative, as required by the principle of respect for persons and their autonomy, rather than construing that narrative as a mere instance of a grand pattern of life/death/rebirth or of a set of substantive beliefs, such as a religious community's core convictions. This point holds even if the individual explicitly identifies in some way with the larger narrative. The implications are significant: we have to respect, for instance, a particular Jehovah's Witness's position on blood transfusions, even if it is wholly rejected by his/ her larger religious community—it is his or her own position that matters. (See the discussion in chapter 1 in this volume.) Or, to take another example, caregivers should respect a particular Navajo's own views about negative information and treatment decisions, rather than simply inferring them from the traditional Navajo narrative or worldview, which holds that language creates rather than reflects reality. After all, a particular Navajo may largely reject that grand narrative or worldview.[32]

While May's narrative perspective can help us see what went wrong, from the standpoint of both care and respect, over the first ten months of treatment of Donald Cowart, that is, up to the time of *Please Let Me Die*, it may be unjustifiably paternalistic or imperialistic to interpret a particular patient's story through a larger narrative pattern that blurs his or her own identity and individuality. That this is a serious risk in May's arguments is evident in his comments about Dax as a "new man," with a new identity. May bases his claim in part on the narrative patterns of life/death/rebirth previously noted and in part on the fact that Donald Cowart changed his name to Dax Cowart. While conceding that Cowart had a manifest, functional reason for changing his name—he couldn't write his full name again (and he also stated that he could hear Dax more clearly than Don)—May finds latent, symbolic meaning in this act: Cowart "knows that Donald Cowart has, if not biologically, existentially died; he must assume a new identity."[33] It is not clear, however, that Dax constituted a new identity for Donald—he still insists that he was wrongly treated against his will, even though he is happy to be alive now. At most, as Sumner Twiss rightly notes, Cowart "appears only to have deepened his original sense of willful independence and determination to live his life on the terms that he chooses. To interpret the forced changes in his life-plan as a reconstruction or even revision of identity may be to impose on

Cowart a moral vision that he does not share and that misinterprets his existential response to his ordeal."[34]

What finally is the upshot of the proposed shift in perspective from norm to narrative, from quality of life to life/death/rebirth, or from a "'right-to-die' story" to a "'chronic illness' story"? What should Cowart's caregivers have done when deciding whether to allow him to choose to die at the point of the original videotape, that is, ten months after the accident? Should they have acquiesced to his stated desire to die, or should they have forcibly treated him against his stated preference? Focusing on narratives, as May does, may simply push the procedural question of decision authority to a different level—away from the patient's particular decision to the patient's own story—without fundamentally altering the question or even the appropriate answer. "On the face of things," Lonnie Kliever writes, "the Cowart story is a classic case of autonomy versus paternalism. Certainly that clash is the perceived message of the film *Dax's Case* and represents Dax's own construal of his experience as a patient."[35] Even though Dax's own story is not incorrigible, and even though respect does not require others to accept it at face value, the shift to narrative simply rewrites the fundamental question so that it now becomes "whose story is it anyway?"[36] Problems of respect for persons and beneficence arise on the level of narrative, just as they do on the level of concrete decision-making.

The case of Donald/Dax Cowart thus raises some important issues about ethics in the narrative encounter—not only about *narration*, such as whose perspective and whose story, but also about *listening*, a term that I will use to encompass all forms of receiving narration. Without being able to develop the important points here, I will simply note that both narration and listening are performative. Analyses of narrative often draw, explicitly or implicitly, on J. L. Austin's analysis of performative speech and suggest that "narration" is the "performative function of story telling."[37] J. Hillis Miller writes that

> storytelling, the putting together of data to make a coherent tale, is performative. Oedipus the King is a story about the awful danger of storytelling. Storytelling in this case makes something happen with a vengeance. It leads the storyteller to condemn, blind, and exile himself, and it leads his mother-wife, Jocasta, to kill herself.[38]

As Miller's example suggests, listening, like narration, is performative. At the very least, listening is active, not merely passive, because it involves interpretation. It is very important to ask exactly what constitutes ethical listening when the healthcare professional listens to the narrative of "the wounded storyteller."[39] To listen ethically means to listen with respect, but respectful listening does not entail that the listener merely accept at face value the narrative that he or she hears. Campbell and I suggested the difficulty of interpreting what is heard, especially when we recognize the temporal and communal dimensions of the self and his or her stories. Furthermore, when the patient is ambivalent, it may be very difficult to determine exactly where to put the interpretive weight.

Ethical listening is indispensable, whether we start with narratives or start with norms, such as beneficence and respect for persons and their autonomous choices. Within either approach, the listener cannot avoid interpretive frameworks but, nevertheless, must be as careful as possible to hear what this particular person is saying, what his or her story is, rather than forcing it into a larger story that putatively illuminates the patient's particular story.

Narrative Experience: Proximity and Distance

In the last section of this chapter I want to consider the authority of particular narrative experiences, especially in setting and resolving moral problems and conflicts, over against general moral norms, often grounded in a tradition's story. This level of the debate about narratives versus norms often focuses on different construals of reality, on what, in an oversimplified formulation, constitutes "moral reality"—individual lived experience or communal moral norms developed over time or both?

Bioethicists often encounter resistance on the grounds that they are removed from practice, or that, even when they are also clinicians, they are still distant from the actual case for which other agents have primary responsibility. More broadly, this resistance sometimes denies that general norms fit or illuminate practical reality. Military metaphors enliven some statements of resistance. Critics protest that only those who are in the trenches or who stand on the firing line can really understand and appreciate the moral problems in healthcare, which may even take the form of what narrators call "war stories." Although such encounters in healthcare regularly embody the conflict between narratives and norms, a closer look suggests a different question: Whose narrative experience and what kind of narrative experience authoritatively sets problems for ethical reflection and indicates directions for resolution?[40]

In order to sharpen this question, and identify a couple of major possible answers to it, I will move outside biomedical ethics altogether and consider a remarkable exchange about the authority of different narratives in evaluating the US decision to drop the first atomic bomb on Hiroshima. Paul Fussell, a distinguished literary critic and author of a fine book on World War I, *The Great War and Modern Memory*,[41] wrote an article entitled "Hiroshima: A Soldier's View" for *The New Republic* near an anniversary of the dropping of the atomic bombs.[42] Echoing those who thanked God for the atomic bomb, Fussell charges that critics of the bombing betray their "remoteness from experience." By contrast, when the bombs were dropped, Fussell was in the infantry in Europe, awaiting transfer to the Pacific to continue the war there. He wants to show how his and many others' views about the first use of the bomb are influenced by "experience, sheer vulgar experience." This experience is evident, too, in his other writings—that is the experience "of having come to grips, face to face, with any enemy who designs your death," the experience of having your ass shot at, if not shot off, the experience of infantry and Marines and line Navy and all those who were told over and over again "to close with the enemy and destroy him."[43] In this discussion of Fussell's claims, I will view his appeal to experience as "a sort of story telling," and view the forcefulness of his appeal to experience as an unsurprising result of "the persuasive power of a coherent narrative."[44]

Presenting these narratives of experience is necessary, Fussell suggests, because "historical memory" tends unwittingly "to resolve ambiguity" about the decision to use atomic weapons, but we can restore ambiguity by considering the way "testimonies emanating from experience complicate attitudes about the cruel ending of that cruel war." These frontline people would have had to carry the war in the Pacific, island by island, if the bombs had not been dropped. In the context of such experiences, he quotes the Naval officer who said of Hiroshima: "Those were the best burned women and children I ever saw." Fussell himself says that it is a pity not that the bomb was used to end the war with Japan, but that it wasn't ready earlier to end the war with Germany. That is the story from "down there"—in the trenches, particularly from one who has been seriously wounded, as Fussell was. "Down there" is "the place where coarse self-interest is the rule."[45]

By contrast, another remarkable book on war, *The Warriors*, by J. Glenn Gray, a philosopher, reports that the US soldiers he was with in Europe were saddled with guilt and shame when they heard about our first use of the atomic bombs.[46] In response, Fussell sarcastically observes that Gray was not in the infantry, but was only an interrogator: *The Warriors* "gives every sign of remoteness from experience. Division headquarters is miles behind the places where the soldiers experience terror and madness and relieve those pressures by sadism."[47] Fussell deflects several other criticisms of the decision by the United States to use the atomic bomb because they too display "a similar remoteness from experience." For instance, he dismisses John Kenneth Galbraith's criticisms by noting that Galbraith served in administrative offices during World War II.[48]

In contrast to Fussell's claims for the primary authority of particular narratives of lived experience, there are good reasons to value the distance expressed in general moral norms embodied in a community's narrative traditions. One sharp criticism of the decision to drop the bomb comes from another thinker with a strong, but different, narrative orientation—Michael Walzer, whose superb book *Just and Unjust Wars* has the subtitle: *A Moral Argument with Historical Illustrations*.[49] When Walzer was preparing his book, which is, in my judgment, the best single twentieth-century work on just war theory and practice, he realized that his lack of experience in war put him at a disadvantage, and he thus read widely in memoirs of war in order to understand and appreciate its experiences and its traditions: "It is important to my own sense of my enterprise that I am reporting on experiences that men and women have really had and on arguments that they have really made."[50] For example, when Walzer attempts to interpret the norm of noncombatant immunity from direct attack as a matter of justice, he begins with the stories told by soldiers who were usually quite willing to fire at enemy soldiers but who refrained from doing so in some quite specific circumstances. In one narrative, George Orwell reported that he had refrained from shooting at an enemy soldier who was running along holding up his trousers: "I had come here to shoot at 'Fascists.' But a man who is holding up his trousers isn't a 'Fascist,' he is visibly a fellow-creature, similar to yourself, and you don't feel like shooting at him."[51]

Beyond particular memoirs, Walzer concentrates on what he calls "the moral reality of war," which involves moral norms, arguments, and judgments: "Reiterated over time, our arguments and judgments shape what I want to call *the moral reality of war*—that is, all those experiences of which moral language is descriptive and within which it is necessarily employed." Over against the claims for authority of certain particular narratives, Walzer insists "that the moral reality of war is not fixed by the actual activities of soldiers but by the opinions of mankind."[52] Yet this moral reality is expressed in arguments about particular narratives, that is, cases, and Walzer's approach is thoroughly casuistical, that is, focused on the examination of cases: "The proper method of practical morality is casuistic in character."[53]

From this perspective, Walzer vigorously challenges Fussell's assertion that in war "there are no limits at all; anything goes, so long as it helps to bring the boys home." There are some limits in war, Walzer argues. The "bombing of Hiroshima was an act of terrorism; its purpose was political, not military." It was murder, as defined by general moral norms, which include the immunity of noncombatants from direct attack. Such norms should and often do shape military choices. Even if these norms, and the arguments associated with them, are "most often expounded by those professors far from the battlefield," for whom Fussell has "such contempt," the moral argument "is an argument as old as war itself and one that many soldiers have believed and struggled to live by." And it is one that should guide those who make decisions apart from the heat of battle itself about the use of weapons. We have responsibilities, Walzer insists, to the "huddled masses" of civilians on their side, as well as to the soldiers on ours. Furthermore, he contends that, to be morally responsible, a decision such as the one to drop the atomic bomb must take account of "all the future victims of a politics and a warfare from which restraint has been banished."[54]

The norm Walzer articulates is not stripped from history, from a larger narrative—instead, his argument draws on that narrative. His conception of "historical memory" has to do not only with individual or collective recollections of World War II, as in Fussell's approach, but also with the traditions of moral reflection conveyed in various ways, including individual narratives, such as memoirs, and debates about particular cases. Of course there are several traditions of reflection on war, and the moral tradition of just war is itself an ongoing argument.[55] However, some important norms receive widespread and virtually universal acceptance in the just war tradition, and judgments we make about particular incidents in war, including exceptional cases, further contribute to the tradition of reflection.

In response to Walzer's critique, Fussell doubts that he and Walzer can ever agree, because their dispute is really "one between sensibilities," between "two different emotional and moral styles." He designates his own style as "the ironic and ambiguous (or even the tragic, if you like)"—it is "the literary-artistic historical" style—and Walzer's as "the certain" sensibility.[56]

To continue the contrast, the one sensibility or style "complicates problems, leaving them messier than before and making you feel terrible. The other solves problems and cleans up the place, making you feel tidy and satisfied." His own aim in writing about Hiroshima "was to complicate, even mess up, the moral picture" in order to dispute the critics. "I observed," Fussell continues,

> that those who deplore the dropping of the bomb absolutely turn out to be largely too young to have been killed if it hadn't been used. I don't want to be needlessly offensive, nor to insist that no person whose life was not saved by the A-bomb can come to a clear—by which I mean a complicated— understanding of the moral balance-sheet. But I note that in 1945 Michael Walzer, for all the emotional warmth of his current argument, was ten years old.

Hence, Walzer really couldn't appreciate what was involved because "understanding the past means feeling its pressure on your pulses." Furthermore, according to Fussell,

> [t]hose who actually fought on the line in the war, especially if they were wounded, constitute an in-group forever separate from those who did not. Praise or blame does not attach: rather, there is the accidental possession of a special empirical knowledge, a feeling of a mysterious shared ironic awareness manifesting itself in an instinctive skepticism about preten- sion, publicly enunciated truths, the vanities of learning, and the pomp of authority.[57]

I have told the story of this debate in some detail because it captures so well tensions between claims of authority for particular experiences—which, as Paul Lauritzen notes, are "narrative experiences"—and broader soci- ocultural narratives as well as between the claims of authority for partic- ular casuistical judgments and for general moral norms, which may also be grounded in and expressed in narratives. However, it is a mistake to try to settle the question of moral authority apart from complex arguments, which often include narratives in various forms. Once we recognize that narratives take many different forms, as do norms, then we can see that the interesting question is how they can and should relate. But in order to make progress on this debate we need much greater clarity, more than I have provided in this chapter, about what is involved in both narrative(s) and norm(s), two complex areas of human discourse.

Conclusion

In conclusion, the debate about norm and narrative in ethics, especially practical ethics, including bioethics, is (largely) misplaced. The norm camp and the narrative camp encompass so many different positions as to be virtually meaningless. Some positions that emphasize norms are much closer to some positions that emphasize narratives than they are to other normists. If we start with either norms or narratives, we are driven to the other.[58] We need both in any adequate ethics. Each plays a corrective, enriching, enhancing role in relation to the other—one by moving to the more general, the other by moving to the more particular. However we conceive their relation—dialectic, conversation, dialogue, and so on—the important but difficult task is to determine how they function together in a rigorous and imaginative ethical perspective, framework, or approach and how they illuminate the choices we have to make about both practices and public policies.

Notes

1. In light of criticisms of principlism based on narrative approaches, as well as my own strong personal interest in stories as I responded to my late wife's illness and death in 1994 and her fervent desire that her grandchildren remember her (both of which entailed attention to narratives), I arranged with Larry Bouchard, a University of Virginia colleague who specializes in religion and literature, to coteach a new graduate seminar in the spring of 1995 on "Narrative in Theology and Ethics." This seminar helped me better understand the possibilities and limitations of narrative in ethics, and I am grateful to my coteacher and to the students in that seminar (as well as in the two later versions of this seminar).

2. James M. Gustafson, "Context versus Principles: A Misplaced Debate in Christian Ethics," *Harvard Theological Review* 58 (1965); reprinted in James M. Gustafson, *Christian Ethics and the Community* (Philadelphia: Pilgrim Press, 1971), pp. 101–126. All references will be to the latter.

3. William David Solomon, "Rules and Principles," in *Encyclopedia of Bioethics*, ed. Warren T. Reich (New York: Free Press, 1978), vol. 1, pp. 407–413.

4. See various works by Alasdair MacIntyre and Stanley Hauerwas, which indicate their differences as well as their similarities. For more discussion of narrative in ethics, see also John Arras, "Nice Story, But So What? Narrative and Justification in Ethics," in *Stories and*

Their Limits: Narrative Approaches to Bioethics, ed. Hilde Lindemann Nelson (New York and London: Routledge, 1997), pp. 65–89, where the current chapter first appeared.

5. See, for example, various works by William F. May, including the ones referred to later.

6. I will often use the term "norms" and the label "normist" in order to avoid the associations triggered by the term "principles" and the label "principlist," particularly because the label was coined by critics. See K. Danner Clouser and Bernard Gert, "A Critique of Principlism," *Journal of Medicine and Philosophy* 15 (1990): 219–236.

7. For example, particularly in the first three editions of *Principles of Biomedical Ethics* (1st ed., 1979; 2nd ed., 1983; 3rd ed. 1989; 4th ed., 1994; 5th ed., 2001; 6th ed., 2009; 7th ed., 2013; 8th ed., in 2019), Tom Beauchamp and I used formulations and charts that were susceptible to the top-down interpretation.

8. Albert R. Jonsen and Steven Toulmin, *The Abuse of Casuistry* (Berkeley: University of California Press, 1988). See also Steven Toulmin, "The Tyranny of Principles," *Hastings Center Report* 11 (December 1981): 31–39.

9. See Robert Scholes and Robert Kellogg, *The Nature of Narrative* (New York: Oxford University Press, 1968), p. 4, for these criteria for narrative literary works.

10. The contributions of casuists often overlap with those of other contemporary perspectives, such as feminist ethics.

11. See the approach taken in Albert R. Jonsen, Mark Siegler, and William J. Winslade, *Clinical Ethics* (2nd edition; New York: Macmillan, 1986; 7th edition; New York: McGraw-Hill, 2010).

12. Richard B. Miller, "Narrative and Casuistry: A Response to John Arras," *Indiana Law Journal* 69 (Fall 1994): 1015–1019, written in response to John Arras, "Principles and Particularity: The Roles of Case in Bioethics," *Indiana Law Journal* 69 (Fall 1994): 983–1014. For one of the best analyses and assessments of casuistry, see John D. Arras, "Getting Down to Cases: The Revival of Casuistry in Bioethics," *Journal of Medicine and Philosophy* 16 (1991): 29–51.

13. Miller, "Narrative and Casuistry," pp. 1015–1019, which is also the source of the quotations in the remainder of this paragraph. For Miller's fuller perspective, see *Casuistry and Modern Ethics: A Poetics of Practical Reasoning* (Chicago: University of Chicago Press, 1996).

14. The next several paragraphs draw freely from James F. Childress, "Ethical Theories, Principles, and Casuistry in Bioethics: An Interpretation and Defense of Principlism," in *Religious Methods and Resources in Bioethics*, ed. Paul Camenisch (Boston: Kluwer, 1994), pp. 181–201.

15. R. M. Hare, "Principles," *Essays in Ethical Theory* (Oxford: Clarendon Press, 1989), pp. 49–65.

16. Henry Richardson, "Specifying Norms as a Way to Resolve Concrete Ethical Problems," *Philosophy and Public Affairs* 19 (1990): 279–320.

17. Beauchamp and Childress, *Principles of Biomedical Ethics*, 4th ed., pp. 33–37. See similar formulations in subsequent editions.

18. Hare, "Principles."

19. See Beauchamp and Childress, *Principles of Biomedical Ethics*, 4th ed., chap. 1. See also subsequent editions.

20. Judith Jarvis Thomson, "A Defense of Abortion," *Philosophy and Public Affairs* 1 (1971): 47–66.
21. See, for example, Susan Mattingly, "Viewing Abortion from the Perspective of Transplantation: The Ethics of the Gift of Life," *Soundings* 67 (1984): 399–410, and Patricia Beattie Jung. "Abortion and Organ Donation: Christian Reflections on Bodily Life Support," *Journal of Religious Ethics* 16 (1988): 273–305.
22. See the important work by Tod S. Chambers, including "The Bioethicist as Author: The Medical Ethics Case as Rhetorical Device," *Literature and Medicine* 13, no. 1 (Spring 1994): 60–78. For a partial response, see James F. Childress, *Practical Reasoning in Bioethics* (Bloomington: Indiana University Press, 1997), chap. 5. See also Tod Chambers, *The Fiction of Bioethics* (New York and London: Routledge, 1999).
23. Dena Davis, "Rich Cases: The Ethics of Thick Description," *Hastings Center Report* 21 (July/August, 1991): 12–17.
24. See William F. May, *The Patient's Ordeal* (Bloomington: Indiana University Press, 1991), chap. 1, which presents a revised version of his chapter "Dealing with Catastrophe," which appeared earlier in *Dax's Case: Essays in Medical Ethics and Human Meaning*, ed. Lonnie D. Kliever (Dallas: Southern Methodist University Press, 1989), pp. 131–150. The essay by James F. Childress and Courtney Campbell titled " 'Who Is a Doctor to Decide Whether a Person Lives or Dies?' " also appeared in *Dax's Case*, and is reprinted in Childress, *Practical Reasoning in Bioethics*, chap. 7. For further commentary, see Sumner B. Twiss, "Alternative Approaches to Patient and Family Medical Ethics: Review and Assessment," *Religious Studies Review* 21 (October 1995): 263–276; and Paul Lauritzen, "Ethics and Experience: The Case of the Curious Response," *Hastings Center Report* 26 (January/February 1996): 6–15. See also "Confronting Death: Who Chooses? Who Controls? A Dialogue between Dax Cowart and Robert Burt," *Hastings Center Report* 28 (January/February 1998).
25. Lauritzen, "Ethics and Experience."
26. A transcript of the videotape *Please Let Me Die*, which consists mainly of psychiatrist Robert B. White's interview of Donald Cowart, appears in Robert A. Burt, *Taking Care of Strangers: The Rule of Law in Doctor-Patient Relations* (New York: Free Press, 1979), pp.174–180. It is unclear whether that videotape is still available for purchase. The follow-up videotape, *Dax's Case* (1985), which includes interviews with many of the participants in the original case, is available from the Filmmakers Library, 124 East 40th St., New York, NY 10107. The later video is also discussed in Kliever, ed., *Dax's Case*.
27. May, *The Patient's Ordeal*.
28. See also James F. Childress, *Who Should Decide? Paternalism in Health Care* (New York: Oxford University Press, 1982), p. ix.
29. See Lauritzen, "Ethics and Experience."
30. May, *The Patient's Ordeal*, pp. 34–35.
31. Sumner Twiss makes a similar argument in "Alternative Approaches," but then he uses categories that may be excessively rationalistic, such as "life plan."

32. See Joseph A. Carrese and Lorna A. Rhodes, "Western Bioethics on the Navajo Reservation: Benefit or Harm?" *Journal of the American Medical Association* 274 (September 13, 1995): 820–825.

33. May, *The Patient's Ordeal*, p. 16.

34. See Twiss, "Alternative Approaches," p. 274. I have similar reservations about Lonnie Kliever's important and somewhat similar effort to re-envision "Dax's case" as a "'chronic illness' story" rather than a "'right-to-die' story." See Kliever, "Rage and Grief: Another Look at Dax's Case," in *Chronic Illness: From Experience to Policy*, ed. S. Kay Toombs, David Barnard, and Ronald A. Carson (Bloomington: Indiana University Press, 1995), pp. 58–76.

35. Kliever, "Rage and Grief," p. 73.

36. I borrow this question from Sue E. Estroff, who uses it for a different purpose in "Whose Story Is It Anyway? Authority, Voice, and Responsibility in Narratives of Chronic Illness," in Toombs, Barnard, and Carson, eds., *Chronic Illness: From Experience to Policy*, chap. 5.

37. Adam Zachary Newton, *Narrative Ethics* (Cambridge: Harvard University Press, 1995), p. 58.

38. J. Hillis Miller, "Narrative," in *Critical Terms for Literary Study*, ed. Frank Lentriccia and Thomas McLaughlin (Chicago: University of Chicago Press, 1990), p. 74.

39. The phrase "wounded storyteller" comes from the title of Arthur W. Frank's book, *The Wounded Storyteller: Body, Illness, and Ethics* (Chicago: University of Chicago Press, 1995).

40. It is not critical to try to resolve whether experience is necessarily narrative or only communicated narratively.

41. Paul Fussell, *The Great War and Modern Memory* (New York: Oxford University Press, 1975).

42. Paul Fussell, "Hiroshima: A Soldier's View," *The New Republic* (22 & 29, August 1981): 26–30. This article is reprinted in Fussell, *Thank God for the Atom Bomb and Other Essays* (New York: Oxford University Press, 1988). See also Fussell, "My War: How I Got Irony in the Infantry," *Harper's* (January 1982): 40–48, and, more recently, Fussell, *Doing Battle: The Making of a Skeptic* (Boston: Little, Brown, 1996), which recycles part of the essay "My War" in the context of his memoir. Another important expression of Fussell's perspective appears in his *Wartime: Understanding and Behavior in the Second World War* (New York: Oxford University Press, 1989), which examines the immediate impact of the war on both soldiers and civilians.

43. Fussell, "Hiroshima: A Soldier's View."

44. See Lauritzen, "Ethics and Experience," pp. 6–15, from which these quoted phrases are drawn.

45. Fussell, "Hiroshima: A Soldier's View," and "My War."

46. J. Glenn Gray, *The Warriors* (New York: Harper and Row, Torchbook edition, 1967), chap. 6, "The Ache of Guilt."

47. Fussell, "Hiroshima: A Soldier's View," p. 29.

48. Ibid., p. 27.

49. Michael Walzer, *Just and Unjust Wars: A Moral Argument with Historical Illustrations* (New York: Basic Books, 1977; 2nd ed., 1992; 3rd ed., 2000; 4th ed., 2006).

50. Ibid., 1st ed., p. xvi. This role of the memoirs Walzer read was particularly evident in his lectures on just war prior to the completion of his book. I had the pleasure of auditing these lectures while I was a postdoctoral Fellow in Law and Religion at the Harvard Law School in 1972–1973.

51. Walzer, *Just and Unjust Wars*, 1st ed., p. 140.

52. Ibid., p. 15.

53. Ibid., p. xvii. This is another example of the compatibility of norms and (particular) narratives, i.e., cases.

54. Walzer, "An Exchange on Hiroshima," *The New Republic* (September 23, 1981): 13–14.

55. On tradition as an ongoing argument, see Alasdair MacIntyre, *Whose Justice, Which Rationality?* (Notre Dame, IN: University of Notre Dame Press, 1988), p. 12 et passim.

56. See Fussell, "An Exchange on Hiroshima," 14. Elsewhere Fussell notes that "World War II produced his sense of irony." See "My War," and *Doing Battle: The Making of a Skeptic*.

57. Fussell, "My War."

58. This was also part of Gustafson's argument about principles and context in his classic essay.

PART II

RELIGION, BIOETHICS, AND PUBLIC POLICY

4

Religion, Bioethics, and Public Policy

Debates about Secularization

In the United States—and elsewhere—religious beliefs, values, and norms frequently occupy an ambiguous place in bioethical discourse, particularly in the context of public policy. Despite claims that a process of secularization has occurred in bioethics, religion has been and remains both a source of meaning, value, and content in bioethics—for example, in shaping some bioethical frameworks—and a source of problems for bioethics—for example, in generating or exacerbating some bioethical conflicts. Several types of conflict arise: (1) between benefiting patients and respecting their choices, often religiously based choices, in clinical contexts; (2) between protecting health professionals' consciences and protecting patients' interests; and (3) in determining the appropriate place, if any, for religious convictions in the formulation of public policy in a pluralistic, democratic society. The last conflict is the focus of this chapter and the next one. The second conflict is the subject of a subsequent chapter in this section that considers conscience-based exemptions from duties articulated in certain public policies, while the first conflict is addressed in the first chapter of this volume.

I begin by analyzing and evaluating two stories of the origins and secularization of bioethics. These emphasize different, though related, conceptions of religion, and they both neglect the range and diversity of bioethics in the United States. Then I critically examine a prominent and illuminating but ultimately flawed interpretation of the secularization of public bioethics. Much of the controversy featured in this chapter hinges on claims about the role of principles in bioethics, particularly whether their enlarged role contributed to or reflected the process of secularization.

Two Stories of Bioethics' Origins and Development

Historically, professional codes and religion-based directives have constituted the two major sources of ethical guidance for physicians (and other
healthcare providers). These two sources have not always been distinguished
or separated—for instance, a religion-influenced neo-Pythagorean cult probably formulated the original Hippocratic oath.[1] Religious communities and
traditions have also long provided ethical guidance for their adherents when
they are patients as well as when they are familial or professional caregivers.

A new field of ethical reflection—"biomedical ethics" or "bioethics"[2]—
emerged in the late 1960s and early 1970s to address the moral perplexities
occasioned by new medical technologies that could prolong life far beyond
previous limits and expectations, transplant organs from one person to another, detect some fetal problems in utero, offer new reproductive opportunities, and the like. From the beginning, this reflective activity has been
multidisciplinary and multiprofessional—its participants have included
clinicians, scientists, lawyers, philosophers, theologians, and other religious
thinkers. Two stories or myths[3] of origin of bioethics assign different roles to
religion, particularly theology and religious thought, in the emergence and
evolution of bioethics. They also provide different accounts of a process of
secularization.

Story # 1

According to the first myth of origins, theologians, along with philosophers,
scientists, and clinicians who were religiously oriented, fueled a "renaissance of medical ethics"[4] and created modern bioethics. Examples of this
myth abound. "Theologians were the first to appear on the scene," writes
Albert Jonsen, himself a former Jesuit as well as an early contributor to bioethics, in comparing the contributions of philosophers and theologians at
the beginning of the field.[5] And one of the field's acknowledged founders,
the Hasting Center's Daniel Callahan, a philosopher with a strong background in religion, stresses: "When I first became interested in bioethics in
the mid-1960's, the only resources were theological or those drawn from
within the traditions of medicine, themselves heavily shaped by religion."[6]
Major early contributors to the field included Joseph Fletcher (whose first
works in medical ethics displayed religious influences); John Fletcher (then

an Episcopal priest); Paul Ramsey; James Gustafson; Richard McCormick, S.J.; Immanuel Jakobovits; William F. May; and Leon Kass (a scientist, physician, and philosopher attentive to religious perspectives). Many of these and other early bioethicists "delved into their religious traditions," as Jonsen puts it, "rediscovering within them directions for bioethics."[7]

Narrators of this story of bioethics' origins then describe and frequently decry its subsequent secularization. Writing in 1990, Callahan observed, "the most striking change over the past two decades or so has been the secularization of bioethics."[8] Echoing Callahan's observation, two theological critics of the secularization of bioethics trace the decline of religion's and theology's roles:

> after the "renaissance of medical ethics" came the "enlightenment" of medical ethics. In the next decade, interest in religious traditions moved from the center to the margins of scholarly attention in medical ethics. The theologians who continued to contribute to the field seldom made an explicit appeal to their theological convictions or to their religious traditions.[9]

As Albert Jonsen summarizes the received wisdom about bioethics, "Bioethics began in religion, but religion has faded from bioethics."[10]

This putative process of secularization, as interpreted by various commentators, was marked by the "marginalization" of religious voices in the conversation; the decline of interest within the field of bioethics in what religious traditions had to offer; the limited appeal to religious traditions and beliefs even in the work of theologians and scholars in religious ethics; and so forth. Among the supposed causes of this process of secularization were the perceived difficulty of doing bioethics in an increasingly pluralistic society, whether at the bedside or in the public square, and the increased interest in bioethical issues in public policy in a democratic society. Hence, principles, rights, and procedures received more and more attention in bioethics discourse and practice. (We will return later to controversies about principles-based ethical frameworks in this putative process of secularization.)

Daniel Callahan summarizes some perceived negative effects of secularization in bioethics:

> Though I am not myself religious, I consider the decline of religious contributions a misfortune, leading to a paucity of concepts, a thin

imagination, and the ignorance of traditions, practices, and forms of moral analysis of great value.[11]

Furthermore, in language that closely connects with the second story, Howard Brody stresses that

what bioethics leaves out, when it tries to go about its business without cross-talk with religion, is a sense of *awe* and of *mystery*—the basic human response to what we perceive to be larger than ourselves. Bioethics, like medicine, tends to want to turn all mysteries into puzzles, so that solutions will be forthcoming.[12]

He also notes religion's function of attaching *meaning* to what happens.

Story #2

In their competing story of the origins and development of bioethics, sociologists Carla M. Messikomer, Renée C. Fox, and Judith P. Swazey challenge the "description of the 'religious-to-secular' trajectory of bio- ethics," claiming that it is "not quite accurate" and is "over-simplified in a number of ways."[13] They charge that the first story greatly exaggerates the historical role of religion and theology in the origins of bioethics. To be sure, these sociologists recognize the early contributions to bioethics by profes- sional theologians and religious ethicists, among others. However, they contend, religion's shaping influence on the conceptual framework of bio- ethics, its issues, its substance and form, and its relationship to public policy deliberations was "modest at best."

According to their analysis, most theologians and religious ethicists in bi- oethics were "already conforming to what quickly became [the field's] pre- dominant, rational secular mode of thought." The field's overall conceptual framework featured individual rights, in part because of the historical con- text of the origins of American bioethics in the era of the civil rights and antiwar movements, and the felt need to find consensus in the public square through principles and procedures. According to these interpreters, the field of bioethics has had a strong and persistent tendency to "screen out" religious questions or "to 'ethicize' them by reducing them to the field's circumscribed definition of ethics and ethical."

Assessing These Stories

How can we explain and evaluate these two different narratives? One partial explanation is that their narrators employ different conceptions of religion. Story #1 relies on a conception of religion that focuses on identifiable religious traditions, and on religious thinkers who mine those traditional resources for bioethical reflection. It presupposes that religion as embedded in these traditions addresses the divine, the sacred, the holy, and the like.

By contrast, in narrating story #2, Messikomer and colleagues do not concentrate on "religious doctrine, practice, or membership in a particular faith community." Their conception attends not to religious traditions or religious thinkers but, instead, to

> basic and transcendent aspects of the human condition, and enduring problems of meaning, to questions about human origins, identity, and destiny; the "why's" of pain and suffering, injustice and evil; the mysteries of life and death; and the wonders and enigmas of hope and endurance, compassion and caring, forgiveness and love.

Furthermore, various "metathemes," particularly ones that concern human birth and mortality, personhood, and finitude, are "religiously resonant, independently of how they are viewed by the articulators and practitioners of bioethics."

According to Messikomer and colleagues, religion in this broad sense has never really been significant in bioethics apart from a few exceptions. Instead, bioethics, at least through its first three decades, "characteristically 'ethicized' and secularized, rationalized and marginalized religion, and thereby restricted its influence on the mode of reflection and discourse, and the purview of the field." In story #2, then, "secularization" was evident from bioethics' birth. The authors wonder whether more recent developments, such as the increasing attention to religion and spirituality in medicine, healthcare, and health, might foretell some shifts in the ways bioethics accommodates religion.

Even though bioethics is a relatively new field, with many contributors, there is remarkable fascination with its origins. Different stories of the origins of bioethics often reflect more than historical or descriptive interests. Instead of aiming only to ensure an accurate historical record, these stories, as Fox and Swazey stress, generally buttress the narrators' claims about what bioethics should be.[14] Nevertheless, it is necessary and important to examine any story of origin for its accuracy and adequacy, apart from its normative goals or implications.

Neither of the two stories of the origins of bioethics is fully satisfactory. Each derives its initial plausibility from its conception of religion and its conception of what counts as bioethics. Particularly problematic is the conception of religion offered in the second story by Messikomer and colleagues, who posit a definition of religion according to which "aspects," "problems," and "questions" are construed as religious, regardless of the interpretations, solutions, or answers offered by those who address them. This definition obviously encompasses a broader span of human activities than a substantive definition focused on sacred or transcendent powers or focused on particular identifiable religious communities and traditions. However, somewhat paradoxically, the broad definition of religion in the story Messikomer and colleagues tell excludes some positions that adherents deem to be religious and that relate bioethics to sacred or transcendent beliefs, norms, and rituals, as interpreted in particular traditions. More importantly, it allows the authors to hold that religion has played only a modest role throughout the history of bioethics because bioethicists from the beginning paid only limited attention to certain problems and questions. For instance, they charge that in *Ethical Issues in Human Stem Cell Research*[15] by the National Bioethics Advisory Commission (NBAC) religion was "*expunged* by being reduced to 'diverse perspectives,' 'ethical issues,' and 'moral concerns.'" To be sure, NBAC, as a *bioethics* commission, attended to *ethical* positions taken by religious traditions and thinkers who usually defended those ethical positions by appealing to their fundamental religious beliefs. Of course, "ethics" does not exhaust a religion. But to hold that attending to a religious tradition's or thinker's *ethical* claims for purposes of deliberation about public policy *expunges* religion itself fails to recognize that religion consists of several interrelated components, ethics being one of them.

In short, this second story suffers from a definition of religion that makes certain positions religious, even if they claim to be secular, because of the problems or questions they address, and that excludes some positions that their adherents view as religious or at least as religiously informed, such as religiously based *ethical* judgments. This argument about the trajectory of bioethics would have been more persuasive if it had avoided the religious-secular polarity altogether and instead held that bioethics has not adequately addressed certain problems and questions, whatever label is used for those problems and questions.

Regardless of the conception of religion employed, it is important not to exaggerate the process of secularization. From the late 1960s/early 1970s to the present, academic bioethics has included both secular and religious, philosophical and theological, perspectives, and it has coexisted alongside—sometimes in interaction with—vibrant religious communities, in which theologians, priests, rabbis, and other interpreters of their traditions have continued to address bioethical issues, in light of their accepted sources of authority, in order to guide professional and nonprofessional caregivers and patients as well as, in some cases, to influence the broader public culture and public policy. Bioethics is not a monolithic field, and stories about its origin and development are misleading when they take part of the field to represent the whole.

Nevertheless, there are signs of increased attention to religious convictions and practices in bioethics as a whole. Many people continue to view religion as a source of bioethical wisdom and guidance for individuals, for particular communities, and for the larger society. Not surprisingly, then, respecting patients' choices often requires understanding their religious perspectives. In this context, as well as others, religion often creates or at least complicates and sometimes exacerbates bioethical problems and dilemmas and must be considered in any efforts to resolve them. Hence, the renewed attention to religion in bioethics partially reflects religion's perceived ambiguity. On the one hand, it is a source of wisdom and insight for addressing ethical problems, as well as a source of important moral values and virtues in healthcare. On the other hand—and at the same time—it is a source of significant conflicts in clinical care and public policy.

Whether they affirm the first or second story of the origins and development of bioethics, those who lament the limited role of religion and theology in American bioethics often connect the process of secularization with the emergence and development of what has been called principlism or principles-based ethical frameworks, featuring "intermediate" and "thin" principles, such as respect for autonomy, beneficence, nonmaleficence, and justice.[16] Not surprisingly, however, they describe this connection in quite different ways. In versions of both of the stories of origin and secularization presented previously, principles-based ethical frameworks are viewed sometimes as causes, sometimes as symptoms, and sometimes as potential, though usually inadequate, solutions to the process of secularization. One such formulation of bioethical principles, *Principles of Biomedical Ethics*, has increasingly appealed to the "common morality." Nevertheless, these principles are quite similar to norms emphasized by different religious traditions.[17] Arguably these principles are justifiable from the standpoint of different religious and secular traditions or represent an overlap or convergence of those traditions. These principles are thin and require specification as well as balancing. Hence, particular religious and secular traditions may flesh them out by thicker and richer interpretations of personhood, harms, benefits, and the like, and defend different priorities when these principles come into conflict.

Such differences sometimes erupt in social and political conflicts, depicted for the last few decades in the United States as "culture wars." However, it is important not to view these putative "culture wars" as only conflicts between *religious* and *secular* views over such bioethical issues as abortion, assisted suicide, and human embryonic stem cell research. Studies by the sociologist James Hunter and others indicate that liberals (or conservatives) in Protestantism, Roman Catholicism, and Judaism, to take three traditions, may share more with liberals (or conservatives) in the other traditions than with their own religious colleagues who do not share their liberal (or conservative) orientation. As Hunter summarizes the results of his research, "The theologically orthodox of each faith and the theologically progressive of each faith divided consistently along the anticipated lines on a wide range of issues," such as sexual morality, family issues, and capitalism.[18] Hence, despite some media interpretations, these "culture wars"—if they can be called that—have not been waged only by combatants identified by specific religious or secular labels. And the opposing sides have often shifted, depending on the particular bioethical issue being addressed. It is quite striking, for instance, that the pattern Hunter and others describe does not hold uniformly for human cloning or human embryonic stem cell research.

To take one illustration, the organizers of a conference for the conservative Center for Jewish and Christian Values, held in the US Capitol and sponsored by conservatives in Congress, were visibly uncomfortable when their expected united front of Protestant, Catholic, and Jewish opposition to human reproductive cloning turned out to be a mirage. The expected consensus broke down when Rabbi Bryon Sherwin, a conservative rabbi, indicated that Orthodox and Conservative Jewish thinkers, on the basis of their legal tradition, find it difficult to condemn human cloning per se, and that much Jewish opposition to human cloning, particularly in Reform Judaism, reflects categories outside Jewish law. "In my view," Sherwin argued, "Jewish theological, ethical and legal tradition can endorse the propriety of cloning human beings, albeit with certain restrictions."[19]

Another example of the lack of uniformity among conservatives (or liberals) across traditions appears in the debate about the status of the embryo in the petri dish or freezer that might be a source of stem cells. The Church of Jesus Christ of the Latter Day Saints—often called "Mormons," a label that the church now officially opposes—usually takes a stand on abortion and abortion policy close to that of the Roman Catholic Church, but its position on human embryonic stem cell research, as articulated by many of its members including several in Congress, has often differed substantially from the official Roman Catholic position because of its very different theological understanding of the creation of human beings.[20]

Playing God: Secularization of Bioethics-Related Public Policy

The book *Playing God: Human Genetic Engineering and the Rationalization of Public Bioethical Debate* (2002),[21] by the sociologist John Evans, offers a very important interpretation and critique of public bioethics in the United States, with particular attention to the diminished role of religious discourse in public policy debates. It focuses on secularization as the marginalization of theologians and religious discourse in a shift to what the sociologist Max Weber called formal rationality, that is, reasoning about means in relation to assumed ends.[22] Despite its insights, *Playing God* has major conceptual, methodological, and analytic flaws. I will focus on three major issues: Evans's criteria for bioethics/bioethicists, his interpretation and critique of principlism, and his understanding of public bioethics, specifically the role and function of bioethics commissions.

Bioethics and Bioethicists

Evans argues that debates about human genetic engineering (HGE) and a number of other bioethical issues are now generally "thin" (formally rational) rather than "thick" (substantively rational) in that they calculate effective and efficient means to assumed ends that are few in number and are considered commensurable and universal. This shift from substantive rationality to formal rationality in bioethical debates resulted from the competition of professions, not from a process of modernization or from democratic pluralism, which some interpretations of the turn to principles emphasize. More specifically, this shift resulted from the emergence and increasing power of the profession of bioethics in the struggle for jurisdiction over the definition of the ethics of HGE. According to Evans, the profession of bioethics, with its distinctive mode of argumentation (principlism), benefited in this competition from the removal of bioethical debate away from the public and legislatures and its reassignment to the state bureaucracy operating through government advisory commissions, a relocation that was supported by scientists seeking to protect their freedom. In this process, the bioethics profession displaced the theological community as a primary influence on public bioethics.

This interesting but problematic thesis hinges, in part, on Evans's criteria for identifying bioethicists and distinguishing them from others who may also engage in bioethical reflection. In popular parlance, people who participate in bioethical debates from a variety of professional and disciplinary backgrounds are often called "bioethicists," but Evans restricts the term "bioethicist" to those who are members of the "bioethics profession." However, it is not clear that bioethics is—or even should be—a profession. Unfortunately, Evans's implicit and explicit criteria for identifying bioethicists are problematic in part because an individual doing bioethics may satisfy one criterion but not another, thereby complicating Evans's classification and argument.

At least three criteria play some role in Evans's discussion. First, being a bioethicist may be a matter of self-designation or self-identification—someone may simply claim, "I am a bioethicist." At one point Evans writes about those "who called themselves bioethicists—rather than theologians, philosophers, or members of any other existing profession" (p. 35). However, this first criterion is not as significant in his analysis as the other two criteria.

Second, Evens holds that "'bioethicists' are those authors whose *primary identification* [also called primary academic appointment] is with a 'bioethics' or 'medical ethics' department or center, whether within a medical school or outside it" (p. 211, italics added). He points to the late John C. Fletcher as a prime example because of Fletcher's pivotal role in the debate about human genetic engineering. Using this second criterion, Evans can say that Fletcher moved from being a theology professional to a bioethics professional when he moved to the National Institutes of Health and subsequently to the University of Virginia. However, the limitations of this criterion are evident when we observe that, in fact, Fletcher's appointment to the faculty of the University of Virginia in the late 1980s was evenly split between the Department of Religious Studies in College of Arts and Sciences and the School of Medicine, where he established the new Center for Biomedical Ethics.

On a personal note, I write in the field of bioethics, but do not consider myself to be a bioethicist. Furthermore, my primary academic appointment was in the Department of Religious Studies, rather than in a bioethics or medical ethics department or center; I founded and directed a university-wide Institute for Practical Ethics and Public Life; and, for my last several years on the faculty, I held the title of University Professor. So I do not satisfy either of Evans's first two criteria. Nevertheless, he views *Principles of Biomedical Ethics*, which I coauthored with Tom Beauchamp (whose primary academic appointment has been in a department of philosophy), as a crucial text for his interpretation of bioethicists' mode of argumentation. As it turns out, then, "primary identification" with a " 'bioethics' or 'medical ethics' department or center" may not be as clear-cut, helpful, or inclusive as Evans supposes. It may reflect historical accidents, such as available opportunities or sources of funding.

Evans also has a third criterion: "the only professionals considered to be bioethicists are those who use the profession's form of argumentation" (p. 35). This criterion reflects an interpretation of profession that differs from ordinary discourse, which tends to focus on a specialized educational degree or organization. And it is also in tension with the first two criteria. According to Evans, we should define a profession "by the abstract knowledge that it uses in its work" (p. 29). By this criterion, people are bioethicists based on their mode of argumentation, whatever their self-designation or affiliation. Evans claims that his "empirical research finds that those whom [he identifies] as bioethicists do use a different form of argumentation than the members of other professions. In short, members of other professions participate in public bioethical debate, but they are not bioethicists unless they use the system of argumentation of the bioethics profession" (p. 35). According to Evans, some people who called themselves bioethicists "created a distinct form of argumentation for this [public bioethical debate]. In so doing they also created a profession, making distinctly different arguments than other professions did" (p. 35). Despite Evans's claim, many of us considered—and still consider—ourselves to be philosophers, theologians, or ethicists, rather than bioethicists.

Before exploring this putatively distinctive mode of argumentation, I would stress the tension among Evans's criteria for bioethicists. For instance, according to Evans, "it seems unlikely that the bioethics profession will move away from a formally rational type of argumentation, because its core jurisdiction of clinical bioethics now depends upon it" (p. 194). This claim is odd, given Evans's link between the profession and its "abstract knowledge." If the bioethics profession is defined by a formally rational type of argumentation, and moves away from that type of abstract knowledge, the logic of Evans's argument is that it would cease to be the bioethics profession. We could, of course, avoid this logical implication by employing one or both of the other two criteria. We could then say that the bioethics profession had changed its "abstract knowledge," instead of ceasing to exist. This example is indicative of the confusion that plagues Evans's criteria.

Principlism as Bioethicists' Mode of Argumentation

The mode of argumentation that Evans claims to find among bioethicists is "principlism," which, as we have seen, is often viewed as a cause or symptom or expression of secularization in bioethics. Unfortunately, Evans exaggerates principlism's role, influence, and significance by virtually ignoring competing approaches, and he greatly oversimplifies principlism as a form of argumentation.

First, Evans takes what has been a prominent bioethical framework since the late 1970s and identifies it as the exclusive framework for bioethics: One is a bioethicist, according to the third criterion, if and only if one uses that framework. However, this argument has the odd consequence that those who are bioethics professionals, according to his definition of primary appointment, cease to be such if they employ a case-oriented framework, such as the influential framework offered by Albert Jonsen, Mark Siegler, and William Winslade in their various editions of *Clinical Ethics*, a work curiously missing from Evans's bibliography. This is a major omission because Evans is making claims about the role of principlism in clinical ethics as well as in public policy.[23]

Second, Evans greatly oversimplifies principlism. His analysis tends to conflate the *Belmont Report* of the National Commission for the Protection of Human Subjects of Biomedical and Behavioral Research (1979) with the principles presented in various editions of Beauchamp and Childress,

Principles of Biomedical Ethics (PBE).[24] Belmont's three principles (respect for persons, beneficence, and justice) are similar to Beauchamp and Childress's four principles (respect for autonomy, beneficence, nonmaleficence, and justice). But there are important differences in terms and in content, some of which emerge in *PBE*'s presentation of principles for bioethics as a whole, not merely for research involving human subjects (the topic for the *Belmont Report*). Other differences include derivative principles or rules such as truthfulness and fidelity that are featured in *Principles of Biomedical Ethics*, as well as methods of justification, specification, and constrained balancing.

Third, Evans distorts many, perhaps most, versions of principlism by filtering it through his ends/means analytic categories. These categories fail to capture the nuances of positions that have broader and, dare I say, richer and thicker frameworks of moral, social, and political reasoning about science and other matters. Part of the ambiguity concerns "means," a term that sometimes refers to technologies and sometimes to actions toward ends. For instance, Evans notes that the thin ends allegedly favored by the principlists "could be applied to every potential debate about a *technological means*, such as HGE, abortion, or the cessation of life support" (p. 18, italics added). But then he writes, "for the formally rational debater, no means is inherently wrong, but is only wrong if it does not maximize the end pursued" (p. 21). Few principlists would hold that "technological means" such as HGE are inherently wrong, but they can and often do consider some actions using those means as morally unjustifiable not because they fail as means to realize an end or produce good consequences but because of their inherent or intrinsic features.

Principlists may hold consequentialist, deontological, or mixed views. Most principlists, unless they are thorough-going consequentialists, hold that some features of acts tend to make them right or wrong, independent of agents' ends and their actions' consequences. Such a view does necessarily not commit principlists to saying that acts with those features are absolutely wrong, and hence never justified; after all, those features could conceivably be overridden by other features of those acts. Nevertheless, for most principlists, "respect for autonomy" is a strong (even if only a prima facie) constraint, a limiting principle, not merely an end. A similar point holds for justice—hence, for most principlists, an act can be wrong because it involves the exploitation of individuals. And deception is at least prima facie wrong. These examples indicate that Evans's means/ends analytic framework fails to illuminate most principlist positions.

Indeed, Evans tends to reduce formal rationality, attributed to principlism, to consequentialist reasoning. Such reasoning is a "hallmark of formal rationality" (p. 15). Because of his reductionist interpretation of principlism, Evans can use the metaphor of *calculation* to replace principlists' metaphors of *weighing* and *balancing* principles. In short, Evans's analysis oversimplifies and distorts principlism by making formal rationality consequentialist and then assimilating principlism to this model.

Fourth, Evans fails to see how significant alternatives to principlism function in public bioethics. For instance, Albert Jonsen and Stephen Toulmin (the former a member of the National Commission for the Protection of Human Subjects, and the latter a member of that commission's staff) have argued that the commissioners reached their judgments about such topics as research involving children through their ethical analysis of types of cases without recourse to principles and that the Belmont principles emerged late in their discussion, toward the end of the commission's term, in part because of a mandate in the original legislation. As Jonsen and Toulmin interpret the work of the National Commission, "the locus of certitude in the commissioners' discussions did not lie in an agreed set of intrinsically convincing general rules or principles, as they shared no commitment to any such body of agreed principles. Rather, it lay in a shared perception of what was specifically at stake in the particular kinds of human situations."[25] Whether we agree or disagree with Jonsen and Toulmin's claim—and I would dispute part of their overall argument[26]—it needs to be seriously considered, because casuistry may have functioned more than principlism in some governmental bioethics commissions.

Evans's Normative Stance on Public Discourse and Governmental Bioethics Bodies

Evans takes a "normative position," influenced by Jurgen Habermas, that "the public debate about HGE should not be artificially limited when such limitation favors the interest of one group over others," and he understands a group's interest in public bioethics as the promotion of that group's moral vision against what it considers as other groups' bad arguments (p. 5). Evans makes in passing, rather than arguing for, another normative—or perhaps metaethical—claim, similar to one offered by Leon Kass, that "visceral reactions" represent "unarticulated wisdom from which we can learn" (p. 3).

Given these points, it is not surprising that he contends that the public bioethics debate in the United States has been "eviscerated" or that "a bigger, deeper, more fundamental, or 'thicker' debate has been replaced by a smaller, shallower, more superficial, or 'thinner' one" (p. 4). While conceding that a thin morality may have a place in public debates, Evans fails to consider why it might sometimes become dominant apart from particular professional groups' interests. Indeed, at times and for various reasons, the public may prefer a thin debate over a thick one. Perhaps public policy in a democracy even depends more on the breadth of argument and agreement among the populace than on depth of argument among debaters. Even though Evans notes what he believes his book "has shown about how people *should* make collective moral decisions in pluralistic societies" (p. 9, italics added), he has not offered a complete or cogent argument for such "collective moral decisions" on all bioethical issues, much less why public bioethics commissions should be construed only as "means commissions," given their limited authority.

Three further observations may be pertinent. First, among the whole range of bioethical issues that could receive attention, it is not clear that all of them—or which ones—should be subjected to thick rather than thin debate. Evans apparently believes that human genetic engineering should have been a matter of thick debate but it is not clear why. At other points he seems to suggest that issues that evoke strong emotional reactions should be subjected to thick debate, but this point also needs further development and argument.

Second, even those who might argue for thin debate in some contexts of *public policy* usually recognize the place and importance of thick debate in the *public culture*, which often has an impact on public policy. According to Evans, the shift of public bioethics to governmental advisory commissions, away from the public and legislatures, led to the exclusion of theologians (p. 196 et passim). However, theologians have remained active in shaping public culture, and they have not been ignored in public policy. It is difficult to establish that the emergence of governmental bioethics commissions or the "profession" of bioethics undermined their role—indeed, evidence suggests a resurgence of interest in religiously based bioethics.

Third, bioethical debates may focus on acts and practices, on the one hand, or on public policies, on the other hand. Public policies typically concern whether to permit, prohibit, or regulate acts or practices or whether to provide or withhold government funds, and within what limits, as the debates about both human cloning and human embryonic stem cell research indicate. In deliberation about coercive public policies, which regulate or prohibit acts, certain moral presumptions are built into our society's constitution, laws, and policies, and they provide starting points for the arguments that follow. Arguments have to rebut those presumptions, for example, about scientific freedom or reproductive liberty.

A failure to recognize such points perhaps in part accounts for Evans's inadequate account of public bioethics commissions, but his account also suffers from other conceptual and empirical problems. Having served on such commissions, including the National Bioethics Advisory Commission (NBAC; 1996–2001) and the short-lived Biomedical Ethics Advisory Committee of Congressional Biomedical Ethics Board (1988–1989), as well as several more specific bodies, such as the Human Fetal Tissue Transplantation Research Panel, the national Organ Transplantation Task Force, and the Recombinant DNA Advisory Committee (RAC), I believe that Evans's interpretation of bioethics advisory commissions and their function is seriously flawed in ways that undermine his analysis and argument.

First, he uses the language of "decide" or "decision" over and over again for what these bioethics bodies do—he views these "commissions as decision-makers" (p. 37 et passim). Of course, they "decide" and make "decisions" in a certain but very limited sense—that is, they decide to make recommendations to policy-makers. But for the most part they do not make policy decisions—in general, just as he proposes, accountable public officials make policy decisions, and they may or may not heed the recommendations offered by bioethics bodies, as a cursory examination of the bioethics bodies I mentioned earlier would indicate. Such bodies have to present analyses and arguments that are convincing to those in positions of accountability. Evans seems to recognize this in his language of "advisory commissions," but if bioethics commissions only have an advisory role, then some of his interpretations and judgments require more qualifications than he provides.

Evans could respond that his points hold for bioethics commissions that advise the bureaucracy—for instance, the RAC—but in fact he focuses mainly on the work of the President's Commission for the Study of Ethical Problems in Medicine and Biomedical and Behavioral Research and also attends in the final chapter to NBAC, another body accountable to the White House. In short, Evans provides no evidence for his claim that "advisory commissions became the *ultimate arbiter* of whether HGE was ethical and thus whether it would occur" (p. 6, italics added).

Just as Evans's analysis distorts what public bioethics commissions do, and can do, it also distorts the major counterexample he offers: abortion. Several times he refers to the "thick" debate about abortion as a counterexample to the "thin" debate about HGE. Human genetic engineering, he contends, was shifted away from the public "toward government advisory commissions," while abortion remains in the public's domain: "the abortion debate has retained the public as the ultimate decision-maker and the HGE debate has not" (p. 178). That analysis is seriously misleading because, as a matter of fact, the US Supreme Court in *Roe v. Wade* in 1973 preempted evolving state decisions about abortion, thereby taking much of the decision-making about abortion laws out of the hands of state legislatures and thus away from the public. This court decision, many argue, short-circuited the public debate about abortion laws, one result being the emergence of a vigorous right-to-life movement. Despite shifts among justices on the Supreme Court, different rationales in subsequent decisions, and other changes in legal rules surrounding women's abortion decisions, the core of *Roe v. Wade* still holds. Of course, this core could change with further changes in the composition of the Supreme Court.

Furthermore, Evans is able to claim that the public is still "the ultimate decision-maker" about abortion only by expanding his interpretation of democratic decision-making: "politicians at the state and federal levels determine whether abortion is going to occur—whether through votes or the appointment of justices" (p. 178). If Evans can accommodate "the appointment of justices" in the exercise of democratic authority, accountable to the public, then he can surely accommodate the appointment of bioethics advisory commissions that have no power other than to offer advice, which accountable agents, such as legislatures and presidents, can follow or not.

In addition, the debates about abortion and about HGE are not fully comparable, in part because of the central place of the embryo/fetus in the abortion debate (as well as in the human embryonic stem cell research debate over the last fifteen years or so) but its marginal role in the debate about HGE. This is important because the debate about abortion and human embryonic stem cell research requires judgments about moral status, which cannot be resolved through moral principles. Instead, judgments about moral status determine how principles, such as respect for persons and nonmaleficence, are applied; moral principles cannot themselves resolve moral status. (For this reason the 6th, 7th, and 8th editions of Beauchamp and Childress, *Principles of Biomedical Ethics* include a chapter on moral status.)

In the final chapter of *Playing God*, Evans discusses "the 1997 debate over human cloning and how the process of the cloning debate provides further evidence for the claims made in this book" (p. 9). Although he concedes that, at first glance, the furor over human cloning might appear to "contradict" his findings, he claims that there is no contradiction: "The answer is that, for this issue, and unlike most other decisions by government advisory commissions, the ultimate arbiter of the ethical decision was the public" (p. 189). In short, some "democratically elected official would be held accountable for the decision on this issue—be it the president or the Congress" (p. 169). In contrast to Evans's claims, that point would also hold for most bioethical debates, including HGE—the public may choose to hold elected officials accountable.

Some of Evans's observations about the context, process, and content of NBAC's 1997 report *Cloning Human Beings* need qualification.[27] He notes that NBAC invited several theologians and philosophers, among others, to testify in what amounted to a thick discussion, but he seems to suppose that the theologians were invited because the public had defined the problem through its expression of repugnance over the prospect of human reproductive cloning (p. 191). It is a mistake to contend as Evans does that "theologians were no longer seen as serious contributors to the debate itself but rather served as spokespersons for communities within a pluralistic public that was closely watching the cloning debate" (p. 189). As I know from my participation in NBAC's deliberations, there was serious interest among commissioners in these theological positions. After all, over the previous twenty-five or so years theologians had analyzed and debated human cloning more extensively than philosophers. Moreover, in different places in its report, NBAC gives several reasons for attending to positions taken by thinkers within religious communities and traditions—some had to do with the wisdom embedded in those traditions, some had to do with feasibility of public policy, and so forth. (See the discussion in the next chapter.)

Despite NBAC's incorporation of theological perspectives into its deliberative process, Evans contends that NBAC's report is not as "thick" as it first appears: "when it came to actually reaching ethical conclusions about what to do about cloning, the broader, substantive debate receded into the background" (p. 191). In fact, NBAC unanimously recommended a federal ban of three to five years on efforts to clone human beings and, at the same time, called for an extended national dialogue ("widespread and continuing deliberation") on human cloning about precisely the kinds of issues that Evans wants debated.

The Commission concludes that at this time it is morally unacceptable for anyone in the public or private sector, whether in a research or clinical settings, to attempt to create a child using somatic cell nuclear transfer cloning. The Commission reached a consensus on this point because current scientific information indicates that this technique is not safe to use in humans at this point. Indeed, the Commission believes that it would violate important ethical obligations were clinicians or research to attempt to create a child using these particular technologies, which are likely to involve unacceptable risks to the fetus and/or potential child. Moreover, in addition to safety concerns, many other serious ethical concerns have been identified which require much more widespread and careful public deliberation before this technology may be used.[28]

It is important to distinguish what NBAC offered as reasons for its recommendations from what individual commissioners may have considered their reasons. All agreed that safety was relevant; perhaps it was sufficient at the time for many or most to reach the unanimous recommendation—certainly it was for me—but some commissioners may have found the other reasons about individuality, threats to the family, and so forth, to be persuasive. And all these reasons require broad public attention.

Some states have banned human reproductive cloning, but there is no federal ban, perhaps in part because of continuing "thick" debates in which a number of participants, including a majority in the House of Representatives, have proposed at the same time to ban human cloning for research purposes. There is widespread agreement among the public and legislators that we should ban human cloning to produce children—in short, we have an overlapping consensus about ethical public policy based on a variety of secular and religious reasons. However, the thick debate about the moral status of the early embryo, in the context of cloning-for-research, reveals deep and perhaps irreconcilable differences among religious communities and traditions, as well as the public at large. This division was evident in the debates, deliberations, and recommendations of the President's Council on Bioethics, established by President George W. Bush under the chairmanship of Leon Kass.[29]

In short, despite some valuable insights, Evans's interpretation of public bioethical discourse suffers from several conceptual, methodological, and analytic flaws, including those noted in this chapter. But there are others as well—for instance, his heavy and problematic social scientific apparatus (e.g., the use of the citation index) fails to generate the insights he supposes. All in all, *Playing God* missed a great opportunity to illuminate the roles of religion and ethical principles in public bioethics. Instead, it left untouched several persistent and prevalent confusions about religion and secularization in bioethics, especially public bioethics, and, for good measure, added several of its own.

Notes

1. For a summary of some of the evidence, see Robert M. Veatch, "Medical Codes and Oaths: History," in *Encyclopedia of Bioethics*, 2nd edition, ed. in chief, Warren T. Reich (New York: MacMillan Library Reference, 1995), vol. 3, p. 1420.
2. Van Rensselaer Potter coined the term "bioethics" in 1970, with a broader meaning than it came to have in common discourse. Potter, "Bioethics: The Science of Survival," *Perspectives in Biology and Medicine* 14 (1970): 127–153.
3. Here I use the terms "story" and "myth" interchangeably and without any implication of the story's or myth's lack of accuracy and trustworthiness. I presented a briefer version of these two myths of the origins of bioethics in my "Religion, Theology, and Bioethics," in *The Nature and Prospects of Bioethics: Interdisciplinary Perspectives*, ed. Franklin G. Miller, John C. Fletcher, and James M. Humber (Totowa, NJ: Humana Press, 2010), pp. 44–47.
4. LeRoy Walters, "Religion and the Renaissance of Medical Ethics in the United States: 1965–1975," in *Theology and Bioethics: Exploring Foundations and Frontiers*, ed. Earl E. Shelp (Dordrecht, Holland: D. Reidel, 1985), pp. 3–16.
5. Albert R. Jonsen, *The Birth of Bioethics* (New York: Oxford University Press, 1994), p. 34.
6. Daniel Callahan, "Religion and the Secularization of Bioethics," *Hastings Center Report* 20 (July/August 1990): 2.
7. Jonsen, *The Birth of Bioethics*, p. 35.
8. Callahan, "Religion and the Secularization of Bioethics," p. 2.
9. Allen Verhey and Stephen E. Lammers, "Introduction: Rediscovering Religious Traditions in Medical Ethics," in *Theological Voices in Medical Ethics*, ed. Verhey and Lammers (Grand Rapids, MI: Eerdmans, 1993), p. 3. See also Allen Verhey, ed., *Religion and Medical Ethics: Looking Back, Looking Forward* (Grand Rapids, MI: Eerdmans, 1996), particularly the chapters by David H. Smith, "Religion and the Roots of the Bioethics Revival," and by Stephen E. Lammers, "The Marginalization of Religious Voices in Bioethics." Throughout bioethics, in academic, clinical, and policy settings, philosophers played increasingly significant roles. See Stephen Toulmin, "How Medicine Saved the Life of Ethics," *Perspectives in Biology and Medicine* 25, No. 4 (1982): 736–750. Kevin Wm. Wildes notes that theological ethics was marginalized because "philosophical ethics offered the hope of resolving such questions [related

to the explosion of technological powers in medicine] without appealing to the faith of a particular community." See Wildes, "Religion in Bioethics: A Rebirth," *Christian Bioethics* 8, No. 2 (August 2002): 163–164.

10. Albert R. Jonsen, "A History of Religion and Bioethics," in *Handbook of Bioethics and Religion*, ed. David E. Guinn (New York: Oxford University Press, 2006), p. 23. Jonsen accepts this received wisdom only with "some qualifications." (p. 33).

11. Daniel Callahan, "The Social Sciences and the Task of Bioethics," *Daedalus* 128 (1999): 280.

12. Howard Brody, *The Future of Bioethics* (New York: Oxford University Press, 2009), p. 34.

13. Carla M. Messikomer, Renée C. Fox, and Judith P. Swazey, "The Presence and Influence of Religion in American Bioethics," *Perspectives in Biology and Medicine* 44, No. 4 (Autumn, 2001): 485–508, at p. 489. Subsequent references to their work in the text are to this article.

14. See Renée C. Fox and Judith P. Swazey, *Observing Bioethics* (New York: Oxford University Press, 2008).

15. National Bioethics Advisory Commission, *Ethical Issues in Human Stem Cell Research*, Vol. 1: *Report and Recommendations* (Rockville, MD: NBAC, September 1999).

16. For example, Tom L. Beauchamp and James F. Childress, *Principles of Biomedical Ethics* 1st edition (New York: Oxford University Press, 1979). Subsequent editions have been published: 1983, 1989, 1994, 2001, 2009, 2013, and 2019.

17. See several of the chapters in Raanan Gillon, ed., *Principles of Health Care Ethics* (New York: Wiley, 1994).

18. James Davison Hunter, *Culture Wars: The Struggle to Define America* (New York: BasicBooks, 1991), p. 96.

19. Bryon L. Sherwin, "Religious Perspectives on Cloning: A Jewish View," Presentation at the US Capitol, June 24, 1997. See also Byron L. Sherwin, *Jewish Ethics for the Twenty-First Century: Living in the Image of God* (Syracuse, NY: Syracuse University Press, 2000), chap. 6, "Cloning and Reproductive Biotechnology." The theme of human partnership with God is prominent in Sherwin's writings; see *In Partnership with God: Contemporary Jewish Law and Ethics* (Syracuse, NY: Syracuse University Press, 1990).

20. See Drew Clark, "The Mormon Stem-Cell Choir," *Slate*, August 3, 2001.

21. John H. Evans, *Playing God? Human Genetic Engineering and the Rationalization of Public Bioethical Debate* (Chicago: University of Chicago Press, 2002). In the remainder of this chapter, page numbers in parentheses will indicate a reference to this work. Evans has published other works that develop some of these themes; see, for example, John H. Evans, "A Sociological Account of the Growth of Principlism," *Hastings Center Report* 30, No. 3 (2000): 31–38; "Max Weber Meets the *Belmont Report*," in *Belmont Revisited: Ethical Principles for Research with Human Subjects*, ed. James F. Childress, Eric M. Meslin, and Harold T. Shapiro (Washington, DC: Georgetown University Press, 2005), pp. 228–243; and "Progressive Bioethics and Religion," in *Progress in Bioethics: Science, Policy, and Politics*, ed. Jonathan D. Moreno and Sam Berger (Cambridge, MA: MIT Press, 2010). These themes also appear in the

first two chapters of Evans, *The History and Future of Bioethics: A Sociological View* (New York: Oxford University Press, 2012).

22. Much of the debate about religion in bioethics and bioethical public policy hinges on definitions of secularization. For different definitions, see, for example, James F. Childress and David B. Harned, eds., *Secularization and the Protestant Prospect* (Philadelphia: Westminster Press, 1970).

23. Albert R. Jonsen, Mark Siegler, William J. Winslade, *Clinical Ethics: A Practical Approach to Ethical Decisions in Clinical Medicine*, 7th edition (New York: McGraw-Hill, 2010).

24. National Commission for the Protection of Human Subjects of Biomedical and Behavioral Research, *The Belmont Report: Ethical Principles and Guidelines for the Protection of Human Subjects of Research* (*Federal Register*, April 18, 1979). Reprinted in Childress, Meslin, and Shapiro, eds., *Belmont Revisited: Ethical Principles for Research with Human Subjects*, Appendix, pp. 253–265. It was also published in late 1978 as a separate volume. *National Commission for the Protection of Human Subjects of Biomedical and Behavioral Research, The Belmont Report: Ethical Principles and Guidelines for the Protection of Human Subjects of Research* (Washington, DC: DHEW Publication OS 78-0012), along with two appendices that provided the background papers considered by the National Commission. For the relation between the *Belmont Report* and Beauchamp and Childress, *Principles of Biomedical Ethics*, see Childress, Meslin, and Shapiro, eds., *Belmont Revisited*, especially chap. 2 by Tom Beauchamp.

25. Albert R. Jonsen and Stephen Toulmin, *The Abuse of Casuistry: A History of Moral Reasoning* (Berkeley and Los Angeles: University of California Press, 1988), p. 18

26. See James F. Childress, *Practical Reasoning in Bioethics* (Bloomington: Indiana University Press, 1997), chap. 2.

27. National Bioethics Advisory Commission (NBAC), *Cloning Human Beings*, Vol. 1: *Report and Recommendations* (Rockville, MD: NBAC, 1997).

28. NBAC, *Cloning Human Beings*, p. iii.

29. For a very positive assessment of the Kass council, see Adam Briggle, *A Rich Bioethics: Public Policy, Biotechnology, and the Kass Council* (Notre Dame, IN: University of Notre Dame Press, 2010).

5

Religion, Morality, and Public Policy

The Controversy about Human Cloning

Introduction

What is the proper role for religious convictions in the formation and for-mulation of bioethical public policy in a liberal, pluralistic democracy? To address this question, I will focus on the controversy about human cloning that erupted upon the announcement, in late February 1997, of the birth of a cloned sheep, "Dolly," several months earlier. I will treat this as a histor-ical case study, because of major scientific and technological changes since then. Hence, rather than updating the debate, I will present the arguments that arose at the time, particularly in the context of the National Bioethics Advisory Commission's (NBAC's) deliberations and report on cloning human beings, but I will add some points about NBAC's deliberations about and report on human embryonic stem cell research that further illuminate the main question of this chapter.[1]

In response to the announcement of Dolly's birth, President Clinton declared a ban on the use of federal funds for research to clone humans, called for a voluntary moratorium in the private arena, and asked NBAC, which had been appointed in late 1996 to deal with issues in genetics and in research involving human subjects, to prepare a report and recommend appropriate public policies within ninety days. The debate about appropriate public policies toward human cloning, both within NBAC and in the society at large, affords one way to examine how religious convictions may legitimately contribute to the formulation of public policy in a liberal, pluralistic democracy, which involves reasoning and giving reasons to other citizens in a deliberative forum.[2] Instead of addressing constitutional issues, which obviously set the background for such debates, I will consider only the public morality or social ethics of speaking in and listening to religious voices in public reasoning and justification.

The National Bioethics Advisory Commission

Even though my reflections draw on my participation in NBAC, I do not profess to speak for the commission—others inside and outside the commission may have quite different interpretations, as some of our critics certainly do.[3]

NBAC's report, *Cloning Human Beings*, released in June 1997, recommended continuing the moratorium that President Clinton had imposed on the use of federal funds for research related to human reproductive cloning, repeating the call for a voluntary moratorium in the private arena, and, in addition, passing federal legislation to prohibit somatic cell nuclear transfer to create children. NBAC rested its recommendations to a great extent on the following argument—"at this time it is morally unacceptable for anyone . . . to attempt to create a child using somatic cell nuclear transfer cloning . . . because current scientific information indicates that this technique is not safe to use in humans at this time."[4] Why? "Dolly" was the only birth out of 277 attempts, even though twenty-eight other fusions developed to the blastocyst stage, and there were at least theoretical reasons to worry, for example, about the effects of the mutations accumulated by the aging somatic cells that are used in cloning—will such mutations lead to cancer and other diseases?[5] (I will use the phrases "human cloning" or "cloning humans" or "cloning human beings" to refer to somatic cell nuclear transfer cloning to create children, unless otherwise indicated.)

Some critics charge that NBAC, a "bioethics" commission, copped out because it based its recommendations largely on a *scientific* argument about safety rather than on an *ethical* argument. That charge is misdirected— indeed, it reflects an inadequate understanding of ethics. More accurately, NBAC, in light of the available scientific evidence, reached a *moral* conclusion, based at least in part on the ethical obligation not to harm, or impose serious risks of harm on, potential children. Safety is a fundamental ethical consideration. It is not merely a scientific consideration, even though judgments about safety obviously rely on scientific evidence. Any procedure that creates a substantial risk of harm to children is morally problematic.

There is no reason to believe that safety problems are permanently insurmountable in cloning mammals. Hence, this ethical barrier will probably be overcome at some point. It is thus crucial to consider other important ethical issues that also arise from the prospect of human cloning, such as the probable impact on the family. Such issues require careful, thoughtful, and imaginative reflection over time so that the society will be ready to respond appropriately to human cloning if and when the technique appears to be safe.

For these reasons, NBAC recommended a sunset clause in federal legislation, review by "an appropriate oversight body" prior to the expiration of the sunset period, and "widespread and continuing [public] deliberation"—in short, a national dialogue—on the whole range of ethical and social issues so that the society could formulate appropriate long-term policies toward human cloning. And it attempted to identify, at least in a preliminary way, some of these issues and to begin to construct a framework for addressing them. However, it did not attempt at the time to resolve—nor is it likely that it could have resolved—the other ethical and social issues that would emerge once the safety threshold is crossed.[6]

The Role of Religious Convictions in the Debate about Public Policies toward Human Cloning

After President Clinton asked NBAC to consider the cloning of human beings, he later commented that "any discovery that touches upon human creation is not simply a matter of scientific inquiry, it is a matter of *morality* and *spirituality* as well."[7] The commission had reached a similar conclusion and set up two days of hearings, with particular attention to scientific, ethical, and religious perspectives.

Why religious perspectives? Some were surprised that NBAC solicited religious perspectives along with the customary philosophical perspectives. However, attention to religious perspectives is not unprecedented in debates about public policies for new technologies—for instance, in the early 1980s the President's Commission's report *Splicing Life* included religious perspectives in its discussion of genetic engineering.[8] In particular, it focused on "playing God," which often has secular as well as specifically religious significance. (President Clinton also invoked that language, which frequently focuses on unwarranted human claims of unlimited power and limited accountability.)

NBAC recognized that public policy in the United States cannot be based on purely religious considerations—that its own reasons for its recommendations could not and should not be religious. But NBAC still believed that it was important to examine religious perspectives, along with philosophical perspectives, on human cloning, in its process of analyzing and assessing moral arguments. In two places in its report NBAC listed several reasons, in slightly different language, for its attention to religious perspectives:

- Religious traditions "influence and shape the moral views of many U.S. citizens and religious teachings over the centuries have provided an important source of ideas and inspiration";
- Policy-makers "should understand and show respect for diverse moral ideas regarding the acceptability of cloning of human beings in this new manner";
- Often religious ideas "can be stated forcefully in terms understandable and persuasive to all persons, irrespective of specific religious beliefs";
- NBAC wanted to determine whether "various religious traditions, despite their distinctive sources of authority and argumentation, reach similar conclusions about this type of human cloning" since a convergence among them, as well as among secular traditions, would be instructive for public policy;
- "[A]ll voices should be welcome to the conversation"; and
- A range of moral views need to be considered in determining the feasibility and costs of different policies, which might be affected, for example, by vigorous moral opposition.[9]

I want to develop in a more systematic way some of these reasons, along with others that did not appear in NBAC's report. In the process, I will challenge some conceptions of "public reason" in a liberal, pluralistic democracy that seem—or even seek—to exclude religious convictions from the process of developing bioethical public policies.

Emotion and Imaginative Deliberation

When "Dolly" made human cloning a more realistic prospect, passionate outcries were heard everywhere—"repugnant," "offensive," and "revolting." Even Ian Wilmut, "Dolly's" creator, found the prospect of cloning a human "offensive." NBAC, according to one analysis, needed to understand "why people reacted with such passion"—their "gut reactions," in chairman Harold Shapiro's words—and so they "started with religion."[10] This oversimplifies why religious perspectives were important to NBAC, even though some religious spokespersons had certainly responded passionately, emotionally, in condemning human cloning, and their responses clearly played some role in the rush to propose legislation.

Religious perspectives not only help *explain* emotional and passionate responses. In public discourse, they may also *instruct* or *inform* emotions and passions. The Harvard law professor Martha Minow gives an instructive example: A trial court judge approved a couple's petition to become the legal guardians of a child with Down syndrome when the biological parents refused to authorize medical treatments that were considered necessary to save the child's life. Judge Fernandez granted their petition, against the biological parents' objections, and in a footnote cited "the Holy Bible, 1 Kings 3:26," which tells the story of King Solomon's threat to cut a child in two when he couldn't determine which of the two women who claimed be the mother actually was the mother. This biblical story instructed Judge Fernandez's emotions, as the judge himself noted, and it offered a way for him to reflect on his own anguish as a decision-maker in a most difficult case.[11]

The biblical story or stories of creation in Genesis may have functioned in a similar way for some commissioners, even if, in Max Weber's language, they were "religiously unmusical," and even though religious thinkers used these biblical passages to reach quite different conclusions. Of particular importance in the discussion of the possibility of human cloning is Genesis 1: 27–28 (New RSV): "So God created humankind in his image, in the image of God he created them; male and female he created them. And God blessed them, and God said to them, 'Be fruitful and multiply, and fill the earth and subdue it; and have dominion over the fish of the sea and over the birds of the air and over every living thing that moves upon the earth.'"

Such stories, whether they are religious or secular, may also be important in public imagination, as part of public reasoning closely connected with the emotions. A strictly rationalistic model of public reasoning neglects the important role of imagination and reimagination in public policy, just as it neglects the role of the emotions. As a result, such a model usually demands that religious views, when offered, be restated or translated into common, secular language. In fact, commissioners on NBAC sometimes asked religious thinkers if they could restate their views in secular terms. And some commissioners "later complained that whenever they asked religious people [in the hearings] to translate their feelings into terms that were more accessible to nonbelievers, they received hate mail accusing them of demeaning spiritual faith."[12]

However, a strictly rationalistic model that requires translation of religious language for public reasoning is inadequate. As Martha Minow reminds us, it forces religious people to make constant efforts "to check their religious language and conceptions at the door." This parallels what some towns in the Old West apparently required—people had to check their guns at the door of meeting places, such as bars. According to Minow, "That seems to be how lots of people talk about excluding religion from public discourse."[13]

However, religion is not the only "gun" in town; there are other "comprehensive views" as John Rawls called them. Furthermore, religious views are not always "weapons." Rather than functioning only as conversation stoppers, they may be quite relevant to the conversation inside the meeting hall, especially if the task is to imagine or reimagine, as is certainly the case when the topic is a dramatically new technology, such as cloning humans.

One NBAC member (Laurie Flynn) reported that she "had been especially moved by [the theologian Gilbert] Meilaender's description of children as a gift" in his testimony to NBAC.[14] Meilaender's description came in the context of his use of the biblical story of creation and his distinction between children as gifts and children as products. It also came in the context of his distinction, drawing on the Nicene creed, between "begetting" and "making."[15] These were heady religious concepts for public discourse about human cloning. As I remember our conversation, Meilaender had asked me, when I called on behalf of NBAC to invite him to testify at the hearing, whether his *theological* approach would be appropriate, and I assured him that it would. Nevertheless, in the discussion at the meeting, individual commissioners asked for translation into secular language, with one commissioner wondering whether it was necessary to use religious categories to express "principled" views, such as the distinction between "making" babies and "begetting" them.[16]

If public reasoning includes imagination, and not only rational deduction from shared secular premises, then even religious stories and theological concepts may enable us to imagine and reimagine in ways that are fruitful for public policy: What does human cloning mean? What are its potential negative and positive effects? And so forth. Rather than excluding religious views, we should consider them on their own terms to see what we might learn from them. They may yield insights[17] through imagination and reimagination, enabling us to see the technology for cloning humans from different perspectives. This re-visioning may be important for public policy, even if in the end policy-makers or advisors reject the positions that the religious stories and concepts support, or if they shape and justify a proposed policy on secular grounds. Such re-visioning may also occur even when the religious positions diverge, as they did in many respects in testimony before NBAC on human reproductive cloning (and on another of its topics—human embryonic stem cell research).

One argument for the possible positive role of biblical stories and other religious categories in public imagination focuses on the place of the bible in American culture. John Coleman suggests that "biblical religion" often provides a "powerful and pervasive symbolic resource" for public ethics in the United States. He notes that major contributors to American public life, such as Abraham Lincoln, Reinhold Niebuhr, and Martin Luther King Jr., all appealed to biblical religion, not as revelation but rather as an important source of "insights and symbols [that] convey a deeper human wisdom. . . . Biblical imagery . . . lies at the heart of the American self-understanding. It is neither parochial nor extrinsic."[18] From this standpoint, then, appeals to a biblical story may sometimes be less provincial than even some secular appeals.[19] Similar points may hold for various other concepts and norms that originated in specific religious traditions but now function independently of those traditions.[20]

Even if the bible is not as significant in the background culture in the United States as Coleman supposes, biblical stories may by their difference or oddness still stimulate the imagination, just as any good story might. Indeed, as Martha Nussbaum stresses, literary imagination can be an important part of public rationality.[21]

Many of us on the commission wanted to hear religious positions in their own terms—in part because they might help us imagine and reimagine—and yet we also wanted to learn whether there might be secular equivalents. In my judgment, such an inquiry does not impose an unfair burden on religious thinkers and traditions.[22] Listening fairly and attentively to religious positions in their own integrity does not preclude also seeking translation, or—if translation is too strong—seeking to determine whether there might be an overlapping consensus.

Overlapping Consensus

Religious communities and traditions often present moral positions and arguments that are not merely or exclusively religious in nature. Their conclusions may rest on premises that are not religious, or not specifically religious, even when they fit within a larger religious framework. For instance, a judgment about human cloning may appeal to "nature" or "basic human values" or "family values," all categories that are not reducible to particular faith commitments and that may be accessible to citizens of different or no faith commitments. Some may serve as "middle axioms," which religious communities may share with nonreligious ones.

A good example appears in the prima facie moral requirement not to harm others. Even if, in particular traditions, this moral principle is connected to specific theological convictions, its meaning and significance are not limited to those connections. And this principle provides a moral basis for holding that human cloning is wrong, and should be seriously restricted or even prohibited, at least until the procedure is safer, because of the potential harm to children so created. To be sure, particular religious traditions will develop fuller, thicker conceptions of this principle, especially with regard to the nature and significance of various harms (as well as the moral status of entities that can be harmed).

In arguing against Christian ethicists who hold that we can identify only scattered moral fragments of past traditions in our society, Lisa Cahill points "to the *fact* of intercultural and interreligious understanding and social cooperation—however halting, partial, and ambivalent." This fact challenges the claim that "universal human experiences, values, and virtues are simply illusory." Cahill uses as an example "the recommendation . . . of the National Bioethics Advisory Commission to provisionally ban human cloning, reached after fairly inclusive hearings and debates by an interdisciplinary committee formed from various religious and political traditions."[23]

To determine whether there is a de facto consensus about public policy toward human cloning, someone might propose a survey to find out what religious people as well as nonreligious people think. However, for purposes of public policy, it is also important to understand the reasons behind any overlapping consensus. On the one hand, knowing the reasons might enable policy-makers to gauge the depth and intensity of views on human cloning. This might be important, for example, as part of a cost-benefit analysis of different possible public policies—for instance, predictable serious and sustained opposition might count as a major cost. On the other hand, the reasons that religious and other thinkers support a particular policy could point in quite different directions under different circumstances—for example, if human cloning proves to be safe for the children so created—and that is important to understand as well.

Even though some religious thinkers, especially within the Roman Catholic tradition with its emphasis on natural law, focus on universal principles or values, a more historicist interpretation of the overlapping consensus is also possible. Sometimes a consensus may emerge because important social-cultural norms are historical deposits of religious traditions. In the secularization debates a number of years ago, the sociologist Talcott Parsons among others offered a very positive interpretation of secularization as the institutionalization of religious norms in the wider social-cultural context. Originating within particular religious traditions, these norms, such as equality, have become secular—they have become embedded in the society and culture.[24] Whatever their historical origins, such norms may now operate on their own tracks, to use one of Max Weber's metaphors, as part of the background culture or the public political culture.

Moral Reasoning about Public Policy in a Particular Political Context

It was not always easy for the commission to determine and keep in clear view its primary target, which I would describe as proposing and justifying a prohibitive, a restrictive, or a permissive public policy with regard to somatic cell nuclear transfer cloning to create a child. In doing public ethics or public bioethics, it is necessary to explicate the premises and presumptions of moral discourse in a particular society, without neglecting universal principles such as human rights. Commissioners need to ask which acts and policies are justifiable within the society's evolving moral framework, not merely which ones they as individuals view as morally justifiable. For several commissioners, the premises and presumptions of a liberal, pluralistic democratic society placed the burden of proof on those who argued for restrictive or prohibitive legislation directed against human cloning. For these commissioners, that burden of proof was met by the safety argument, or by the concerns about other ethical issues, or by both in combination, whether these were viewed as equally significant or as primary/secondary.

Another point about context is also crucial. Many liberal political theorists who debate the role of religion in public policy focus on the nature of liberal democracy as such, or liberal, pluralistic democracy as such. However, too many factors about a particular liberal, pluralistic democracy are relevant to permit such a high level of generalization. Hence, the debate about the appropriateness of religious convictions best occurs within a particular liberal, pluralistic democracy, such as the United States, with its own specific history, traditions, institutions, and practices.[25]

Within this specific context, the following additional points are also important. First, arguments for and against a significant role for religious convictions in public policy appeal to two different fears, each of which may be more or less plausible depending on the particular liberal, pluralistic democracy at a particular time. On the one hand, opponents often fear religion's divisiveness. John Rawls begins his book on political liberalism with the story of religious conflict in the West, and we know all too well religion's role in conflicts around the world.[26] Many who argue for a reduced role—or no role at all—for religious convictions in public policy share this fear, and it is not unreasonable. On the other hand, many who argue for an increased role for religious convictions find the "public square" in the United States too naked or empty, and believe that religious contributions could enhance the moral quality of our deliberative process. This too is plausible in particular circumstances.

The appropriateness of appeals to religious convictions may also depend on particular institutions and roles within a democracy. For instance, many liberal theorists view the courts as the paradigmatic institution in a democracy that should not make decisions on religious grounds or give religious justifications for their decisions. Liberal theorists' views vary more widely when they consider legislators, executives, and citizens. NBAC consisted of citizens, appointed by the president, to advise the White House Office of Science and Technology Policy, and President Clinton specifically asked for advice on policies toward cloning humans, which he then used to propose federal legislation. The kind of information gathering, analysis, and reasoning that NBAC pursued could, in principle, be much more open to religious perspectives than would be appropriate for some other institutions and roles within our democracy.

Appreciating and understanding significant disagreements among religious (and also nonreligious) individuals, communities, and traditions can also be important. One NBAC member, Arturo Brito, a pediatrician, who voted for NBAC's recommendations on human embryonic stem cell research—that the federal government provide funds for both the derivation of and research on derived stem cell lines—was quite unsure about his decision throughout much of the commission's deliberative process. He was aware of the great promise of human embryonic stem cell research, but he was uncomfortable with the destruction of human embryos in the process of creating stem cell lines (and with the use of fetal tissue following deliberate abortions). And he was very concerned about "symbolic complicity" in the destruction of human life (as he viewed the human embryo). "Sometimes I can't sleep at night," he said, because the decision was "haunting" him. However, he continued, "We live in a pluralistic society. I have to consider more than my own views on this topic. There are so many different views about the moral status of the early embryo. Who's to say who's right?"[27] Brito indicated to fellow NBAC members that, as anguished as he was, a "turning point" for him was the public meeting NBAC held with several thinkers from Roman Catholic, Eastern Orthodox, Protestant, Jewish, and Muslim traditions.[28] The disagreements within and across these religious traditions led him to believe that NBAC's position was a defensible compromise.

It is, in my view, appropriate to attend to religious perspectives in the *process* of formulating public policies, as NBAC attempted to do in its advisory capacity, even if it is necessary to limit their role in the *content* and *justification* of proposed policies. The *process* of reaching a decision—or, in NBAC's case, a recommendation—should attend to the widest possible range of positions and reasons for those positions, but the *outcome* in substance and public justification needs to involve a *sufficient* or *adequate* secular, that is, nonreligious, reason.[29] This is especially true when the policy involves coercive measures, as so many do—for example, NBAC proposed a temporally limited ban on cloning humans, and the legislation that the White House subsequently proposed included criminal sanctions.

In critiquing how religion appears in contemporary bioethical discourse, Messikomer, Fox, and Swazey criticize the way NBAC handled religion in its report on *Human Stem Cell Research*. They charge that religion was "expunged by being reduced to 'diverse perspectives,' 'ethical issues,' and 'moral concerns.'"[30] However, their alternative is unclear. A religiously based justification of the passage of coercive laws or the use of federal funds is problematic, unfair, and disrespectful of fellow citizens in this liberal, pluralistic democracy. It would also encounter serious constitutional challenges.

Even the strongest critics of a place for religious convictions in public reasoning about public policies, particularly policies that involve coercion, tend to recognize a legitimate place for religious convictions in the "background culture," which according to Rawls includes "nonpublic reasons . . . the many reasons of civil society" and which obviously shapes how a new technology such as cloning may be viewed.[31] However, it is very difficult to draw a hard and fast line between "background culture" and public policy debates, particularly on new technologies such as human cloning. Since the "background culture" tends to spill over into the public debate about appropriate policies, it is better simply to welcome all arguments and assess their worth in public.

Public Scrutiny of Religious-Moral Reasons

One version of this last argument for inviting religious contributions to debates about public policy also rests on specific features of the background culture and political life in the United States. This argument holds that, since religious convictions inevitably play a role in citizens' proposals for public policies, at least in the United States, those reasons need to be brought into public view so that they can be subjected to appropriate testing.

Richard Rorty once stated that it is appropriate to make religion private and keep it away from "the public square," even to the extent of "making it seem bad taste to bring religion into discussions of public policy."[32] In response, Michael Perry contends that we need to "public-ize" religion not privatize it: "We should welcome religiously based moral arguments into the public square (where we can then test them), not try to keep them out."[33] Perry's argument proceeds this way: Given the fact—and he takes it as a fact based on opinion surveys and other data—that so many Americans are religious, it is "inevitable" that some legislators and some citizens will rely on religious arguments in making political choices. "Because of the role that religiously based moral arguments inevitably play in the political process," he continues, "it is important that such arguments, no less than secular moral arguments, be presented in, so that they can be tested in, public political debate."[34] Perry is not very clear about how this testing might proceed. He suggests at one point that it occurs, at least ideally, "by competing scripture- or tradition-based religious arguments," but that surely is too limited for public political debate. In addition, it is not clear that or how public bioethics bodies can or should undertake such a task of sorting out and assessing the range of interpretations of scripture and traditions.

Another possible approach, which attends to consistency, presuppositions, implications, and so forth, appears in NBAC's report on human embryonic stem cell research. In a discussion that staff philosopher Andrew Siegel initially proposed and drafted, the report notes that

> The abortion debate offers an illustration of the complex middle ground that might be found in ethically and politically contentious areas of public policy. Philosopher Ronald Dworkin maintains that, despite their rhetoric, many who oppose abortion do not actually believe that the fetus is a person with a right to life. This is revealed, he claims, through a consideration of the exceptions that they often permit to their proposed prohibitions on abortion.
>
> For example, some hold that abortion is morally permissible when a pregnancy is the result of rape or incest. Yet, as Dworkin comments, "[i]t would be contradictory to insist that a fetus has right to live that is strong enough to justify prohibiting abortion when the childbirth would ruin a mother's or a family's life, but that ceases to exist when the pregnancy is the result of a sexual crime of which the fetus is, of course, wholly innocent."
> [...]
> The importance of reflecting on the meaning of such exceptions in the context of the research uses of embryos is that they suggest that even in an area of great moral controversy it may be possible to identify some common ground. If it is possible to find common ground in the case of elective abortions, we might be able to identify when it would be permissible in the case of destroying embryos.[35]

When religious convictions are brought into the public square they too are subject to—and should be subjected to—close public scrutiny, just as any other reasons should be. For instance, some of them may be mutually contradictory. The fact that a position is religiously based gives it no special claim or privilege in public political debate. Just as a position shouldn't be excluded or rejected merely because it is religious, so it shouldn't gain any special advantage just because it is religious. The model of "religious and moral engagement" (in Michael Sandel's language) that appears appropriate, as a form of "mutual respect" in a deliberative democracy, entails inclusion but also scrutiny.[36]

The fundamental concern about religious convictions and arguments in public political debate, Perry argues, is not *that* they are brought to bear, but rather *how* they are brought to bear—for example, they may be asserted dogmatically. But concerns about *how* fundamental convictions are brought to bear extend to secular convictions no less than to religious convictions.[37] This point is often neglected.

To take one example, R. C. Lewontin, in criticizing NBAC for "inviting" religious discussants to the table, fails to see that both religious and secular arguments, including philosophical ones, may display similar flaws and deficiencies in this regard.[38] He claims that theologians attempt to "abolish hard ethical problems" and avoid "painful tensions." (I will ignore his phrase "internal contradictions," which he includes along with "painful tensions," because both philosophers and theologians try to avoid "internal contradictions" in order to develop defensible positions.) Many theologians as well as many philosophers, in testimony to NBAC and elsewhere, have recognized these "painful tensions." Neither group as a whole fails to appreciate the moral conflicts involved in cloning humans, in various scenarios, or in different public policies toward cloning humans, even if different thinkers resolve them differently. NBAC's own reflections benefited greatly from both theological and philosophical perspectives and considerations. In contrast to Lewontin's interpretation, those religiously related reflections appear not only in NBAC's chapter "Religious Perspectives," but are also interwoven into the chapter "Ethical Considerations," along with philosophical reflections.[39]

Theologians and other thinkers within religious traditions had already engaged in sustained moral analysis and assessment of the prospect of human cloning, beginning as early as the late 1960s and early 1970s. At that time, in response to scientifically premature proposals for human cloning, the ethicist Paul Ramsey, a Methodist, responded negatively, worrying about its dehumanization, while Joseph Fletcher, who taught ethics at the Episcopal Divinity School in Cambridge, Massachusetts, but who by then thought mainly within a secular framework, responded positively by viewing human cloning, along with other reproductive technologies, as more human than normal, sexual reproduction—according to Fletcher we are most human when we create and use technologies, rather than simply yielding to "nature."[40] These thinkers and others mined resources in different religious (and philosophical) traditions to arrive at their judgments and recommendations. In some ways, then, religiously based or religiously related thinking was at least as far along as, and may have had more to build on, than much philosophical reflection for ethical analysis and assessment of human cloning.

For the reasons just elucidated, it was appropriate and even important for NBAC to invite testimony from several religious thinkers. It heard from scholars in Jewish, Protestant, Roman Catholic, and Islamic traditions, and it contracted with Professor Courtney Campbell of Oregon State University for a paper on these and other religious perspectives, including, for example, Eastern Orthodox, Buddhist, Hindu, and Native American perspectives.[41] In addition, public testimony often reflected religious perspectives. Furthermore, as a follow-up to NBAC's report, Senator William Frist organized a hearing before the US Senate Labor and Human Resources Subcommittee on Public Health and Safety entitled "Ethics and Theology: A Continuation of the National Discussion on Human Cloning."[42]

Selected Religious Positions in the Debate about Public Policy toward Human Cloning

Presenters of religious perspectives identified several relevant ethical concerns about cloning humans, as did presenters of philosophical perspectives. They didn't always agree on the significance of those concerns, perhaps in part because some problems would not emerge unless human cloning became a widespread practice—and asexual reproduction does not seem likely to replace sexual reproduction! Their concerns included physical harm to children so created (the safety issue), psychosocial harm to children, wrongs to children and others through objectification and commodification, harms to the family, and injustice in the allocation of resources.

There is disagreement among particular religious traditions, and in the society at large, about whether, in light of these different ethical concerns, no conceivable acts of human cloning could ever be justified if the technique were safe for the children so created. On the one hand, some thinkers, especially but not only in the Roman Catholic tradition, hold that cloning humans is wrong in and of itself (i.e., intrinsically wrong), and that it would thus be wrong under any conceivable circumstances. Any use would violate human dignity, the natural law, the natural order, or some other fundamental principle or value, and revulsion would be the appropriate emotional response to this violation.[43]

On the other hand, many hold that human cloning would be wrong in some, perhaps in most, circumstances but not in others that could be imagined. Although there are numerous variations, several Protestant and Jewish thinkers, along with many secular thinkers, take this second position and worry about inappropriate uses or abuses of human cloning rather than about every single possible use. Some who take this second position view human cloning as a morally "neutral" technology, as Rabbi Elliot Dorff does, while others, such as the Protestant ethicist Nancy Duff, view it as morally problematic but not intrinsically wrong.[44]

Several possible scenarios need consideration: Cloning because of problems of infertility; cloning to provide a compatible source of biological material, such as bone marrow, for treatment of a dying child's leukemia; and cloning a dying child. Many who hold that human cloning could be justified under some circumstances would not view all these scenarios as ethically acceptable. In any event, virtually all religious and secular positions that ethically accept some possible cases of human cloning presuppose that the procedure is sufficiently safe for the child created by cloning and that the child's rights and interests will be adequately protected. Otherwise human cloning even for legitimate purposes would be morally unjustifiable.

At one point a strong consensus exists among Jewish, Roman Catholic, and Protestant thinkers: A child created through somatic cell nuclear transfer cloning would still be created in the image of God.[45] This point is important because some commentators on religious views on cloning overlook it. One distinguished political scientist even suggested that religious thinkers would obviously oppose cloning because the children so created would be "soulless."[46]

Such a misunderstanding may result from the claim, made by some religious traditions and thinkers, that cloning would *violate* the dignity of the child created this way. However, *violation* may occur without *destruction*. While stressing that cloning would *violate* a child's dignity, a Roman Catholic theologian further emphasizes that it would not *diminish* that child's dignity.[47] In different language, Rabbi Dorff stresses that cloning would create "a new person, an integrated body and mind, with unique experiences," however difficult it may be for such persons to "establish their own identity and for their creators to acknowledge and respect it."[48] And Rabbi Bryon Sherwin notes that none of the Jewish sources "suggest that the clone would not have his or her own unique individual human identity."[49] (These comments reflect two views of the *violation* of human dignity: on the one hand, human dignity involves being brought into being through sexual intercourse of a married couple; on the other hand, it involves independent identity and respect for that identity.)[50]

Religious thinkers who reject all human cloning as immoral tend to favor a permanent legislative ban. By contrast, those who believe that human cloning could sometimes be ethically justified may argue for a ban (perhaps temporary), or regulation, or permission, depending on the circumstances. At the time of NBAC's report, in view of the great uncertainty about the safety of human cloning, a temporary ban or strict regulation seemed plausible to many. Nevertheless, concerns quite properly arose about the range and scope of any ban or regulation as well as about its potential effectiveness.

The sociologist James Hunter has observed that conservatives (orthodox) in a particular religious tradition may share more with conservatives (orthodox) in other religious traditions than with liberals (progressives) in their own tradition; the same point also applies to liberals (progressives).[51] It is quite striking, however, that this pattern does not hold as uniformly for human cloning as for some other bioethical topics. For example, Rabbi Bryon Sherwin, a conservative rabbi, stresses that Orthodox and Conservative Jewish thinkers, on the basis of the Jewish legal tradition, find it difficult to condemn human cloning per se, and that much Jewish opposition to human cloning, particularly in Reform Judaism, reflects categories outside Jewish law. "In my view," Sherwin argued, "Jewish theological, ethical and legal tradition can endorse the propriety of cloning human beings, albeit with certain restrictions."[52]

Religious and secular thinkers alike insist, in what is clearly an overlapping consensus about the moral minimum, that it is morally obligatory not to inflict serious harm on children created through human cloning. One such harm is physical. Cloning would be wrong at least for the present, according to many religious thinkers, because cloners could not be sure that they would not be doing unacceptable harm to children. This is also the position NBAC took, based on broad societal moral norms, in holding that safety is a fundamental ethical issue, though not the only one, and that, at least for the time being, human cloning to create a child should not be undertaken and should be prohibited through legislation. Such prohibitive legislation would also provide a window of opportunity for the society to determine whether safe human cloning would have unacceptable moral costs and should be severely restricted or even banned.

Consensus on these arguments meant, however, that NBAC did not have to try to resolve the larger debate about the probable impact of acts and especially of widespread practices of human cloning on social values that are not reducible to harms or wrongs to individuals—under a temporary prohibition there would be time for the society to address the other ethical concerns. One such major concern is human cloning's potential impact on the family, especially if it were to become a widespread practice rather than an occasional, isolated act. Among the risks, which some commissioners considered speculative, are threats to fundamental responsibilities within the family, including intergenerational relationships. Certainly questions arise about how to understand relationships—for example, between the source of the cloned tissue and the child created (delayed identical twin)—but our language about family also identifies different responsibilities.

NBAC sought to engender and sustain in its own meetings and in its report serious moral discourse about human cloning and about public policies toward human cloning. Hence, it listened to and attempted to understand as fully as possible various religious and philosophical positions. And it called for a similar national process over time.

Postscript (2019)

In the version of this chapter published in 1999, I concluded, "It is not clear what to expect from a period of sustained 'moral and religious engagement.' Unfortunately, it appears that this engagement may occur without the deliberative space created by a temporary ban."[53] Even now in 2019, there is no federal ban on human reproductive cloning, even though various states have such bans. This is, in part, the result of vigorous disagreements about the *scope* of a possible ban: Some want to ban what the President's Council on Bioethics called "cloning-for-biomedical research" along with "cloning-to-produce children."

In announcing (August 9, 2001) his administration's policy on the use of federal funds in stem cell research, President George W. Bush indicated that he would also appoint a presidential bioethics council, chaired by Leon Kass, to monitor stem cell research and to recommend guidelines and regulations as well as to consider the implications of biomedical innovation. The new council would "give our nation a forum to continue to discuss and evaluate these important issues." However, the Bush administration had not established such a council when, at the end of September 2001, NBAC's charter expired—the terrible events of 9/11 had understandably redirected the administration's attention. At the end of November 2001, at least partly in response to a biotechnology company's announcement that it had cloned embryos, President Bush issued an Executive Order to establish the new council. In July 2002, following six months of deliberations, the President's Council on Bioethics (PCB) issued its first report, *Human Cloning and Human Dignity*.[54] The PCB's selection of this first topic was not surprising, in view of the lack of a federal ban on human reproductive cloning and the spirited, often rancorous, debate about "cloning-for-biomedical research." Indeed, it would have been surprising if the PCB had started with some other topic. After all, at the PCB's first meeting, President Bush said: "Let me say two other things and then I will listen. One, you need to monitor the stem cell issue. That was the charge I gave on national TV that day [August 9, 2001]...., And the other thing is that I have spoken clearly on cloning. I just don't think it's right. On the other hand, there is going to be a lot of nuance and subtlety to the issue, I presume. And I think this is very important for you all to help the nation understand what this means."

The PCB designed its first report to "inform" public policy through a thorough, deep, and broad examination of human cloning in its larger contexts. The council recognized that it is difficult to move "from moral assessment to public policy" (p. 195). The relationship between ethics and policy is not a one-way street. Indeed, where moral assessments differ as much as they do in American society, and in this report, informing public policy in a very loose sense is the most that can be expected.

The PCB also did not want its "moral analysis" to be skewed by specific legal or policy questions, in part because the moral analysis, for example, of the various human goods at stake, has greater and broader significance. Nevertheless, in my judgment, the report fails to develop adequately the moral dimensions of formulating public policy in a liberal, pluralistic society marked by presumptions in favor of reproductive and scientific freedom and by a variety of acknowledged human goods and conceptions of human flourishing. An approach, similar to the one NBAC took, might ask, for instance, when the societal presumption in favor of reproductive and scientific freedom—and it is only a presumption—can be justifiably rebutted. Such an approach would focus on the ethics of public policy in a liberal, pluralistic, democratic society.

All PCB members (except one who did not vote because he did not participate in several meetings) unanimously agreed that cloning-to-produce-children should be prohibited by federal law. However, the commission was sharply divided about cloning-for-biomedical research. In the final tally, a ten-member majority called for a four-year federal moratorium on cloning-for-biomedical research. Even though seven of those ten members actually favored a ban, they compromised with the three members who endorsed a moratorium in order to constitute a majority against members who favored a regulatory approach. Not surprisingly, the spirit of the academic seminar that the PCB had sought evaporated in its effort to develop recommendations that a majority could back.

The philosopher Daniel Callahan and others have drawn a distinction between regulatory and prophetic bioethics. Clearly governmental bodies, established to address public bioethics, are more likely to be regulatory in nature, that is, aimed at formulating desirable and feasible public policies. Even though the PCB prioritized shaping public culture, it was not as prophetic as many observers desired, particularly when the policy recommended by the majority was perceived by critics as a morally ambiguous compromise. In any event, the first PCB report suffered the same fate as NBAC's earlier reports on *Cloning Human Beings* and *Human Stem Cell Research*: their recommendations were not adopted as public policy.

It was reasonable for the PCB to anticipate political uses of its report and policy recommendations. The PCB knew that President Bush opposed all human cloning, whatever its aim. Hence, it is not surprising that the White House indicated that the PCB report would not alter the president's position, a position that "is based on principle. Any attempt to clone a human being is morally wrong." Senator Sam Brownback, a vigorous opponent of all human cloning, emphasized the PCB's majority support for a four-year moratorium. By contrast, Senator Edward Kennedy, a supporter of research cloning, noted: "It's significant that even the president's hand-picked panel of advisers rejected an outright ban on this promising medical research."

What about the role of religion and religious convictions in the PCB's work? In his opening remarks to the President's Council on Bioethics at its first meeting January 17, 2002, Leon Kass, the chair, made points similar to some that NBAC made in justifying attention to religious perspectives:

All serious relevant opinions, carefully considered, are welcome. Any that may not now be represented on the Council we will seek out through invited testimony. Moral positions rooted in religious faith or in philosophy or in ordinary personal experience of life are equally relevant, provided that the arguments and insights offered enter our public discourse in ways that do not appeal to special privilege or authority. Respect for American pluralism does not mean neutering the deeply held religious or other views of our fellow citizens. On the contrary, with the deepest human questions on the table, we should be eager to avail ourselves of the wisdom contained in the great religious, literary, and philosophical traditions.[55]

More so than NBAC and most other commissions, the PCB included theologians, such as William F. May and Gilbert Meilaender, as well as other members explicitly and closely tied to particular religious traditions and positions. Although the PCB was widely perceived to be more attuned and receptive to religious perspectives than NBAC, the PCB, in fact, did not devote as much attention to the views of particular religious traditions as NBAC did. In addressing the controversial areas of human cloning and human embryonic stem cell research, NBAC specifically requested input from spokespersons for and interpreters of particular religious traditions, both in public meetings and in commissioned reports. Perhaps the PCB attended less to particular religious traditions because a religious or theological sensibility was more pervasive among its members or because its working assumptions already incorporated broad religious convictions.

Rather than attending to the views of particular religious traditions, the PCB's reports often appealed to broad concepts, particularly "human dignity," which, according to some critics, masked religious commitments. One such critic, Stephen Marks, observed that the PCB report *Human Cloning and Human Dignity* "did not define the term [human dignity] and tended to use it as a code for a theological commitment to the sanctity of life."[56]

Questions about faith-based views arose in a very specific context for the next commission too, the Presidential Commission for the Study of Bioethical Issues (PCSBI), established by President Barack Obama. We saw that for NBAC and, to some extent, for the PCB, these questions emerged mainly in the context of debates about technologies that involved human reproductive cloning and human embryonic stem cell research. For the PCSBI, religious positions became a subject of interest as it deliberated on developments in synthetic biology, as specifically requested by President Obama. Scientists at the J. Craig Venter Institute inserted a copied and modified genome of a small bacterial cell into a living cell of another species; the result was a new, synthetic organism. In preparing *New Directions: The Ethics of Synthetic Biology and Emerging Technologies*, its inaugural report, the PCSBI "took special efforts to learn the views of major faith-based communities, including those of Christianity, Judaism, and Islam," and considered the arguments of both "faith-based and secular ethicists."[57] These efforts included a session devoted to "philosophical and theological perspectives." In contrast to faith-based intrinsic arguments for unqualified opposition to certain specific scientific activities, such as human reproductive cloning and human embryonic stem cell research, the PCSBI did not encounter such objections to synthetic biology, in part because most recognized that the reported research did not involve the creation of life solely from inorganic chemicals. In the absence of faith-based intrinsic objections to this research, the PCSBI did not need to offer an extended examination of religious views in the deliberative democratic process leading to its report and recommendations. Its later topics, including research involving human subjects, privacy in whole genome sequencing, public health, and neuroscience, did not encounter major divisions among faith-based communities and thinkers and thus could easily be addressed without regard to particular religious views.

Notes

1. The author is indebted to several institutions and individuals, particularly members of the NBAC, as will be evident throughout the essay. An earlier version of this essay was delivered as the 1997 Sorensen Lecture at Yale University Divinity School, a portion was given as testimony at a Hearing before the US Senate Subcommittee on Public Health and Safety of the Committee on Labor and Human Resources, and some of the materials appeared in the *Hastings Center Report* 27, No. 5 (September–October 1997). The author is grateful for helpful discussions at Yale University Divinity School, as well as with the Hastings Center working group on religion and biotechnology. Discussions with Courtney Campbell have also been very valuable.

2. For a helpful depiction of "deliberative democracy," especially in relation to bioethical issues, see Amy Gutmann and Dennis Thompson, "Deliberating about Bioethics," *Hastings Center Report* 27, No. 3 (May–June 1997): 38–41. See also their *Democracy and Disagreement* (Cambridge, MA: Belknap Press of Harvard University Press, 1998) and *Why Deliberative Democracy?* (Princeton, NJ: Princeton University Press, 2004). The Presidential Commission for the Study of Bioethical Issues (PCSBI) (2009–2016), which was established by President Barack Obama and was chaired

by Amy Gutmann, adopted, as one of its basic ethical principles for assessing emerging technologies, the principle of "democratic deliberation." See PCSBI, *New Directions: The Ethics of Synthetic Biology and Emerging Technologies* (Washington, DC: PCSBI, December 2010), pp. 4–5.

3. See *Cloning Human Beings: Report and Recommendations of the National Bioethics Advisory Commission* (Rockville, MD: NBAC, June 1997). For a critical review, see R. C. Lewontin, "The Confusion over Cloning," *New York Review of Books* (October 23, 1997). See also the criticisms offered by John Evans in *Playing God? Human Genetic Engineering and the Rationalization of Public Bioethical Debate* (Chicago: University of Chicago Press, 2002) and my response to those criticisms in the previous chapter in the current volume.
4. *Cloning Human Beings*, p. iii.
5. Ibid., chap. 2, pp. 22–24.
6. Subsequent discussions among individual commissioners suggest that there is some disagreement about whether (1) the recommended temporally limited ban rested equally on safety and the other ethical concerns, or (2) it rested primarily on safety with the ban presenting further opportunity to address other ethical concerns. Individual commissioners may have had different reasons for supporting the ban, and there is some textual evidence for both (1) and (2).
7. *Cloning Human Beings*, p. 12.
8. President's Commission for the Study of Ethical Problems in Biomedical and Behavioral Research, *Splicing Life* (Washington, DC: US Government Printing Office, November 1982).
9. *Cloning Human Beings*, pp. 7–8, 39–40.
10. Susan Cohen, "A House Divided," *Washington Post Magazine*, October 12, 1997, p. 15
11. "Political Liberalism: Religion and Public Reason" (A Symposium), *Religion and Values in Public Life* 3, No. 4 (Summer, 1995): 4–5.
12. Cohen, "A House Divided," p. 15.
13. This paragraph and the next one are greatly influenced by Martha Minnow's comments and language in "Political Liberalism: Religion and Public Reason" (A Symposium), pp. 4–5, 11.
14. Cohen, "A House Divided," p. 16.
15. Gilbert Meilaender, "Remarks on Human Cloning to the National Bioethics Advisory Commission," March 13, 1997, reprinted in *BioLaw* II, No. 6 (June 1997): S:114–118.
16. Cohen, "A House Divided," p. 15.
17. As Meilaender puts it, the theological language he used seeks "to uncover what is universal and human." "Remarks on Human Cloning," S:114.
18. John A. Coleman, SJ, *An American Strategic Theology* (1982), pp. 192–195; quoted in Michael J. Perry, *Religion in Politics: Constitutional and Moral Perspectives* (New York: Oxford University Press, 1997), p. 48.
19. Of course, proponents of religious positions may decry the loss of the distinctiveness of religious positions in public debate when stories function as part of the background culture, but it is outside the scope of this chapter to explore such concerns.

20. For instance, one of the major shifts in public policy toward the allocation of organs for transplantation occurred when the national Task Force on Organ Transplantation held that donated organs belong not to the procurement teams and transplant surgeons that remove them from the cadaver but rather to the public, to the community at large, and that procurement teams and transplant surgeons only hold those organs in trust, as stewards, for the community. This fundamental shift in perspective occurred in part through language influenced by biblical accounts of stewardship. See US Department of Health and Human Services, Report of Task Force on Organ Transplantation, *Organ Transplantation: Issues and Recommendations* (Washington, DC: Department of Health and Human Services, 1986).

21. See Martha C. Nussbaum, *Poetic Justice: The Literary Imagination and Public Life* (Boston: Beacon Press, 1995).

22. Contrast Courtney Campbell's discussion in "Prophecy and Policy," *Hastings Center Report* 27, No. 5 (September–October 1997): 15–17.

23. Lisa Sowle Cahill, "Beyond MacIntyre," *Religion and Values in Public Life* 5 (1997), p. 7.

24. Talcott Parsons, "Christianity and Modern Industrial Society," in *Secularization and the Protestant Prospect*, ed. James F. Childress and David B. Harned (Philadelphia: Westminster Press, 1970).

25. See Kent Greenawalt, *Private Consciences and Public Reasons* (New York: Oxford University Press, 1995).

26. John Rawls, *Political Liberalism* (New York: Columbia University Press, 1993).

27. Diane M. Gianelli, "Panel Takes Middle Road on Stem Cell Research," *American Medical News*, August 2, 1999, http://www.ama-assn.org/amednews/1999/pick_99/prfa0802.htm (accessed September 16, 2007).

28. NBAC, *Ethical Issues in Human Stem Cell Research*, Vol. 3: *Religious Perspectives* (Rockville, MD: NBAC, 2000).

29. In this formulation, I am indebted to Robert Audi, "Liberal Democracy and the Place of Religion in Politics," in Robert Audi and Nicholas Wolterstorff, *Religion in the Public Square: The Place of Religious Convictions in Political Debate* (Lanham, MD: Rowman & Littlefield, 1997), pp. 24–33. The principles of (adequate) secular rationale and (adequate) secular motivation are part of Audi's conception of civic virtue.

30. Carla M. Messikomer, Renée C. Fox, and Judith P. Swazey, "The Presence and Influence of Religion in American Bioethics," *Perspectives in Biology and Medicine* 44, No. 4 (Autumn 2001): 485–508, at p. 505. See my discussion and critique of their interpretation and arguments in chapter 4 in this volume.

31. Rawls, *Political Liberalism*, p. 220, fn. 42.

32. Richard Rorty, "Religion as Conversation-Stopper," *Common Knowledge* 1 (1994): 3, quoted in Michael J. Perry, *Religion in Politics*, p. 49.

33. Perry, *Religion in Politics*, p. 49. Emphasis added. Elsewhere he writes that it is "important that religious arguments be presented—principally, so that they can be tested—in public political debate" (p. 6).

34. Ibid., p. 45.

35. NBAC, *Ethical Issues in Human Stem Cell Research*, Vol. I: *Report and Recommendations of the National Bioethics Advisory Commission* (Rockville, MD: NBAC, 1999), p. 52.
36. See Michael Sandel's comments in "Political Liberalism: Religion and Public Reason," especially p. 3. He argues for an expansive conception of public reason, "a public reason of moral and religious engagement," which expresses the idea "that mutual respect among citizens means *addressing* our fellow citizens, not just talking at them or appealing to reasons that can't possibly engage them in moral argument."
37. Perry, *Religion in Politics*, p. 49.
38. Lewontin, "The Confusion over Cloning."
39. This observation also serves in part to rebut Courtney Campbell's objection that "in the NBAC hearings, the contributions of religious perspectives were deemed politically important and ethically insignificant." Campbell, "Prophecy and Policy," p. 17.
40. See Paul Ramsey, *The Fabricated Man: The Ethics of Genetic Control* (New Haven, CT: Yale University Press, 1970), and Joseph Fletcher, *The Ethics of Genetic Control* (Garden City, NY: Anchor Press, 1974).
41. Courtney Campbell, "Religious Perspectives on Human Cloning," *Cloning Human Beings: Report and Recommendations of the National Bioethics Advisory Commission*, Vol. II: *Commissioned Papers* (Rockville, MD: NBAC, June 1997).
42. "Ethics and Theology: A Continuation of the National Discussion on Human Cloning," Hearing before the Subcommittee on Public Health and Safety of the Committee on Labor and Human Resources, U.S. Senate, 105th Congress, First Session, June 17, 1997.
43. See, for example, Lisa Sowle Cahill, "Hearings on Cloning: Religion-Based Perspectives," and Father Albert S. Moraczewski, OP, "Cloning and the Church," Testimony before NBAC, March 13, 1997, both reprinted in *BioLaw* 2, No. 6 (June 1997): S:100–105. For an emphasis on repugnance and revulsion, see Leon Kass, "The Wisdom of Repugnance: Why We Should Ban the Cloning of Humans," *New Republic*, June 2, 1997, pp. 17–26.
44. Nancy J. Duff, "Theological Reflections on Human Cloning," Testimony before NBAC, March 13, 1997, and Rabbi Elliot Dorff, "Human Cloning: A Jewish Perspective," both reprinted in *BioLaw* II, No. 6 (June 1997): S:106–113, 118–125.
45. Nevertheless, in discussion at NBAC and at the Hastings Center, Gilbert Meilaender thought that the status of the child created by cloning at least merited more reflection.
46. See James Q. Wilson, "The Paradox of Cloning," in Leon R. Kass and James Q. Wilson, *The Ethics of Human Cloning* (Washington, DC: AEI Press, 1999).
47. Moraczewski, "Cloning and the Church."
48. Dorff, "Human Cloning: A Jewish Perspective."
49. Bryon L. Sherwin, "Religious Perspectives on Cloning: A Jewish View," Presentation at the US Capitol, June 24, 1997, p. 6.
50. The NBAC report rightly avoided all uses of the term "clone" or related terms to refer to the children created by this process, on the grounds, as one commissioner put it, that we should not create a new social category that could create mischief,

provide the basis for discrimination, and so forth. It does appear in some writings, including some that condemn cloning. For example, Leon Kass in "The Wisdom of Repugnance" refers to the "clonant" (p. 20).

51. See James Davison Hunter, *Culture Wars: The Struggle to Define America* (New York: BasicBooks, 1991), p. 96: "The theologically orthodox of each faith and the theologically progressive of each faith divided consistently along the anticipated lines on a wide range of issues," such as sexual morality, family issues, and capitalism.

52. Sherwin, "Religious Perspectives on Cloning: A Jewish View," p. 2.

53. "Religion, Morality, and Public Policy: The Controversy about Human Cloning," in *Notes from a Narrow Ridge: Religion and Bioethics*, ed. Dena S. Davis and Laurie Zoloth (Hagerstown, MD: University Publishing Group, 1999), pp. 65–85.

54. The President's Council on Bioethics, *Human Cloning and Human Dignity* (New York: Public Affairs Press, 2002).

55. Leon Kass, Opening Remarks to the President's Council on Bioethics, Thursday, January 17, 2002, http://biotech.law.lsu.edu/research/pbc/transcripts/jan02/opening01.html (last accessed March 5, 2019) See also the slightly different transcript version at http://bioethics.georgetown.edu/pcbe/transcripts/jan02/jan17session1.html (last accessed March 5, 2019).

56. Stephen P. Marks, "Human Rights Assumptions of Restrictive and Permissive Approaches to Human Reproductive Cloning," *Health and Human Rights* 6, No. 1 (2002): 81–100.

57. See PCSBI, *New Directions: The Ethics of Synthetic Biology and Emerging Technologies*, pp. 137 and 3.

6

Conscientious Refusals in Healthcare

Protecting Health Professionals' Consciences and Patients' Interests

Introduction

My aim is to address the following question: Should the state, society, institutions, and professions exempt healthcare professionals from expectations and requirements to perform procedures or provide services or products that they deem to be morally objectionable, even though they are legal and patient-sought?[1] In setting the context for addressing this question, I will first note the wide variety of cases of conscientious refusal (CR) in or related to healthcare, examine the controversy generated by a professional society's ethics committee's report on the *limits* of CR (which resulted in conflicting policies by the Bush, Obama, and Trump administrations), and consider an empirical study of physicians' views of their obligations when they conscientiously object to performing or providing some procedure, service, or product.

Cases of Conscientious Refusal by Health Professionals

Following are several actual cases of CR by health professionals and others involved in providing legal health-related services, procedures, and products sought by individuals[2]:

- Refusal to perform abortions or sterilizations
- Refusal to participate in assisted dying in states where physician-assisted dying is legal
- Refusal to provide pain medication
- Refusal to withhold or withdraw artificial nutrition and hydration from dying patients or from patients in a permanent vegetative condition

- Refusal to provide further treatment because it would be a "waste" of medical resources
- Refusal to follow official rationing policies (in United Kingdom)
- Refusal to do prenatal diagnosis on grounds of disability rights
- Refusal to do sex selection on grounds of gender equality
- Refusal to provide reproductive services to single persons, to gays, to lesbians, to unmarried couples, and so forth
- Refusal to remove organs, with permission, from people declared brain-dead
- Refusal to use animals in education or research
- Refusal to tell parents about the varicella vaccine because it was developed using tissue from aborted fetuses
- A pharmacist's refusal to fill a hormonal contraception prescription (because of a belief that it amounts to abortion)
- A pharmacist's refusal to return the prescription or transfer it
- Refusal to participate in capital punishment through lethal injections

Other examples include:

- A medical transporter refuses to take a woman to an abortion clinic
- Somali Muslim taxi drivers in Minneapolis-St. Paul refuse to transport blind persons because they are accompanied by (unclean) seeing eye dogs
- A Jehovah's Witness anesthesiologist refuses to provide a blood transfusion to a non–Jehovah's Witness patient who is bleeding out
- A nurse refuses to participate in male infant circumcision
- A secretary refuses to type a letter of referral for an abortion
- A nephrology team refuses to care for a patient who received his kidney transplant abroad because they suspect his "transplant tourism" included the purchase of a kidney
- A Jewish physician in Germany who was preparing to perform surgery on a patient was shocked to discover the patient's swastika tattoos and other indications that the patient was a neo-Nazi and withdrew from the operating room to secure a substitute surgeon
- A student in a counseling program refuses to counsel a gay man because of her biblically based opposition to unmarried sex

This somewhat random array of cases involves a broad range of agents who, on grounds of conscience, refuse to participate in a wide array of activities. Some of these conscience-based refusals are considered both legally and professionally acceptable; hence, conscientious objectors are already exempted from performing or providing some objectionable services, procedures, or products. These include, for example, protections of conscientious refusals to perform abortions or sterilizations in most nonemergency cases or to participate in physician-assisted dying in states in the United States, where it has been legalized. However, some CRs lack such protection and may subject the agents to professional, institutional, civil, or legal penalties. Some CRs may actually be efforts to change laws or policies.[3]

In view of the wide range of conscientious refusals, and the need to indicate the kinds of cases that will be the focus of this analysis, I will use the symbol "X" to refer to legal and patient-sought services, procedures, and products that some providers find ethically wrong to perform or provide.

ACOG Ethics Committee on the Limits of Conscientious Refusal

In 2007, the American College of Obstetricians and Gynecologists (ACOG) issued Opinion #385, prepared by its Committee on Ethics and titled "The Limits of Conscientious Refusal in Reproductive Medicine."[4] The ACOG has an understandably strong interest in the limits of conscience-based refusal because so many refusals constrain women's reproductive choices and may negatively impact their reproductive health. This is true in other countries as well as in the United States.[5] Opinion #385 delineated several criteria for determining appropriate limits: the potential of the refusal to impose the provider's values on the patient; the refusal's effect on patient health—the paramount criterion; the scientific integrity of the refusal (e.g., whether an objection to a particular contraception as an abortifacient is scientifically sound); and the potential for discrimination (e.g., against women as a group or against classes of women).

The opinion then offered fairly standard recommendations for the physician's advance notice, disclosure, referral, and treatment in an emergency. Indeed, these recommendations are close to what has been called the "conventional compromise" in our society on CRs.[6] Perhaps most controversial was the opinion's recommendation that conscientious objectors practice in close proximity to nonobjectors or otherwise ensure effective referral processes. While hardly radical, this opinion set off an enormous firestorm. In retrospect, it appears that the major sparks came from the opinion's emphasis on setting *limits* and its focus on the phenomenon of appeals to conscience rather than on the grounding of CRs, as well as its recommendation about practice locations, combined with the mistaken belief that the American Board on Obstetrics and Gynecology uses compliance with ACOG Ethics Committee Opinions as a basis for certifying obstetricians and gynecologists.

Over several months, the Department of Health and Human Services (HHS) had two different responses to this controversy under two different presidents. With the vocal participation of HHS Secretary Michael Leavitt, under President George W. Bush, HHS proposed new certification rules for institutions to ensure the protection of healthcare providers from coercion and discrimination if they conscientiously refuse to perform or provide X. It viewed these certification rules as merely ensuring the implementation of the well-established "conscience clauses" in different federal legislation, particularly relating to abortion and sterilization. It concentrated on the value of protecting conscience, combined with a consequentialist argument that protecting healthcare providers' conscience is needed to ensure an adequate supply of providers, in view of the pending shortage of providers, especially in underserved areas.[7]

In announcing its proposal to rescind these rules, the Obama administration indicated its (tentative) judgment that these rules were unnecessary and confusing and would probably have a negative impact on patients' access to services and information. But it requested more information before taking a final action.[8] Then, in March 2011, the Obama administration in part revised and in part rescinded these rules.[9]

Empirical Evidence about Physicians' Views of Obligations in Conscientious Refusal

Despite the variety of cases I mentioned and the controversy about the ACOG Ethics Committee's attempts to delineate limits of CR in reproductive medicine, it is possible that the conflicts and tensions about CO are exaggerated. In an effort to generate relevant data, Farr Curlin and colleagues studied 1,144 responses to a questionnaire sent to 2,000 physicians—a 63% response rate.[10] The researchers asked physicians from all specialties whether they personally objected to three currently contested clinical practices: (1) 17% objected to providing terminal sedation (sedating dying patients to the point of unconsciousness); (2) 42% objected to prescribing birth control to teenagers without their parents' consent; and (3) 52% objected to performing abortion for failed contraception. What the researchers most wanted to determine, however, was what physicians feel obligated to do when they conscientiously oppose performing or providing X. Specifically, the researchers were interested in whether the respondents believed that objecting physicians should "present all possible options" to the patient and "have an obligation to refer the patient" to a nonobjecting physician, as well as whether objecting physicians may explain to patients the religious/moral basis of their objection.

Their results were striking. When asked, "Does the [objecting] physician have an obligation to present all possible options to the patient, including information about obtaining the requested procedure?" 86% said yes, while 8% said no, and 6% were undecided. In response to the question "Does the [objecting] physician have an obligation to refer the patient to someone who does not object to the requested procedure?" 71% indicated yes, while 18% answered no, and 11% were undecided. Moreover, most respondents were very clear that objecting physicians have no obligation to refrain from sharing their religious and/or moral reasons for their objection to the requested procedure. When asked, "Would it be ethical for the [objecting] physician to plainly describe to the patient why he or she objects to the requested procedure?" 63% answered yes, 22% no, and 15% undecided.

Curlin and colleagues stress that these data have several significant practical implications for patients:

> If physicians' ideas translate into their practices, then 14% of patients—more than 40 million Americans—may be cared for by physicians who do not believe they are obligated to disclose information about medically available treatments they consider objectionable.
>
> In addition, 29% of patients—or nearly 100 million Americans—may be cared for by physicians who do not believe they have an obligation to refer the patient to another provider for such treatments.[11]

In short, we have the potential for serious and widespread conflicts, particularly between physicians' consciences and patients' interests. Curlin and colleagues further emphasize that their survey data "point to a basic dilemma facing patients and physicians in our plural[istic] democracy. Because patients and physicians come from many different moral traditions, religious and secular, they will sometimes disagree about whether a particular medical intervention is morally permissible."[12] Later we will return to the researchers' conclusions and recommendations, especially to a serious limitation of their proposals for addressing this situation.

In the context of the above cases, the controversy about the ACOG report and recommendations, and the data from the Curlin et al. study, the following question will guide subsequent analyses and arguments: Should the state, society, institutions, and professions *exempt* conscientiously objecting healthcare professionals from performing objectionable procedures or providing objectionable services or products that are legal and patient sought? If so, under what circumstances and within what limits?

The Nature, Contours, and Scope of Conscientious Refusals

Claims of Conscience: Conscience-Based Refusals

How can we understand claims of CO (i.e., objection, on grounds of conscience, to performing or providing X, whether one finally does so or not) and acts of CR (i.e., refusing, on grounds of conscience, to perform or provide X)? (I use the phrases "conscientious refusal" and "conscience-based refusal" interchangeably.) The term "conscience" is more common in some religious and moral traditions than others, but the phenomenon that both CO and CR describe is widespread.[13] It is this: A person believes that he or she should or must not—indeed, perhaps, cannot—perform a particular act because that act would violate his or her core, fundamental values (religious and/or moral) and thus damage his/her integrity and self-respect. And so that person conscientiously objects to or conscientiously refuses to perform the act or provide the service or product in question.[14]

Dramatic language is common in such cases:

- "I couldn't live with myself if I did that."
- "I would hate myself if I did that."
- "I couldn't look at myself in the mirror."
- "I wouldn't be able to sleep at night."

The agent's claims of integrity, often but not always stated in terms of "conscience," stress that the ethical principles and values at stake are fundamental to his or her identity—indeed, so fundamental that their breach would result in a loss of integrity, wholeness, and harmony in the self, accompanied by severe feelings of guilt or shame. Hence, this is what has been described as a "can't help" or a "volitional necessity."[15]

Authentic and Spurious Claims of Conscience

Any claim of conscience may be spurious rather than genuine—for example, it may mask other interests. One question is how we can distinguish authentic from inauthentic conscientious objections and how important it is to do so in healthcare.

In the United States conscientious objectors to conscripted military service have often had to appear before "draft boards" to establish that their claimed conscientious objection meets the relevant standards for exemption in federal law and administrative rules. And they frequently have had to convince these boards that they sincerely held their beliefs, that their claims of conscience were genuine. In reaching their verdicts, these boards considered a variety of factors, including the claimant's behavioral patterns over time.

In military conscription, it is important to examine the sincerity of an individual's objection for two main reasons. First, exempting an objector from military service means that someone else will probably have to serve in his place, and, second, the objector could reasonably be thought to have other motives for not wanting to serve (e.g., a fear of being killed). Are there similar concerns in healthcare? Exempting a particular healthcare provider does mean that someone else will probably have to perform or provide X. It is an empirical question whether there will be enough nonobjectors to perform or provide X in a timely way, and this may depend on what X is. Furthermore, and quite importantly, the exemption may create burdens and harms, including dignitary harms, for patients; we will later discuss possible ways to reduce those burdens and harms. Finally, in some cases, the healthcare provider's refusal to perform or provide X may be motivated more by other factors such as fears (e.g., fears generated by violent protests of X) than by conscience.

In one situation four obstetricians/gynecologists objected to performing a requested second-trimester abortion in a public hospital and signed a declaration of "moral, ethical, or religious objections," as required by state law. However, Christopher Meyers and Robert Woods note that the real reasons behind their declarations did not clearly display moral opposition.[16] Three of the physicians' reasons were (1) a concern about possible loss of patients at a fertility clinic; (2) a personal preference to restrict his practice to gynecology; and (3) a concern about inadequate compensation for providing abortions. The fourth physician found second-trimester abortions to be "complex and frankly ugly"—a reason that could reflect an unarticulated ethical objection.

What policies, if any, should we adopt to distinguish genuine from spurious CO claims in healthcare? We do not yet have a consensus about the exemptible claims of conscience in healthcare, and without that consensus, close scrutiny of the authenticity or sincerity of specific individual claims may not be very helpful. Moreover, it does not appear to be generally necessary at this time to establish or mandate review boards for prospective COs in healthcare, but this could change, depending on the numbers of CRs involved and the effects of widespread CRs on patients' rights and welfare.[17] However, this is not to deny the value of requesting and even requiring moral justification, beyond checking a box or signing a form, for claims of exemption on the part of healthcare professionals who object to performing or providing Xs, even if the review is not highly formal.

Religious and/or Moral Conscience

Curlin and colleagues found that healthcare-related conscientious refusals were more common among participants in religious communities, particularly in Roman Catholic and evangelical Protestant communities.[18] Physicians' reluctance to disclose all options and to refer patients for ethically contested (but legal) procedures correlated with their religiousness, as measured intrinsically and extrinsically (through involvement in religious communities). Hence, Curlin and colleagues titled their article "Religion, Conscience, and Controversial Clinical Practices."[19] Furthermore, as Alta Charo stresses, the battles over CRs in healthcare are in part battles over the role of religion in public and professional life—they are part of our "culture wars."[20]

Nevertheless, it is crucial to stress that the prominence and prevalence of religiously based objections along with the constitutional protections of the free exercise of religion do not necessarily mean that religious conscience is privileged over nonreligious or secular conscience in the American tradition. Indeed, evidence to the contrary appears in US Supreme Court decisions in the context of conscientious objection to military service.

Historically legal exemption from military service in the United States was limited to religious pacifists. Then—to greatly shorten a long and more complicated story—the US Supreme Court in *Welsh v. United States* in 1970 held that under the Selective Service Act

> what is necessary for a registrant's conscientious objection to all war to be "religious," within the meaning of the statute, is . . . that the opposition to war stem from the registrant's moral, ethical, or religious beliefs about what is right and wrong and that these beliefs be *held with the strength of traditional religious convictions*. . . . If an individual deeply and sincerely holds beliefs which are purely ethical or moral in source and content which but which nevertheless *impose upon him a duty of conscience* to refrain from participating in any war at any time, those beliefs certainly *occupy in the life of that individual "a place parallel to that filled by . . . God"* in traditionally religious persons. Because *his beliefs function as a religion in his life,* such an individual is as much entitled to a "religious" conscientious objector exemption under #6 (j) as is someone who derives his conscientious opposition to war from traditional religious convictions.[21]

This decision, building in part on earlier decisions, emphasized the "parallel belief" test and the functional equivalence test for thinking about the comparability of religiously based and nonreligiously based claims of conscience. While developed in the context of conscientious objection to military conscription, these points are pertinent to conscientious refusals in healthcare, and there is no reason to suppose that they would not—or should not—hold in this context too. Nevertheless, the empirical point also holds: CRs in healthcare in the United States statistically correlate with religious beliefs and practices.

Universal and Selective Conscientious Refusals

Another important distinction in CO to military service is pertinent to CO in healthcare. This is the distinction between *universal* CO and *selective* CO.

In the context of military conscription, the United States has granted conscientious objector status, with exemption from military service (but with requirements for either noncombatant service in the military or alternative service outside the military), only to universal objectors (i.e., pacifists who oppose all wars), and not to selective objectors who only oppose particular wars that fail to satisfy their criteria for ethically just or justified wars, for instance, criteria that have been emphasized in the just-war tradition.[22] Although sometimes dismissed as mere political or economic objectors, rather than conscientious objectors, selective objectors may have genuine ethical claims just as much as universal objectors. However, granting exemptions from military service to selective objectors can be politically fraught (because the objection is to "this particular war") and administratively difficult (both because these ethical objections overlap with other kinds of objections and because testing sincerity is more difficult).[23]

In healthcare, universal objection is an objection to performing or providing X as such. For the universal objector, there would be no conditions under which performing or providing X, such as an abortion or sterilization or assistance in dying, could be ethically justifiable for him or her. By contrast, the selective objector is opposed to performing or providing X only under certain circumstances or for certain groups or classes of persons.

The Bush administration's proposed conscience rule for health professionals allowed selective conscientious refusals, what it called "graded refusals."[24] For instance, a physician might refuse to sterilize young women or single women while being willing to sterilize married women. According to the Bush administration, the conscience clauses in statutes related to sterilization and abortion allow conscientious refusal "on any ground." I take this to include general or specific, broad or narrow, grounds, as long as there is a "conscience" claim. Thus, in the case of statutes with "conscience clauses," the HHS continued, "it is the individual's religious beliefs or moral convictions that will control in a particular case, *rather than the frequency of the objection*" (italics added). So, from this standpoint, the objection need not be universal, that is, applying to all Xs, but presumably it should be universalizable in the sense of applying to all Xs of a particular type, such as sterilization of single women.

Selective objection is sufficient for exemption, HHS noted, unless the decision is "based on an individual's characteristics that are federally protected, [which] is impermissible." These include characteristics such as race and gender. However, some other characteristics may be protected by state laws, and some may viewed as morally important even though not legally protected on either the national or the state level.

In a California case, the plaintiff charged that two doctors refused her a fertility treatment on the grounds of her sexual orientation—the fact that she is a lesbian. However, the defendants in this case insisted that what was at issue was her marital status, not her sexual orientation. They objected to performing intrauterine insemination on unmarried women, whether heterosexual or lesbian, because such an action would violate their Christian beliefs. They contended that their refusal was protected by their constitutional right to freedom of religion.

In this 2008 case, the California Supreme Court asked "Do the rights of religious freedom and free speech, as guaranteed in both the federal and the California Constitutions, exempt a medical clinic's physicians from complying with the California Unruh Civil Rights Act's prohibition against discrimination based on a person's sexual orientation?" The court's answer was "no."[25]

The reasons for suspicion of selective CRs in healthcare thus differ from the reasons that operate in the context of military conscription. In healthcare the risk is unjust discrimination against groups or classes of persons.[26]

Scope of CRs: Narrow and Broad Interpretations of Participation

Throughout we have used the language of performing or providing X. That language focuses on the agent's *direct* performance or *direct* provision of X. However, conscientious objectors and refusers often also oppose and resist *indirect* participation. Several terms express this broader range. While "participation" is probably the most common, others are also widely used: "assistance" (in the performance or provision of X), "cooperation," "collaboration," "association," "involvement," and "complicity." The last, "complicity," is the most morally laden; the others have more neutral and even positive versions, but we can only be complicit in something bad.

Agents and observers use several metaphors, particularly physical metaphors, as evaluative descriptions of participation and nonparticipation. The main physical metaphors for participation focus on *dirty hands* and *soiled consciences*, while the main metaphors for nonparticipation are *step away, stand aside, hand off, washing one's hands,* and *distancing.*

Conflicts and tensions between respecting providers' consciences and protecting patients' interests have been exacerbated by expansive conceptions of what counts as "assistance in the performance" or provision of X and "expansive notions of complicity."[27] These expansions amplify and intensify the conflicts and tensions in healthcare because they increase (1) the number of *acts* of "participation," and (2) the number of *agents* who consider themselves "participants."

The debate about "participation"—its scope and limits—also surfaced in the conscience rule adopted by the Bush administration in December 2008. The Department of Health and Human Services, in seeking to provide "broad protection for individuals," chose not to limit the definition of "assist in the performance," drawn from the federal conscience statutes, related particularly to abortion and sterilization, to "direct involvement." Instead, it adopted a definition of "assist in the performance" that included and was limited to "any activity with *a reasonable connection* to a procedure, health service or health service program, or research activity" (italics added). "Assist in the performance" would include "referrals, training, or other arrangements for the procedure, health service, or research activity."[28]

In further clarifying "assist in the performance," HHS included specific examples: (1) a standard example: an operating room nurse would be considered to "assist in the performance" of an operation, and (2) a more contestable example: "an employee whose task it is to clean the instruments used in a particular procedure would also be considered to assist in the performance of the particular procedure under the proposed rule."[29]

We might also extend the second example to include cleaning the room in which the objectionable procedures occurred. In either the original or expanded second example, it is not that the instruments used in abortion or sterilization—or the room itself—are tainted, but that the cleaner's actions would be assisting in the objectionable procedure of abortion or sterilization, whether before or after the fact.

This second example can be viewed retrospectively (i.e., after the objectionable procedure has occurred) or prospectively (i.e., in preparation for the objectionable procedure). If the procedure has been completed, and the abortion or sterilization has been finished, it may appear difficult to view the cleaner's work as "assisting in the performance" of the already-completed objectionable procedure. But an expanded sense of complicity focuses on the overall system required to provide such procedures, a system that includes sterilizing used equipment and instruments. It also includes disposal of medical waste. Yet it would be exceedingly difficult and expensive to sort medical waste according to the types of procedures that produced it.[30]

Focusing on the preparatory sterilization of instruments, Robert Card stresses that "one would have to know that this scalpel was going to be used to (eg) perform a vasectomy as opposed to an appendectomy, which is unlikely."[31] He contends that it would not be workable for hospitals to attempt prospectively to identify instruments for objectionable and unobjectionable procedures in order to protect cleaners' consciences. For instance, an instrument being used in a C-section delivery may have to be used for an emergency hysterectomy because of unforeseen complications during the procedure.

Religious traditions vary in the guidance they offer their adherents about such participation. Catholic moral theologians have developed a complex set of distinctions about cooperation with evil—with attention to the distinction between formal and material cooperation and different degrees of material cooperation. These are reflected in directives for Catholic healthcare professionals and institutions along with attention to the potential for scandal.[32] But this detailed framework is not available to all (even to all religious) conscientious objectors. And an individual's sense of participation as complicity in others' wrongdoing is highly subjective. This further complicates processes of exemption.

Exemptions of COs/CRs: Ethical Balancing

The fundamental ethical question for this chapter is: Should the state, society, institutions, and health professions *exempt* conscientiously objecting physicians, nurses, and others from performing or providing X? This is not only a matter of professional ethics, such as medical or nursing ethics, but also a matter of political and social philosophy and, more specifically, of political, social, institutional, and organizational ethics, in addressing the tensions and conflicts between respecting healthcare providers' CRs and protecting patients' interests.

On the one hand, respecting the healthcare professional's CR is important because of the values of moral integrity, identity, and self-respect identified earlier and because of several important consequentialist considerations. The Bush administration appealed to consequentialist considerations in support of its conscience rule, stressing that many conscientious refusers are also committed to needed medical service in underserved areas. These considerations have been elaborated by others. For instance, White and Brody identify several possible negative consequences of a ban on CRs. It could "negatively influence the type of persons who enter medicine" and "how practicing physicians attend to professional obligations" as well as their faithfulness to their professional responsibilities; it could also foster "callousness" and encourage physicians' "intolerance" of diverse moral beliefs among their patients (and, we might add, among their colleagues as well).[33] Perhaps the main cause of such possible negative consequences would be a ban's lack of respect for the physician's core moral values reflected in some CRs. While some of these possible effects are quite speculative, they merit consideration.

On the other hand, it is important to protect patients' legitimate interests, particularly their interests in (1) timely access, (2) safe and effective care, (3) respectful care, (4) nondiscriminatory treatment, (5) care that is not unduly burdensome, and (5) privacy and confidentiality.

Several metaphors of response recognize, and attempt to include, both interest sets: *balancing, striking a balance* (or an appropriate balance), *finding middle ground, reaching mutual accommodation, reasonable compromise, practical reconciliation,*[34] and so forth. The most common metaphor, by far, is *balancing* or *striking a balance*. Widespread usage, however, does not guarantee clear and helpful guidance. Indeed, the fact that all parties to the debate invoke this metaphor to describe their own positions, over against others, suggests its limitations.[35]

However, this metaphor does exclude two extreme positions. On the one hand, it does not exempt all CRs. The claim, based on conscience, that performing or providing X shall not occur "through me" is not always exemptible on the balancing model. On the other hand, the metaphor does not require the conscientious objector to perform or provide the X in question in every case. Years ago, a long-time medical colleague was stunned when, after telling a patient that he could not in good conscience perform a particular procedure but that he would refer her to a nonobjecting physician, the patient challenged him, "Don't I have a right to *you*?" My colleague was correct: having a right to X does not necessarily entail having a right to its performance or provision by a specific health professional.[36]

Even though the metaphor of balancing does not provide very clear or precise guidance beyond ruling out these extremes, it pervades professional and other proposals for addressing conflicts involving claims of conscience. The ACOG Ethics Committee Opinion on "The Limits of Conscientious Refusals in Reproductive Medicine" proposes that lawmakers "advance policies that *balance* [1] protection of providers' consciences with [2] the critical goal of ensuring timely, effective, evidence-based, and safe access to all women seeking reproductive services."[37] (Italics and bracketed numbers added)

Similarly, the Bioethics Committee of the American Academy of Pediatrics indicates that the Academy "supports a *balance* between the individual physician's moral integrity and his or her fiduciary obligations to patients" (italics added). It goes beyond many invocations of the metaphor of balancing by offering some criteria for this process: "A physician's duty to perform a procedure within the scope of his or her training increases as the availability of alternative providers decreases and the risk to the patient increases."[38] This identifies two factors that are crucial in what we might call structured or constrained balancing:[39] (1) Are alternatives available to a particular health professional's performance/provision of X? (2) What are the risks (both probability and seriousness of harm) to the patient if a particular health professional refuses to perform or provide X? These two factors will figure in our analysis and assessment of different proposals for striking a balance between respecting the healthcare professional's CO and protecting the patient's interests.

Proposals for Striking a Balance: An Assessment

Several proposals recognize conscience claims and seek to safeguard them, without, at the same time, threatening patients' interests in timely, efficacious, safe, and nondiscriminatory access without undue burdens in a context of care and respect. We are again limiting our attention to the performance/provision of legal Xs.

The first model of balancing focuses on the moral implications of the particular health professional's responsibilities in choosing a profession and employment: (1) *An individual should avoid a profession/employment where performance or provision of a conscientiously opposed X is expected; anyone entering that profession/employment is obligated to perform or provide this X.* Of course, it is easy enough to say that a person who is conscientiously opposed to performing/providing X, which is part of the expectations of the profession, should avoid that profession, and this certainly applies, even more strongly, to particular employment contexts. An editorial in the *New York Times* sharply states this view in reference to pharmacists: "Any pharmacist who cannot dispense medicine lawfully prescribed by a doctor should find another line of work."[40]

While important, this admonition is too simple. After all, "professional expectations" may not be sufficiently clear in advance and may change over time, as the following examples make clear: In the United States after being widely banned, abortion was legalized in some states by the early 1970s and then across the country in 1973; reproductive and genetic technologies have undergone major transformations over the last three decades; and physician-assisted dying has been legalized in several states. Even if we say that core duties have been long articulated for health professionals—for instance, care for the sick and injured, relieve patients' pain and suffering, and protect and promote patients' health—these are notoriously broad and unspecific. And their specifications are subject to debate because of unclear and contested primary categories, such as health. Professional expectations under the World Health Organization's broad definition of health as "complete physical, mental, and social well-being"[41] would differ greatly from the expectations under a narrower definition of health focused on the absence of disease. And meanings can change over time, for instance, in the context of changes in technologies. As a result, dissenters in some cases may plausibly deny that they voluntarily accepted certain current expectations when they entered the profession. Nevertheless, this model offers valuable cautionary guidance to prospective professionals for their moral tranquility as well as for their patients' benefit.

A second model focuses on the health professional's advance notice: (2) *Advance notice, by the health professional, that he/she will not perform or provide X so that prospective patients, clients, or consumers can seek alternative providers.* For instance, a few years ago, one of the fourth-year medical students in my Religion and Medicine elective was planning to enter a Christian medical practice that provided to all prospective patients a brochure that indicated its vision as well as some Xs that would not be performed or provided.

This model is very important as far as it goes. But, in stressing matching patients with physicians (and other health professionals), it assumes an ideal set of relationships that may not be available in much modern healthcare, which takes place among strangers. As a result, the trust involved, if it is present at all, is not based on personal knowledge of the different parties and their values. Furthermore, persons seeking services may experience rapid and urgent needs, and may not have alternatives or may have only extremely

burdensome alternatives. For all these reasons, this approach, while important, is inadequate as a solution to conflicts involving conscience.

A third model also emphasizes disclosure in the context of the evolving relationship rather than merely or primarily at the outset. (3) *Nonperformance
or nonprovision of X by a health professional, combined with his/her disclosure
of information to patients, clients, consumers about X and options for obtaining
X.* This model is acceptable if nonburdensome options exist in nonemergency circumstances.

It is important to recall the study by Curlin and colleagues: *only 86%* of
the physician-respondents recognized an affirmative obligation to "present
all possible options to the patient, including information about obtaining the
requested procedure." (It is possible that some respondents interpreted "information about obtaining" as close to "referral," but this is not clear from
the report of the research.) In this context, Curlin and colleagues stress that
patients may need to be *proactive* by informing themselves about options and
then asking their physicians about those options, but Curlin and colleagues
also indicate that the ideal is "respectful dialogue" between physicians and
patients "to anticipate areas of moral disagreement and negotiate acceptable
accommodations before crises develop."[42]

I have elsewhere supported a model of negotiation that can lead to mutual
accommodation, and I believe that such a model, combining advance notice
and ongoing discussion, can be valuable.[43] However, from my standpoint,
Curlin and colleagues fail to emphasize enough physicians' advance notice
and their continuing disclosure of options as well as limits—hence, they place
an undue burden on patients to be proactive. Of course, it would be prudent
for patients to be proactive, but advance notice and continuing disclosure
of options are ethical obligations for health professionals, grounded in their
fiduciary responsibility, the imbalance of power in the medical relationship,
and ethical and legal requirements of informed consent/refusal. Disclosure
of all relevant information is, in my judgment, ethically mandatory (and
should be professionally mandatory too). While some health professionals
view disclosure of options as a form of complicity in subsequent wrongdoing,
I believe this is a nonnegotiable minimum. It may be combined with a health
professional's respectful statement about why on religious/moral grounds he
or she does not perform or provide X.[44]

A fourth model is more controversial because what it requires (referral) is more widely viewed as a form of complicity with wrongdoing.
(4) *Nonperformance/nonprovision of X by a health professional, combined with*

referral or transfer of patients, clients, or consumers to another health professional who will perform or provide X. This too is acceptable if nonburdensome alternatives exist for patients in nonemergency circumstances. But major conflicts erupt because many health professionals are adamantly opposed to referral or transfer as complicity in wrongdoing. According to the study by Curlin and colleagues, only 71% of the respondents to the survey believe that an objecting physician has a duty to refer the patient to a nonobjecting physician. (The rest are either opposed or undecided.)

Conscience is personal: the logic of conscience is that it concerns me and my acts, it concerns what I do or do not do. We say, for example, "My conscience won't let me do X." It would be odd or absurd for me to say: "My conscience indicates that he shouldn't do X," or "I would have a guilty conscience if he did X." However, it would not be odd or absurd to say: "I would have a guilty conscience if I helped him do that."[45]

The personal logic of conscience helps us see why many people consider direct referral problematic and even equivalent to the performance or provision of X. Certainly, referral or transfer can reasonably be seen to *involve* the agent more closely and intimately in the performance/provision of X than disclosure of options, and this means that, if we are serious about striking a balance, we will need to find some way, perhaps through imaginative institutional mechanisms or arrangements, to accommodate health professionals' consciences and patients' interests at precisely this point. And there are some possibilities.

The Bioethics Committee of the American Academy of Pediatrics describes the duty to refer: "In situations of potential harm to patients, physicians have a duty to refer in a timely manner. This duty may be fulfilled by informing patients about referral services such as those provided by hospitals or insurance companies."[46] In a similar vein, Chervenak and McCullough propose what they call indirect referrals rather than direct referrals to a specific physician; such indirect referrals could provide information about "responsible health care organizations" with which the patient could consult.[47]

In view of many health professionals' strong convictions that referral is morally equivalent to performing/providing X, we need to exercise our moral imagination to see whether we can identify ways to protect both the health professional's conscience and the patient's interests. The suggestions that have emerged for handling conscientious objections to referral point to a final model for balancing health professionals' conscientious objections and patients' interests. (5) *The development of systems and mechanisms to ensure the performance/provision of X to meet patients' interests while exempting COs.* While it is clear that these several models are not mutually exclusive but can be combined in various ways, this institutional approach enables the protection of individual health professionals' consciences and patients' interests.

In part as a result of controversy over Plan B, the Washington State Board of Pharmacy developed rules that allowed *pharmacists* not to dispense a medication if they are personally opposed to doing so. However, these rules also required *pharmacies* to deliver lawfully prescribed drugs or devices to patients and distribute Food and Drug Administration approved (but restricted) drugs and devices in a timely manner.[48] This is not a perfect solution because it can pose problems of employment for individual pharmacists in small pharmacies. Nevertheless, it is an important and promising accommodation in the balancing process.

Also vitally important is collective professional responsibility. One strong argument in favor of placing a heavy burden on the health professions, as distinguished from particular health professionals, is that they have a quasi-monopoly status that requires the restriction of the liberties of others.[49] As Alta Charo summarizes, "the power imbalance between the parties, and the special obligations placed upon professionals as a group due to their privileged, quasi-monopoly status as health care providers, form the basis for what is arguably a collective obligation of the profession to provide non-discriminatory access to all lawful services."[50]

Conclusions

In conclusion, it is important to distinguish *conscientious refusal* from *conscientious obstruction*. The logic of personal conscience may have to do not only with refraining from participating in X but also in trying to stop X. But there are firm limits to conscientious obstruction that should be enforced by professional and legal sanctions if necessary. Professionals may try to persuade their patients about right moral actions, but their own *exempted* acts of conscience may not go beyond persuasion and nonparticipation (within the limits previously noted) to manipulation of information or coercion of prospective or actual patients.

To be sure, many health professionals who conscientiously object to performing or providing X also believe that X should not be performed or provided. They are committed to not being or becoming an instrument of some

X's performance or provision but also to stopping some X altogether. And, of course, they may legitimately engage in various efforts to have X banned. However, they should not expect an exemption in taking it on themselves to stop a legal X from being performed or provided for a particular patient. This is obstruction, and even the refusal to provide information about options, including objectionable options, plausibly falls under obstruction.

A CR can function as a "shield" or as a "sword." Douglas White and Baruch Brody write, "Conscience-based refusals should be a 'shield' to protect individual physicians from being compelled to violate their core moral beliefs rather than a 'sword' to force their beliefs onto patients."[51] Using a different physical metaphor, the American Pharmacists Association affirms the pharmacist's right *"to step away, not in the way"* of patients seeking their medication.[52] (italics added).

Finally, it is important to recognize that not all Xs are equal. I have chosen the symbol X for efficiency in this chapter. Yet it would be a mistake to conflate all Xs as though distinctions among them were unimportant. This would also extend and overextend the paradigm of protection of CRs to perform abortions to the entire range of conscientiously opposed acts and practices. There are very strong reasons to exempt conscientious objectors to abortion because they believe that the act constitutes the direct killing of an innocent human being. The moral rule against the direct killing of innocent human beings—however it is worded and whether it is brought under a broader principle of not harming others or neighbor love, for example—is a bedrock of social and medical morality. Disputes hinge in part on the moral status of the fetus, a dispute that is difficult, if not impossible, to resolve in a pluralistic society. But to force a person to kill or to participate in killing a fetus which he or she views as a full human being would be a fundamental breach of moral requirements and horrifying and traumatic for conscientious objectors to abortion. A similar reason (without necessarily involving attributions of "innocence") operates in our society's exemption from military service of conscientious objectors to killing in war. To force people to kill another human being against their conscientious objection is to force such a fundamental violation of their conscience that it should be avoided when at all possible.

Notes

1. In focusing on "conscientious refusals" I am attending to only a dramatic subset of acts, claims, and expressions of conscience in healthcare. This focus neglects conscience as part of patients' interests, as well as many healthcare professionals' conscientious willingness to act on behalf of patients' interests. See, for instance, Elizabeth Sepper, "Conscientious Refusals of Care," in *The Oxford Handbook of U.S. Health Law*, ed. I. Glenn Cohen, Allison Hoffman, and William M. Sage (New York: Oxford University Press, 2017), Chapter 16; and Sepper, "Taking Conscience Seriously," *Virginia Law Review* 98 (2012): 1501–1575. I am also focusing on *individual* conscientious refusals, not on institutional, business, or corporation refusals, an important topic in the debate about the Affordable Care Act and for another occasion.

2. These cases have been drawn from a variety of reports in conversations and the media as well as the following: Alta Charo, "The Celestial Fire of Conscience: Refusing to Deliver Medical Care," *New England Journal of Medicine* 352, No. 24 (June 16, 2005): 2471–2473; Rebecca Dresser, "Professionals, Conformity, and Conscience," *Hastings Center Report* 35, No. 6 (November-December 2005): 9–10; Julian Savulescu, "Conscientious Objection in Medicine," *British Medical Journal* 332 (2006): 294–297; Howard Brody's testimony to the President's Council on Bioethics, September 11, 2008. Available at https://bioethicsarchive.georgetown.edu/pcbe/transcripts/sept08/session3.html (accessed March 17, 2017); and Mark R. Wicclair, *Conscientious Objection in Health Care: An Ethical Analysis* (New York: Cambridge University Press, 2011). Wicclair's book and his many articles represent some of the most thoughtful and illuminating work on the ethics of conscientious objection in healthcare.

3. See Childress, "Civil Disobedience, Conscientious Objection, and Evasive Non-Compliance: A Framework for the Analysis and Assessment of Illegal Action in Health Care," *Journal of Medicine and Philosophy* 10 (February 1985): 63–83.

4. American College of Obstetricians and Gynecologists (ACOG) Committee Opinion 385 (Committee on Ethics), "The Limits of Conscientious Refusal in Reproductive Medicine," *Obstetrics and Gynecology* 110 (2007): 1203–1208. I served on the ACOG ethics committee at the time of this report and certainly did not anticipate the level of controversy it would provoke. The name of this professional organization has since changed; it is now the American Congress of Obstetricians and Gynecologists rather than the American College of Obstetricians and Gynecologists.

5. See, for example, the vigorous debate in the Council of Europe Parliamentary Assembly in 2010. It rejected a committee's recommendation against "unregulated use of conscientious objection" to lawful medical care (focused on the protection of women) and, instead, approved "the right to conscientious objection to lawful medical care." Parliamentary Assembly, "The Right to Conscientious Objection in Lawful Medical Care," Resolution 1763 (2010), Final Version, http://assembly.coe.int/nw/xml/XRef/Xref-XML2HTML-EN.asp?fileid=17909&lang=en.

6. Dan W. Brock, "Conscientious Refusal by Physicians and Pharmacists: Who Is Obligated to Do What, and Why?" *Theoretical Medicine and Bioethics* 29 (2008): 187–200. Brock delineates this "conventional compromise" and defends it as a "reasonable accommodation" (p. 199).

7. *Ensuring That Department of Health and Human Services Funds Do Not Support Coercive or Discriminatory Policies or Practices in Violation of Federal Law; Final Rule,* 45 CFR Part 88, *Federal Register,* December 19, 2008 (Volume 73, Number 245): 78071–78101.

8. For a valuable discussion of the federal conscience clauses including the Bush administration provider conscience regulation and the Obama administration's response, see Kimberly A. Parr, "Beyond Politics: A Social and Cultural History of Federal Healthcare Conscience Protections," *American Journal of Law and Medicine* 35 (2009): 620–646.

9. *Regulation for the Enforcement of Federal Health Care Provider Conscience Protection Laws,* 45 CFR Part 88, *Federal Register,* February 23, 2011 (Volume 76): 9968–9977. For a discussion, see Rob Stein, "Obama Administration Replaces Controversial 'Conscience' Regulation for Health-care Workers," *Washington Post,* February 18, 2011 http://www.washingtonpost.com/wp-dyn/content/article/2011/02/18/AR2011021803251.html.

   While this book was in press, the Trump administration replaced the Obama administration's 2011 regulation with its own final conscience rule—*Protecting Statutory Conscience Rights in Health Care; Delegations of Authority,* 45 CFR Part 88, *Federal Register,* May 21, 2019 (Volume 84): 23170-23272. However, a federal judge vacated this rule before it could be implemented, and its status is unclear as of November 2019. The rule incorporates a number of existing federal laws and regulations, enhances enforcement mechanisms, and also significantly expands the list of agents in health care who can claim rights of religious and conscientious exemption and the kinds of acts for which they can claim exemptions. See Lawrence O. Gostin, "The 'Conscience' Rule: How Will It Affect Patients' Access to Services?" *JAMA* 321, No. 22 (2019): 2152–2153.

10. Farr A Curlin, Ryan E. Lawrence, Marshall H. Chin, and John D. Lantos, "Religion, Conscience, and Controversial Clinical Practices," *New England Journal of Medicine* 356, No. 6 (February 8, 2007): 593–600.

11. Ibid., p. 597.

12. Farr Curlin, quoted in a press release "Conscience, religion alter how doctors tell patients about options," from The University of Chicago News Office, February 7, 2007, http://www-news.uchicago.edu/releases/07/070207.doctorsandreligion.shtml.

13. See James F. Childress, "Appeals to Conscience," *Ethics* 89 (1979): 315–335.

14. "Conscientious" sometimes refers to the *process* of reaching a judgment or decision; my discussion focuses on the final judgment or decision, whether it's based on a complex reasoning process or an immediate intuition or an emotional response or some other process as long as it is moral in nature and connects with the person's core values.

15. See Andrew Koppelman, "Conscience, Volitional Necessity, and Religious Exemptions," *Legal Theory* 15 (2009): 215–244.

16. Christopher Meyers and Robert Woods, "Conscientious Objection? Yes, But Make Sure It Is Genuine," Peer Commentary on "Conscientious Objection and Emergency Contraception," by Robert F. Card, *American Journal of Bioethics* 7, No. 6 (June 2007): 19–21.

17. See Rebecca Dresser's discussion of such boards in "Professionals, Conformity, and Conscience."

18. Curlin et al., "Religion, Conscience, and Controversial Clinical Practices." Not all religious groups may have been well represented in this US survey. A study in the United Kingdom found that nearly half of the medical students from several schools who responded to a survey believed in "the right of doctors to conscientious object to *any* procedure. Demand for the right to conscientiously object is greater in Muslim medical students when compared with other groups of religious medical students." Sophie Strickland, "Conscientious Objection in Medical Students: A Questionnaire Survey," *Journal of Medical Ethics* 38 (2012): 22–25.

19. Curlin et al., "Religion, Conscience, and Controversial Clinical Practices."

20. Charo, "The Celestial Fire of Conscience: Refusing to Deliver Medical Care."

21. *Welsh v. United States*, 398 U.S. 340 (1970). Italics added.

22. See Childress, *Moral Responsibility in Conflicts: Essays on Nonviolence, War, and Conscience* (Baton Rouge: Louisiana State University Press, 1982).

23. See Ibid., chap. 6.

24. *Ensuring That Department of Health and Human Services Funds Do Not Support Coercive or Discriminatory Policies or Practices in Violation of Federal Law; Final Rule*, 45 CFR Part 88, *Federal Register*, December 19, 2008 (Volume 73, Number 245): 78071–78101.

25. *North Coast Women's Care Medical Group, Inc. v. San Diego County Superior Court*, 189 P.3d 959 (Cal. 2008).

26. In view of the large number of cases of CR that involve women patients, some flag these cases as potentially indicative of unjust discrimination against women. See Sepper, "Conscientious Refusals of Care."

27. Charo, "The Celestial Fire of Conscience: Refusing to Deliver Medical Care."

28. *Ensuring That Department of Health and Human Services Funds Do Not Support Coercive or Discriminatory Policies or Practices in Violation of Federal Law; Final Rule.*

29. Ibid.

30. Robert Card, "Federal Provider Conscience Regulation: Unconscionable," *Journal of Medical Ethics* 35 (2009): 471–472.

31. Ibid.

32. US Conference of Catholic Bishops, *Ethical and Religious Directives for Catholic Health Care Services*, 5th edition (Washington, DC: United States Conference of Catholic Bishops, 2009), http://www.usccb.org/issues-and-action/human-life-and-dignity/health-care/upload/Ethical-Religious-Directives-Catholic-Health-Care-Services-fifth-edition-2009.pdf. An earlier edition had a lengthy appendix on cooperation with evil.

33. Douglas B. White and Baruch Brody, "Would Accommodating Some Conscientious Objections by Physicians Promote Quality in Medical Care?" *JAMA* 305, No. 17 (May

4, 2011): 1804–1805. Piers Benn also argues for allowing limited conscientious refusal on the grounds that "the profession flourishes best if there are diverse ethical views to be found within it." "Conscience and Health Care Ethics," in *Principles of Health Care Ethics*, 2nd edition, ed. Richard E. Ashcraft et al. (Chicester, UK: John Wiley & Sons, Ltd., 2007), p. 350.

34. Most of these terms are fairly common; "practical reconciliation" appears in Lynn D. Wardle, "Access and Conscience: Principles of Practical Reconciliation," *Virtual Mentor: American Medical Association Journal of Ethics* 11, No. 10 (October 2009): 783–787.

35. For instance, both ACOG and HHS under the Bush administration invoked the language of "balancing" to describe their positions. An ACOG News Release (September 5, 2008) indicated: "ACOG supports a *reasonable balance* between a physician's right to his or her moral or religious beliefs and a patient's right to needed health care, including reproductive health information and services." And in explaining the Provider Conscience Regulation, HHS wrote:

> The doctor-patient relationship requires a *balancing of interests*. The patient has an interest in obtaining legal health care services—and, in the context of federally funded health care programs, an eligible patient may have the right to obtain certain health care services from certain entities. This must be *balanced against* the statutory right of the provider in the context of a federally funded entity to not be discriminated against based on a refusal to participate in a service to which they have objections, such as abortion. (*Ensuring That Department of Health and Human Services Funds Do Not Support Coercive or Discriminatory Policies or Practices in Violation of Federal Law; Final Rule*; Italics added)

36. It is plausible to hold that negative rights, such as the right to noninterference, hold against all but that positive rights can be discharged by a variety of agents.

37. ACOG Committee Opinion 385, "The Limits of Conscientious Refusal in Reproductive Medicine."

38. American Academy of Pediatrics, Committee on Bioethics, "Policy Statement—Physician Refusal to Provide Information or Treatment on the Basis of Claims of Conscience," *Pediatrics* 124, No. 6 (October 2009).

39. Tom Beauchamp and I use the language and process of "constrained balancing" to move beyond vague calls to balance principles when they conflict. See *Principles of Biomedical Ethics*, 7th edition (New York: Oxford University Press, 2013), pp. 19–24.

40. *New York Times* Editorial, "Moralists at the Pharmacy," April 3, 2005, http://www. nytimes.com/2005/04/03/opinion/moralists-at-the-pharmacy.html?_r=0.

41. *World Health Organization: Basic Documents*, 26th ed. (Geneva: World Health Organization, 1976), p. 1.

42. Curlin et al., "Religion, Conscience, and Controversial Clinical Practices," p. xxx.

43. See Childress and Mark Siegler, "Metaphors and Models of Doctor-Patient Relationships: Their Implications for Autonomy," *Theoretical Medicine* 5 (1984): 17–30.

44. The interpretation offered by HHS of the Provider Conscience Rule under the Bush administration indicates the following: "Providers who object to participation in abortion or a particular health service may provide information on other options, if asked, but are under no obligation to do so." This fails to meet the ethical minimum in at least two ways. First, it only focuses on disclosure about other options in response to a patient's inquiry; this puts all the burden on the patient. Second, it fails to recognize an *obligation* to provide information about other options—providers "may" do so in response to a patient's inquiry, but they have no obligation to do so even when patients ask. This gives too much discretion to health providers both apart from and within the context of a specific patient inquiry about options. *Ensuring That Department of Health and Human Services Funds Do Not Support Coercive or Discriminatory Policies or Practices in Violation of Federal Law; Final Rule.*

45. See Childress, "Appeals to Conscience."

46. American Academy of Pediatrics, Committee on Bioethics, "Policy Statement—Physician Refusal to Provide Information or Treatment on the Basis of Claims of Conscience."

47. See Frank A. Chervenak and Laurence B. McCullough, "The Ethics of Direct and Indirect Referral for Termination of Pregnancy," *American Journal of Obstetrics and Gynecology* 199, No. 3 (2008): 232.e1–232.e3. A supporter of conscientious objection in the United Kingdom suggests that the general practitioner who conscientiously opposes making a direct referral for abortion should ask the pregnant women to see another general practitioner instead. J. W. Gerrard, "Is It Ethical for a General Practitioner to Claim a Conscientious Objection When Asked to Refer for Abortion?" *Journal of Medical Ethics* 35 (2009): 599–602.

48. See Gene Johnson, "Ruling: Washington Can Require Pharmacies to Dispense Plan B," *Seattle Times*, July 23, 2015, updated July 24, 2015, http://www.seattletimes.com/seattle-news/ruling-washington-can-require-pharmacies-to-dispense-plan-b/.

49. See Elizabeth Fenton and Loren Lomasky, "Dispensing with Liberty: Conscientious Refusal and the 'Morning-After Pill'," *Journal of Medicine and Philosophy* 30 (2005): 579–592.

50. Charo, "The Celestial Fire of Conscience: Refusing to Deliver Medical Care."

51. White and Brody, "Would Accommodating Some Conscientious Objections by Physicians Promote Quality in Medical Care?" p. 1804.

52. American Pharmacists Association, Government Affairs, Issue Brief, "Federal Conscience Clause," March 2009, p. 3, https://pol285.blog.gustavus.edu/files/2009/08/APhA-Issue-Brief-on-Conscience-Clauses.pdf.

PART III
DECEASED ORGAN DONATION
AND ALLOCATION

7

Difficulties of Determining Death

What Should We Do about the "Dead Donor Rule"?

Introduction

There is a widespread, perhaps universal, fear of a premature, mistaken declaration of death. Historically, this was expressed in the fear of being buried alive as well as the fear of burying others alive. For example, Edgar Allan Poe, the 19th century originator of the detective story and author of horror stories, among other kinds of works, wrote a story entitled "The Premature Burial." For Poe, this topic was a long-standing fascination and even obsession, based on tales he had heard or read about people being buried or entombed alive. It appears in at least a half-dozen of his stories. "The Premature Burial" itself was probably inspired by the publicity surrounding the exhibition of a "life-preserving coffin" at a fair in New York City in 1843:

> To be buried while alive is, beyond question, the most terrific of [the] extremes which has ever fallen to the lot of mere mortality. That it has frequently, very frequently, so fallen will scarcely be denied by those who think. The boundaries which divide Life from Death, are at best shadowy and vague. Who shall say where the one ends, and where the other begins? We know that there are diseases in which occur total cessations of all the apparent functions of vitality, and yet in which these cessations are merely suspensions, properly so called. They are only temporary pauses in the incomprehensible mechanism. A certain period elapses, and some unseen mysterious principle again sets in motion the magic pinions and the wizard wheels. The silver cord was not forever loosed, nor the golden bowl irreparably broken. But where, meantime, was the soul?[1]

Now, long after the development of technologies that can help us better determine who is on which side of the boundary dividing life from death, fears remain, often in the context of organ procurement.

Modern day versions of Poe's horror story often focus on the removal of organs following a mistaken declaration of death. The following story comes from a state and federal investigation of a 2009 case at St. Joseph's Hospital in Syracuse, New York—the federal investigative report was not made public until 2013. In this case, doctors were about to remove organs from a 41-year-old woman, Colleen Burns, who had already been declared dead but who suddenly opened her eyes under the bright lights of the operating room. Many physicians, nurses, and others made a series of mistakes that led to this fiasco, beginning with the failure to adequately address what had brought her to the hospital (a drug overdose and its effects). Then error on error landed her in the operating room for the removal of her organs. These compounded errors, at least five or six, included insufficient testing to ensure that the drugs had cleared her system, too few brain scans, lack of attention and response to a nurse's suggestion that the woman was still alive, and a failure to examine other signs, such as curled toes and respirator resistance. When hospital personnel informed the family that Ms. Burns was dead (brain dead), the family authorized the removal of life support systems and donation of her organs for transplantation. Later, reviewing the records, an outside physician noted that the woman had been given a sedative "to the point that she would be non-reactive": "If you have to sedate them or give them pain medication, they're not brain dead and you shouldn't be harvesting their organs."[2]

For all these mistakes, the hospital was fined only $6,000.00—perhaps because it appeared that the woman was not harmed. She committed suicide sixteen months later, but there appears to be no connection between her suicide and the hospital's earlier egregious mistakes. Ms. Burns' mother indicated that her daughter was already so depressed that this incident "really didn't make any difference to her."

This case can be viewed as a failure to adhere to established protocols for determining brain death before making a declaration of death and removing organs. It suggests the need for better professional education about determining death by neurological standards. As a result, the state ordered the hospital to hire a consultant neurologist to educate its staff on brain death criteria. But a number of scientists, bioethicists, and others charge that these criteria are themselves unsound and the entire conception of brain death is deeply flawed. If their charges are sound, it is not merely a matter of educating physicians and other health professionals so they can more reliably apply these criteria. Instead, patients may be wrongly declared dead in violation of the Dead Donor Rule even when established protocol is carefully followed. If the neurological standards for determining death and the underlying conception of brain death are flawed, questions arise about how this should affect the process and content of informed consent to donation (as provided in this case by Ms. Burns' mother) and even whether we need to reconsider the ethical and legal status of deceased organ donors.

The Dead Donor Rule (DDR)

The Dead Donor Rule (DDR), as John Robertson sees it, "is a centerpiece of the social order's commitment [including the medical profession's commitment] to respect persons and human life."[3] It also serves as the "ethical linchpin" for the system of voluntary deceased organ donation, based on trust.

The DDR is both permissive and restrictive. It allows us to take vital organs from dead persons with their consent or their next of kin's consent. But it also prohibits taking vital organs from living persons, even with their consent: We may not kill people in order to take their organs, and we may not kill people in the process of taking their organs.

The DDR and its operation presuppose that it is possible to determine the status of persons as living or dead and that, in contrast to Poe's concern, the line between life and death can be reliably drawn for purposes of removing vital organs for transplantation. Being on one side or the other of the line affects people's legal and moral status. If people are dead, they cannot be harmed—vital organ removal does not set back their interests (in Joel Feinberg's language). A declaration of death by appropriate medical personnel is a speech act, performative speech, which changes an individual's moral and/or legal status. The physician or physicians (as authorized by law) can declare or pronounce death (after determining that it has occurred). In describing (or putatively describing) a biological reality, this speech act assigns an individual to a particular status—that of a dead person—and thus alters the structure of the legal/moral rights of and obligations to that individual. A wide variety of actions can follow a declaration of death, from burial to payment of life insurance. The declaration of death also serves a gate-keeping function for organ donation: Post-mortem removal of vital organs for transplantation now becomes a possibility, assuming appropriate consent.

When organ transplantation became possible in the mid-1950s, kidneys could be transplanted from living donors, and vital organs could be removed for transplantation from dead individuals, who at the time were declared dead by conventional cardiopulmonary standards. By the mid- to late 1960s, there was interest in increasing the number of potential organ donors and improving the viability of donated organs by redefining death or updating the criteria for determining death to include brain-oriented formulations.[4] International conversations among physicians and scientists, with some input from other professionals, led to the development of the concept of brain death and criteria and measurements for determining when it occurs.

An important milestone in this process was the 1968 report of the Harvard committee to examine "the definition of brain death," which offered a "new criterion for death" (irreversible coma).[5] It identified two reasons for a new definition and criteria, growing out of recent technological developments. One reason focused on the care of patients: "Improvements in resuscitative and supportive measures have led to increased efforts to save those who are desperately injured," sometimes with "only partial success" and major and irreversible brain damage, creating great burdens for patients, their families, and hospitals, as well as for others in in need of hospital beds.

The second reason focused on the way "obsolete criteria for the definition of death can lead to controversy in obtaining organs for transplantation." This reason, stated gingerly in the report, was discussed among members of the Harvard committee and others in more provocative ways: "Can society afford to lose organs that are now being buried?"[6] Clearly, there was also an interest, as Martin Pernick puts it, in "defend[ing] the entire medical profession against the public perception that transplant surgeons were organ-stealing killers."[7] This second reason presupposed the Dead Donor Rule—we can only remove vital organs from deceased individuals. Hence, it is important to have brain death and other criteria for determining when death occurs. We will examine this reason in detail below.

The first reason concerned what can be called the Dead Patient Rule. At the time, many felt that we needed "a 'dead patient rule' for turning off mechanical ventilators."[8] However, we soon overcame that limitation and set standards and procedures for determining when it is ethically justifiable to withhold or withdraw ventilators and other medical technologies from dying (though not yet dead) patients. Many bioethicists in early 1970s expected, as Robert Veatch has noted, to continue wrangling for a long time about decisions to withhold or withdraw medical procedures in order to let patients die.[9] By contrast, many thought—and I was one of them—that the determination of death in general and for deceased organ donation in particular was more or less settled, perhaps because it seemed to rest on a biological foundation identified and agreed upon by scientists and physicians.

However, in some countries, such as the U.S., the standards and procedures for withholding and withdrawing life-prolonging treatments now enjoy a wider consensus and have greater stability than do the standards and procedures for determining death in the context of deceased organ donation. Indeed, we now face a crisis about the Dead Donor Rule in part because of difficulties in determining death, with the resultant uncertainty about whether we are in fact killing people to take their organs or through taking their organs.

I will use two major poets to partially frame this discussion, and I will return to these frames later. Seamus Heaney described the task of the poet as "undeceiving the world"[10] and in the *Four Quartets* T.S. Eliot observed that "human kind cannot bear very much reality."[11] These themes bear on the ethics of proposals to address problems in the DDR.

Three Practices of Post-Mortem Organ Removal for Transplantation

The crisis about the DDR arises in three different contexts and practices of obtaining deceased donor organs. Each raises somewhat different problems, but all three face significant challenges, on the grounds that they usually or often violate the DDR or that we cannot know with enough certainty that they are not violating that rule.

According to the Uniform Determination of Death Act, "an individual who has sustained either (1) irreversible cessation of circulatory and respiratory functions, or (2) irreversible cessation of all functions of the entire brain, including the brain stem, is dead," as determined by the application of "accepted medical standards."[12] This act has been adopted in some form throughout much of the U.S., and states that have not explicitly adopted it through legislation generally operate with both standards for determining death.

Donation after Neurological Determination
of Death (DNDD)

Most transplanted organs come from brain dead donors, as determined by neurological standards. A large number of kidneys in some countries—for instance, the U.S. and Japan—come from living donors, but most kidneys and all vital organs—hearts, livers, and lungs (except for portions of livers or lungs)—come from donors who are declared dead, usually by neurological standards.

As of August 2013, available statistics indicated that since 1988 in the U.S., there had been just over 283,000 organ donors—just over 124,000 were living donors, while more than 158,000 were deceased donors. Most were declared dead by neurological standards, and all were deemed to meet the Dead Donor Rule. Over that same twenty-five-year period, these donations enabled about 575,000 organ transplants. Just over 124,000 organs, mainly kidneys, came from living donors, and over 450,000 organs came from deceased donors— deceased donors usually provide more than one organ (in the U.S., an average of under three per donor).[13] Thousands of other transplants occurred in the two decades before 1988 and thousands more have occurred around the world since the 1960s, saving many lives and improving the quality of many lives. However, there is a substantial gap between the need for and supply of transplantable organs, and this source of organs (brain dead individuals) is severely limited. It is estimated that, out of about 2.5 million deaths in the U.S. each year, only 12,000–16,000 or so would satisfy the criteria for brain death. Even if we obtained 80% of the organs from this pool, we would not be able to solve the organ shortage.

Some difficulties and challenges in donation after neurological determination of death (DNDD) suggest why the Dead Donor Rule is threatened by controversies surrounding brain death. There is a long-standing minority challenge: whole brain death does not mark the death of the human being if breath and blood circulation continue even with technological assistance. Another challenge is that the conception of whole brain death is deeply flawed. It lacks a coherent, cogent explanation that matches biological facts. In light of the clinical and pathophysiological knowledge that has emerged over the last 45 years (since the Harvard report in 1968), some long-standing assumptions appear to be mistaken.

Consider the claim that brain death is death because of the loss of the brain's integrative, controlling, and other functions. Neurologist Alan Shewmon has shown that patients diagnosed with brain death may have somatic integration, such as some hemodynamic stability and body temperature, immune response to infection, and stress response to incisions.[14] Newer technologies can also prolong the body's survival much longer than previously anticipated based on this conception of brain death. Yet the President's Council on Bioethics (under President George W. Bush) indicated in a White Paper that, in such cases, there is no recovery of capacity to breathe spontaneously or show signs of consciousness.[15]

The council offered an alternative philosophical/biological perspective: focused on "total brain failure"—such a human being is dead because he or she "is no longer able [and irreversibly so] to carry out the fundamental work of a living organism," including "a fundamental openness to the surrounding environment as well as the capacity and drive to act on this environment on his or her own behalf."[16] This interpretation of brain death has not gained widespread acceptance. Indeed, many believe that we do not yet have—and may never have—a satisfactory explanation.

Donation after Circulatory Determination of Death (DCDD)

Cardiopulmonary or circulatory standards were used in post-mortem organ procurement before the development of brain death criteria. Over the last twenty years or so, these standards have emerged again, alongside neurological standards, because of the severe, persistent shortage of organs for transplantation. However, special difficulties arise when we incorporate cardiopulmonary or circulatory standards into the practice of organ procurement, especially because of the need to obtain the organs quickly before they are compromised and often to start measures to preserve organs before death has been declared.

I will use the language of "donation after circulatory determination of death" (DCDD) instead of "donation after cardiac death" (DCD) because the DCDD's focus on the circulatory standard for determining death is less confusing and more informative.[17] There are two kinds of DCDD—*controlled* and *uncontrolled*. In *controlled* DCDD, the patient (perhaps through an advance directive or living will) or the patient's family makes a decision to stop treatments so the patient can die; hence, the patient's death is expected. After this decision to terminate treatments, the appropriate medical personnel make an inquiry about willingness to donate. No effort is made to resuscitate the dying patient. By contrast, in *uncontrolled* DCDD, the individual's death is not expected; he or she suffers a cardiac event and resuscitative efforts are undertaken but are unsuccessful.

Consider, first, controlled donation after circulatory determination of death (cDCDD). Earlier, for instance, in the original Pittsburg protocol, such donors were called "non-heart-beating donors" (as distinguished from "heart-beating donors" in DNDD). Over the last decade, there has been an increase in number of cases of cDCDD in the U.S: from 87 to 848 donors each year.[18] They now constitute slightly over 10% of the deceased organ donations each year. According to one study, "optimal identification and management of potential controlled DCDD could increase the supply of deceased donor organs, but by no more than 25%." If only optimal cDCDD organs were used, then the expansion would probably be no more than 10%.[19] The U.K. and Australia saw substantial increases in cDCDD over the last decade and now more than one third of all deceased organ donors in those countries come from cDCDD.[20]

There are a number of difficulties of and challenges to cDCDD, ranging from a general attack that labels it "an ignoble form of cannibalism" (medical sociologist Renée Fox), which is irreverent as well as medically and ethically problematic,[21] to a variety of more specific criticisms. These include:

- Conceptual problems: in cDCDD "irreversible" has been interpreted to mean "permanent" because of the decision not to provide resuscitation. Hence, resuscitation *will not* be performed in contrast to *cannot* be performed.[22]
- Short waiting time: One problem for many practitioners is the short waiting time—2–5 minutes after cardiac arrest before organ recovery. This time, which is supposedly long enough to avoid the possibility of autoresuscitation, is a matter of concern for a number of clinicians—are these individuals really dead?
- Effect on end-of-life care: Concerns have been raised about possible compromises in the quality of end-of-life care, for instance, in ante-mortem interventions, some of which may cause discomfort or hasten death.

In response to the development and expansion of cDCDD programs in the U.S., several medical associations and professionals, even when somewhat supportive, have registered these and other concerns.[23] Some critics have called for a moratorium on cDCDD programs, particularly those involving children.[24] Running through these concerns and criticisms is a worry that cDCDD circumvents the Dead Donor Rule.

Similar concerns, criticisms, and worries also plague uncontrolled donation following circulatory determination of death. In uDCDD, the individual's death is not planned or expected; a person, often outside the hospital, suffers a cardiac event and resuscitation is unsuccessful. Protocols vary. One in New York City requires 30 minutes of vigorous resuscitative efforts, by well-trained emergency technicians, under on-line direction from a physician. Once the point of futility is reached, efforts are stopped and death is declared. Organ preservation efforts do not begin for 15–20 minutes while "consent to donate is verified and the police and medical examiner clear the body for removal."[25] Spanish protocols do not involve declaring death at the scene, but only at the hospital. Hence, it is possible to wait to ask the family.[26] Given the-opt out system in Spain, it is legitimate to take some measures to prepare the body for donation before the family is asked.

Some uDCDD programs are quite successful—for instance, Spain and France have increased rates of transplantation with good outcomes. (Incidentally, Spain accepts uDCDD but not cDCDD, whereas the US has accepted cDCDD but mainly has pilot programs in uDCDD—these differences reflect a variety of social, cultural, and historical factors.) The 2006 Institute of Medicine report, *Organ Donation: Opportunities for Action*, identified uDCDD as a promising way to increase the supply of transplantable organs, perhaps providing as many as 22,000 additional organ donation opportunities in the U.S.[27] But so far there has been little progress in implementing uDCDD in the U.S.

Following are some difficulties of and challenges to uDCDD. Critics charge that weak tests are used and do not guarantee irreversibility,[28] while proponents insist that "there is actual, demonstrated irreversibility of cardiac, respiratory, and spontaneous circulatory function" and thus conformity with the Dead Donor Rule.[29] Critics further contend that irreversibility cannot be established until the exhaustion of all possible resuscitative measures, because there is evidence of recovery following unconventional resuscitation measures. Hence some of those who become donors in uDCDD could have been saved.

uDCDD doesn't meet the "permanence" standard of cDCDD regarding "circulatory function" when there are efforts, after the determination of death, to institute artificial circulation—by using chest compressions, ventilation, and extracorporeal membrane oxygenation (ECMO). These individuals, some say, become "undead," thereby invalidating the previous circulatory determination of death.[30] But defenders respond that the restoration is far below normal physiologic range.[31] (Some recommend that if ECMO is used, an intra-aortic balloon should be inserted to prevent meaningful circulation to heart and brain.)[32] Issues of trust also arise in the cessation of futile resuscitative efforts in order to commence organ preservation and procurement efforts. Still another criticism is that uDCDD requires a very heavy investment of resources and diverts resources from rescue efforts to organ retrieval.[33]

In short, there are serious on-going controversies about the determination of death in each of these three practices of organ procurement—DNDD, cDCDD, and uDCDD. Hence, it is fair to say that the Dead Donor Rule faces a crisis in part because of the difficulties of determining death and the uncertainties about whether the donor is actually dead when the organs are removed.

What Should We Do about the Dead Donor Rule?

Given this crisis, what should we do about the DDR, which presupposes that we are able to draw a clear line between life and death? What are the ethical implications of different approaches to the DDR in transplantation medicine, and which policies, laws, and practices should we adopt?

Truth or Consequences?

Let's start with "truth or consequences," the title of Dan Brock's article reflecting on his experiences as a philosopher on the staff of the President's Commission for the Study of Ethical Problems in Medicine and Biomedical and Behavioral Research.[34] There is often a tension between what we might call truth, as understood in an academic seminar, and formulating ethically acceptable and feasible public policies, all things considered, in the particular circumstances. Yet the latter is and should be the primary concern in public policy. (Incidentally, my experience on bodies advising governmental policy-makers on organ transplantation and other matters is similar.)

Brock was on the staff of President's Commission in the early 1980s, when it was developing a major and influential report on *Deciding to Forego Life-Sustaining Treatment*.[35] It had become commonplace at the time to say that it is permissible to allow patients to die, to let nature take its course, as long as we do not kill them. Philosophically, Brock held a different view—that the difference between killing and allowing to die "is not in itself morally important, and that stopping life-sustaining treatment is often killing, though justified killing." Brock's view was not held—and was even sharply rejected—by the majority of the members of the President's Commission. Suppose, in the name of truth, Brock could have "undeceived" these commissioners, convincing them that there is no sharp distinction between allowing to die and killing, and that letting die is killing. That likely would have had very unfortunate effects.

The commissioners probably would *not* have said, "Letting die is the same as killing and we should permit both of them." Instead, they probably would have said, "Letting die is just as bad as killing, and we shouldn't permit either of them." Such a conclusion would have produced bad consequences for many patients at the end of their lives. It would have deprived them of their exercise of autonomy and required them to undergo treatments they wanted to refuse. Patients would have been wronged as well as harmed. In short, "undeceiving" the commissioners would have probably have had terrible effects in the real world.

Now what should we do about the dead donor rule? In discussing several possible options, I should note that some of these options might apply only to one or two of the three practices of deceased organ procurement rather than to all of them.

Option 1: Abandon the rule and institute an alternative: living vital organ donation.

Many who propose that we abandon the DDR do so because of the difficulties of determining death. Others apparently would support an alternative approach—living vital organ donation—even if the line between life and death could be reliably drawn. However, the latter thinkers also point to the difficulties in determining death to buttress their arguments. Among the several opponents of the DDR, Frank Miller and Robert Truog have written a number of important and powerful articles and an excellent book *Death,*

Dying, and Organ Transplantation: Reconstructing Medical Ethics at the End of Life that take this approach.[36]

They insist that the DDR "does no genuine moral work in current practices of vital organ donation because 'brain-dead' donors remain alive and donors under DCDD protocols are not known to be dead at the time organs are procured." Hence, we "should be working toward honestly facing the fact that currently we are procuring vital organs from patients who are not known to be dead and that it is ethically legitimate and desirable to do so." According to Miller and Truog, where there are valid decisions to stop life-sustaining treatment and where there is consent to donation, we should be able to use vital organs from these living-though-dying persons. We do not harm them (because they will be dead shortly, in any event); and we have their or their family's consent. "The absence of harm plus appropriate consent legitimate vital organ donation" (112). The upshot is that DDR "must be abandoned" (114). "The ethics of withdrawing LST [life-sustaining treatment], recognizing that this causes death, underlies the justification for vital organ donation from still–living patients" (115).

The Miller/Truog approach fails to connect with the public's (and medical professionals') moral beliefs, symbols, values, and practices, including religious ones, which largely mesh with and support the DDR. If the Miller/Truog position were to be adopted by policy-makers, its consequences would likely be disastrous for organ donation and transplantation. Consent to deceased organ donation, particularly by families, and medical participation in obtaining and transplanting organs often hinge on the beliefs, symbols, and values represented in the DDR. In short, this way of "undeceiving the world" could be disastrous for many potential recipients of donated organs—because many in the public and medical and health professions "cannot bear very much reality," if indeed what is argued is reality.

Option 2: Accept the ascribed status of death in deceased organ donation as a legal fiction that preserves the DDR at least for the time being.

Miller and Truog recognize the possible negative effects of immediately abandoning the DDR. In short, they seem to hold that "human kind cannot [at least yet!] bear very much reality." Hence, they propose an alternative: Maintain the DDR as a legal fiction, as a temporary measure, until the public matures enough to face reality. "Undeceiving" involves education about the legal fiction.[37]

In proposing that we view the DDR as a "legal fiction," Miller and Truog want to evacuate its "moral force," depriving it of any "inherent ethical significance." It does have "ethical significance" as a rule within a larger set of ethical principles, some consequentialist, some deontological. Even though in theory we should drop the DDR, this is practically "difficult to achieve"— again, without harmful consequences. Thus, Miller and Truog view their "legal fictions approach as a halfway house in the evolution of medical ethics and the law"—"halfway to abandoning the dead donor rule." It is a "temporary expedient," "a pragmatic compromise," a "progressive" step in the direction of "greater transparency." It "weakens the link between the ethics of organ transplantation and standards for determining death" (171).

This legal-fictions approach may be a way for critics of the DDR to assign it some temporary instrumental value, without ceasing efforts to abandon it over time. But to make the DDR transparent as a fiction would probably have negative effects similar to those of Option 1 above—though perhaps less dramatic and extensive. Of course, this is an empirical question. In my judgment, Miller and Truog again fail to attend adequately to the moral beliefs, including those in major religious traditions, which would have an impact; these are moral beliefs that it is wrong to kill people in order to take their organs. (Miller and Truog suggest that we need more surveys of beliefs as well as additional educational efforts.)

They further argue that "in a liberal democracy, public policy supported by the law permits practices that some find deeply objectionable" (149). While that is true, one intended function of the DDR is to provide a basis for trust so people will voluntarily donate organs for transplantation. Parallel to Brock's situation, if Miller and Truog were to convince policy-makers and others of the legal fictions approach, there would probably be resistance to deceased organ donation, particularly by families, because this would amount morally to killing their loved ones, whether in DNDD or in DCDD. Many medical practitioners would probably feel the same way—this is already evident in the responses of many physicians and others to cDCDD.[38]

Actually, what Miller and Truog propose would not differ greatly from current practices of selecting donors of vital organs, but the interpretation of the DDR as a "legal fiction," in all probability, would contribute to the delegitimation of deceased organ donation and would be accompanied by a decline in organ donors as well as a reluctance of many physicians, nurses, and other professionals to participate in the process of organ procurement and transplantation.

Option 3: Retain the DDR with expanded individual/familial choices of conceptions and criteria of death.

Another approach, represented in Robert Veatch's writings, maintains the DDR but opens the range of possibilities for determining death. Two states, New York and New Jersey, have set a conventional approach to death but accommodate religious and moral objections to being declared dead by neurological standards.[39] Hence, people can choose to be declared dead by cardiopulmonary standards if they wish rather than by neurological standards.

One advantage of this option is that it allows individual choice (and, where the individual has not chosen, familial choice) of the conception of death and hence, at least, of neurological or circulatory standards for determining death. Veatch draws a distinction between the value questions involved in setting a definition of death at the conceptual level and the technical questions, such as how to test for signs of life, that necessarily involve medical expertise. The value questions should be in the domain of "religious/philosophical/policy choice," not medical science.[40] Given the value diversity in liberal pluralistic societies, recognizing a plurality of value-laden definitions of death is an appropriate step. However, rather than "letting a hundred flowers bloom," as China's Chairman Mao put it, Veatch proposes that the society set a "default definition"—probably, whole brain death—and then grant individuals a reasonable range of options in conceptions of death. Expanding to an unlimited range would create public health, societal, and ethical problems.

The option of conscientious objection to brain death has received support from religious groups, such as Orthodox Jews, Buddhists, and Native Americans, among others, who favor a cardiopulmonary conception. From Veatch's standpoint, this option should also include a higher-brain conception of death for those who might prefer it, as Veatch himself does. This is "the humane, respectful, fair, and pragmatic solution."[41]

Even if a range of tolerable views is established, both professionals and the public will still have to face the difficulties and challenges, already identified, of determining death in the context of organ donation. People's choice of one or more standards over others will need to be adequately informed, and this will entail fuller disclosure of the problems we have already identified in the three major approaches to obtaining organs from deceased individuals. The difficulties of interpreting and applying the standards will remain, whichever standards individuals and families select. Furthermore, medical professionals will have to decide whether they are comfortable participating in organ removal and transplantation based on any or all of the tolerable standards. Some of these points also apply to the fourth option and will be further developed below.

Option 4: Retain and strengthen the DDR and ethically improve its operation.

Given the deep and widespread uncertainties about and challenges to the Dead Donor Rule, in part because of the difficulties of determining the "dead donor," there are serious ethical concerns about our social and medical practices of obtaining organs for transplantation. I propose we retain the rule and seriously consider, not only with professional groups but also through public engagement, how best to sustain the DDR, by improved conceptual, scientific, clinical, and other work and by enhanced ethical practices. This entails attention to both truth *and* consequences, to "undeceiving the world" and also helping human kind—the public and the professionals—"bear reality."

One indispensable condition is improving the process of informed consent. What kind of consent do we want from whom for what? Too often we have been satisfied with a very weak, watered-down version of consent for post-mortem organ donation in both opt-in and opt-out systems. In general, these systems do not require the kind and level of disclosure of information expected in much of medicine and research. Nor do these systems probe potential donors' understanding. For *living* organ donation, consistent with standards elsewhere in medicine and in research, the process of voluntary, informed consent should include (1) disclosure of information to a person, (2) who is deemed to be competent to decide, (3) an assessment of his or her comprehension or understanding, and (4) determination of the voluntariness of his or her decision.[42]

Some of these components are missing or seriously diluted in much, perhaps most, *deceased* organ donation in both opt-out and opt-in countries. For instance, in the U.S. little information is disclosed for first-person consent to deceased organ donation. This consent often occurs when a person is getting a driver's license from a state department of motor vehicles. Only limited information is disclosed in that context, and there is no real opportunity for individuals to inquire more broadly and deeply into what's at stake in making the decision. Specifically, there is no disclosure that a person might be declared dead by either neurological or circulatory standards—only that organs will be removed after death. And no information is provided about the difficulties and challenges of determining death in the three different practices we have examined. Perhaps the process is a little better when families decide, but there is no reason to believe it is adequate. In any event, consent to "deceased organ donation" without further specification is probably not informed consent because of the different practices of determining death, each with its own difficulties and uncertainties.

Why do we have such inadequately informed consent for deceased organ donation? Perhaps because of the common view that the line between life and death can be clearly drawn, the determination of death is a purely objective matter, and the dead body cannot be harmed. But this approach to consent is problematic in view of the known difficulties of and challenges to ways of determining death in the context of organ donation. Whether first-person or family consent, whether opt in or opt out, more information about relevant uncertainties and doubts is needed to ensure prospective donors' understanding and, hence, their adequately informed choice. As matters now stand, fewer than 56% of pediatricians in one survey thought that physicians are being truthful about the death of patients in DCDD.[43]

Beyond these points, how much and what kind of information should be disclosed? In my judgment, disclosure should be guided by the baseline of what reasonable people would want to know, augmented by what particular potential donors want to know.[44] However, determining what reasonable people want to know is not easy. Conversation is needed, and focus groups can be instructive, along with other ways to engage the public.

While vitally important, transparency and public engagement are also badly neglected. Neither has been featured in the development of the conceptions and criteria of death that provide content for the Dead Donor Rule. The Harvard criteria were featured on the front page of *The New York Times* in 1968 but, for the most part, this report "did not foster a public debate."[45] Instead, there was widespread deference to the medical profession. Similarly, some professional and inter-professional discussion, but only limited public discussion, has accompanied the development of cDCDD protocols.[46] Furthermore, policies on uDCDD in Spain and France "were introduced and implemented without previous societal consensus or transparency."[47] In the U.S., efforts have been made to engage public officials and the public about the recent pilot program of uDCDD in New York City and the earlier one in Washington DC.[48] Overall, the record of transparency and public engagement is at best spotty, at worst woefully unsatisfactory.

Earlier, I observed that in the U.S. and several other countries, there was movement beyond the so-called Dead Patient Rule (under which a patient had to be dead before mechanical ventilation could be stopped) to a substantial consensus about standards and procedures for stopping medical treatments of dying-but-not-yet-dead patients in order to allow them to die. In the U.S., this occurred over time, with widespread participation by the public as well as by clinicians, ethicists, governmental advisory bodies, policy-makers, and the like. Legal decisions by the courts were also important, and they often resulted from citizens' challenges. There are serious doubts that today's "political and social climate" will allow a similar process for the Dead Donor Rule and the criteria involved in DNDD, cDCDD, and uDCDD.[49] One defender of the rule finds it hard to imagine "how public deliberation might proceed explicitly to consider whether to retain the incoherencies and obfuscations in the current criteria for death determination."[50] Nevertheless, in my judgment, one of the most urgent, immediate tasks is to figure out how to engage the public in open, transparent, and productive ways. As David Rodríguez-Arias and colleagues rightly emphasize, avoiding such discussions "may lead to an increased inconsistency, rationalization, and obfuscation that could feed public distrust and, ultimately, impede the goal everyone seems to want—more organs to save and improve more lives."[51]

It is obvious that organ donation and transplantation depend on public trust—after all, members of the public donate the organs needed for transplantation. In addition to being ethically problematic, silence about or obfuscation of the difficulties and uncertainties in determining death will probably not sustain public trust in the long run. Even though there are rumblings of unease as well as explicit concerns among healthcare professionals, especially about some DCDD protocols, there has been a notable lack of public outrage or even public disquiet. However, this does not count as passive acceptance, given the dearth of transparency. A systematic review of a number of empirical studies finds "deep-rooted concerns" about DCDD among the general public as well as among medical personnel. These concerns "need to be taken seriously in order to maintain or foster trust in the transplantation system."[52] They provide an important reason for public engagement and deliberation.

In conclusion, this fourth option involves maintaining and strengthening the Dead Donor Rule by further conceptual and scientific work on determining death and by ensuring its ethical interpretation and application. The major ethical concerns are not identical across the three major practices of obtaining organs for transplantation—DNDD, cDCDD, and uDCDD—or across different countries, which have not adopted these practices at the same rate or to the same extent.[53] For each practice, transparency and public engagement and fuller disclosure of information to ensure donors' adequately informed consent are essential, along with measures to eliminate or control conflicts of interest[54] and to safeguard conscientious refusals by healthcare professionals who object to participation in one or more of these practices.[55]

It is also crucial that debates about the Dead Donor Rule and its implications for practices of obtaining organs be morally serious, rather than forms of academic gamesmanship—after all, these are matters of life and death.[56] We cannot totally separate truth *and* consequences. And while we seek to "undeceive" the public, through transparency, public engagement, and disclosure of information to prospective donors, we need, at the same time, to help the public as well as healthcare professionals "bear reality." All this won't be easy.

Notes

1. Poe, "The Premature Burial," in *Complete Stories and Poems of Edgar Allan Poe* (Garden City, NY: Doubleday & Company, Inc., 1966), p. 261.
2. The information about this case, in this and the subsequent paragraph, has been drawn from John O'Brien and James T. Mulder, "St. Joe's 'dead' patient awoke as doc prepared to remove organs," Syracuse.com, updated July 9, 2013. Available at http://www.syracuse.com/news/index.ssf/2013/07/st_joes_fined_over_dead_patien.html Last accessed November 27, 2013.
3. John A. Robertson, "The Dead Donor Rule," *Hastings Center Report* 29, no. 6 (November–December 1999): 6–14.
4. Paul Ramsey, *The Patient as Person* (New Haven, CT: Yale University Press, 1970).
5. Report of the Ad Hoc Committee of the Harvard Medical School of Examine the Definition of Brain Death, "A Definition of Irreversible Coma," *Journal of the American Medical Association* 205, no. 6 (August 5, 1968): 85–88.
6. See Eelco F.M. Wijdicks, *Brain Death*, 2nd ed. (New York: Oxford University Press, 2011), p. 8.

7. Mathew Pernick, "Brain Death in a Cultural Context: The Reconstruction of Death, 1967–1981," in Stuart J. Youngner, Robert M. Arnold, and Renie Schapiro, eds., *The Definition of Death: Contemporary Controversies* (Baltimore, MD: The Johns Hopkins University Press, 1999), pp. 3–33.

8. David Rodríguez-Arias et al., "Casting Light and Doubt on Uncontrolled DCDD Protocols," *Hastings Center Report* 43, no. 1 (2013): 29.

9. Robert M. Veatch, "The Evolution of Death and Dying Controversies," *Hastings Center Report* 39, no. 3 (2009): 16–19.

10. From an interview with Seamus Heaney, published in *The Economist* in 1991, and reprinted by *The Economist*, September 5, 2013 under the title "A soul on the washing line." http://www.economist.com/blogs/prospero/2013/09/poetry Last accessed November 27, 2013.

11. T.S. Eliot, "Burnt Norton," in *Four Quartets* (San Diego, CA: Harcourt Brace and Company, A Harvest Book, 1971), p. 14.

12. National Conference of Commissioners on Uniform State Laws, *Uniform Determination of Death Act* (1980). Available at http://www.uniformlaws.org/shared/docs/determination%20of%20death/udda80.pdf Accessed November 27, 2013.

13. These data have been drawn from the data provided by the Organ Procurement and Transplantation Network (OPTN). For updated data, see http://optn.transplant.hrsa.gov/latestData/rptData.asp

14. Among Alan Shewmon's many relevant publications, see Shewmon, "The Brain and Somatic Integration: Insights into the Standard Biological Rationale for Equating 'Brain Death' with Death," *Journal of Medicine and Philosophy* 26, no. 5 (2001): 457–478; Shewmon, "Recovery from 'Brain Death': A Neurologist's Apologia," *Linacre Quarterly* 64, no. 1 (1997): 30–96.

15. President's Council on Bioethics, *Controversies in the Determination of Death: A White Paper by the President's Council on Bioethics* (Washington, DC: The President's Council, December 2008), p. 45

16. President's Council on Bioethics, *Controversies in the Determination of Death*, p. 90.

17. James F. Childress and Catharyn T. Liverman, eds., for the Committee on Increasing Rates of Organ Donation, Board on Health Sciences Policy, Institute of Medicine, *Organ Donation: Opportunities for Action* (Washington, DC: The National Academies Press, 2006), p. 31. For a cautionary note about the shifting language, see David Rodríguez-Arias and Carissa Véliz, "The Death Debates: A Call for Public Deliberation," *Hastings Center Report* 43, no. 6 (2013): 34.

18. A.S. Klein et al., "Organ Donation and Utilization in the United States, 1999–2008," *American Journal of Transplantation* 10 (2010): 973–986; see also Kevin G. Munjal et al., on behalf of the New York City uDCDD Study Group, "A Rationale in Support of Uncontrolled Donation after Circulatory Determination of Death," *Hastings Center Report* 43, no. 1 (2013): 19–26.

19. Scott D. Halpern et al., "Estimated Supply of Organ Donors after Circulatory Determination of Death: A Population-Based Cohort Study," Research Letter, *Journal of the American Medical Association* 304, no. 23 (2010): 2592–2594.

20. A.R. Manara, P.G. Murphy, and G. O'Callaghan, "Donation after Circulatory Death," *British Journal of Anaesthesia* 108, suppl 1 (2012): i108–i121, at i110.

21. Renée C. Fox, "'An Ignoble Form of Cannibalism': Reflections on the Pittsburg Protocol for Procuring Organs from Non-Heart Beating Cadavers," *Kennedy Institute of Ethics Journal* 3, no. 2 (June 1993): 231–239.

22. For a defense of the standard of permanence, see several works by James L. Bernat, singly or with others. Among these is Bernat, "On Noncongruence between the Concept and Determination of Death," *Hastings Center Report* 43, no. 6 (2013): 25–33.

23. See, for example, the Committee on Bioethics, American Academy of Pediatrics, "Ethical Controversies in Organ Donation after Circulatory Death," *Pediatrics* 131 (2013): 1021–1025.

24. A.R. Joffe et al., "Donations after Cardiocirculatory Death: A Call for a Moratorium Pending Full Public disclosure and Fully Informed Consent," *Philosophy, Ethics, and Humanities in Medicine* 6, no. 17 (2011).

25. Munjal et al., "A Rationale in Support of Uncontrolled Donation after Circulatory Determination of Death," pp. 19–26.

26. Rodríguez-Arias et al., "Casting Light and Doubt on Uncontrolled DCDD Protocols," p. 28.

27. Childress and Liverman, *Organ Donation: Opportunities for Action*, chap. 5.

28. Rodríguez-Arias et al., "Casting Light and Doubt on Uncontrolled DCDD Protocols," p. 28.

29. Munjal et al., "A Rationale in Support of Uncontrolled Donation after Circulatory Determination of Death," p. 23.

30. James L. Bernat, "Determining Death in Uncontrolled DCDD Organ Donors," *Hastings Center Report* 43, no. 1 (2013): 32; Bernat et al., "The Circulatory-Respiratory Determination of Death in Organ Donation," *Critical Care Medicine* 38 (2010): 972–979.

31. Munjal et al., "A Rationale in Support of Uncontrolled Donation after Circulatory Determination of Death," p. 24.

32. Bernat et al., "The Circulatory-Respiratory Determination of Death in Organ Donation," p. 979.

33. Rodríguez-Arias et al., "Casting Light and Doubt on Uncontrolled DCDD Protocols," p. 28.

34. Dan Brock, "Truth or Consequences: The Role of Philosophers in Policy Making," *Ethics* 97, no. 4 (July 1987): 786–791.

35. President's Commission for the Study of Ethical Problems in Medicine and Biomedical and Behavioral Research, *Deciding to Forego Life-Sustaining Treatment: A Report on the Ethical, Medical, and Legal Issues in Treatment Decisions* (Washington, DC: US Government Printing Office, March 1983).

36. Franklin Miller and Robert Truog, *Death, Dying, and Organ Transplantation: Reconstructing Medical Ethics at the End of Life* (New York: Oxford University Press, 2012). All subsequent references to the arguments by Miller and Truog are to this book (often indicated by page numbers in the text), unless otherwise indicated.

37. See also Robert Truog, "Brain Death—Too Flawed to Endure, Too Ingrained to Abandon," *American Journal of Law, Medicine & Ethics* 35, no. 2 (Summer 2007): 273–81.

38. See Committee on Bioethics, American Academy of Pediatrics, "Ethical Controversies in Organ Donation after Circulatory Death."

39. Robert S. Olick, Eli A. Braun, and Joel Potash, "Accommodating Religious and Moral Objections to Neurological Death," *The Journal of Clinical Ethics* 20, no. 2 (Summer 2009): 183–91.

40. Among Veatch's several relevant writings on this topic, see Veatch, "The Conscience Clause: How Much Individual Choice in Defining Death Can Our Society Tolerate?" in Youngner, Arnold, and Schapiro, eds., *The Definition of Death*, pp. 137–160.

41. Veatch, "The Conscience Clause," p. 157.

42. See Tom L. Beauchamp and James F. Childress, *Principles of Biomedical Ethics*, 7th ed. (New York: Oxford University Press, 2013).

43. A.R. Joffe, N.R. Anton, and A.R. de Caen, "Survey of Pediatricians' Opinions on Donation after Cardiac Death: Are the Donors Dead?" *Pediatrics* 122 (2008): e967–e975

44. Beauchamp and Childress, *Principles of Biomedical Ethics*, 7th ed., chap. 1.

45. Wijdicks, *Brain Death*, 2nd ed., p. 12.

46. Robert M. Arnold and Stuart J. Youngner, guest editors, Special Issue: "Ethical, Psychosocial, and Public Policy Implications of Procuring Organs from Non-Heart-Beating Donors," *Kennedy Institute of Ethics Journal* 3, no. 2 (June 1993).

47. Rodríguez-Arias et al., "Casting Light and Doubt on Uncontrolled DCDD Protocols," p. 27.

48. Stephen P. Wall et al., "Derivation of the Uncontrolled Donation after Circulatory Determination of Death Protocol for New York City," *American Journal of Transplantation* 11, no. 7 (2011): 1417–1426; Childress and Liverman, *Organ Donation: Opportunities for Action*, Appendix F, "Washington Hospital Center: Protocol for the Rapid Organ Recovery Program, Transplantation Services."

49. Rodríguez-Arias et al., "Casting Light and Doubt on Uncontrolled DCDD Protocols," p. 29.

50. Robert A. Burt, "Where Do We Go from Here?" in Youngner, Arnold, and Schapiro, eds., *The Definition of Death*, p. 339.

51. Rodríguez-Arias et al., "Casting Light and Doubt on Uncontrolled DCDD Protocols," p. 29.

52. S. Bastami et al., "Systematic Review of Attitudes toward Donation after Cardiac Death among Health Care Providers and the General Public," *Critical Care Medicine* 41, no. 3 (2013): 1–9.

53. Several variations across different countries have been noted in the text. Here I should also add that practices of DCDD are "virtually non-existent" in Germany and Portugal, among other countries. See Manara, Murphy, and O'Callaghan, "Donation after Circulatory Death," p. i110.

54. James F. Childress, "Organ Donation after Circulatory Determination of Death: Lessons and Unresolved Controversies," *Journal of Law, Medicine and Ethics* 36, no. 4 (2008): 766–771.

55. Committee on Bioethics, American Academy of Pediatrics, "Ethical Controversies in Organ Donation after Circulatory Death," p. 1025.

56. For an important though overly strong cautionary note, see James M. DuBois, "The Ethics of Creating and Responding to Doubts about Death Criteria," *Journal of Medicine and Philosophy* 35 (2010): 365–380.

8

The Failure to Give

Facilitating First-Person Deceased Organ Donation

Introduction

This chapter focuses on moral frameworks for evaluating first-person failures to donate organs after death and for selected public policies to overcome these failures.[1] My starting point is the persistent, chronic shortage of organs for transplantation in the United States, where organ procurement was relatively stagnant for over a decade and, even with recent increases, still falls far short of meeting patients' needs. Fewer organ donors (deceased and living) were recovered in 2013 (14,260) than in 2006 (14,750). The number of actual organ transplants was practically the same in 2013 as in 2006: 28,954 to 28,940.[2] In 2015, the number of organ transplants rose significantly to 30,973. This increase appears to have resulted mainly from using more marginal or riskier donor organs and obtaining more organs and discarding or wasting fewer organs from donors since the total number of organ donations (deceased and living) in 2015 was 15,062—only 312 more donations than in in 2006.[3]

Several factors affect organ donation and procurement. One is the pool of potential donors, particularly those who are declared dead by neurological standards. Over several years, a dramatic decline occurred in the number of motor vehicle deaths as a result of increased seat-belt usage, improved automobile safety, and more effective programs to promote better driving. In 2010 traffic fatalities reached their lowest numbers since 1949 in a much larger population.[4] There was also a decline in the number of living donors of kidneys, from 6,435 in 2006 to 5,732 in 2013. The overall transplant figures would have been even worse if the criteria for deceased donor eligibility had not been relaxed—for example, in the increased acceptance and utilization of organs from donors previously considered marginal, such as older donors, or too risky, such as drug users.[5] Indeed, much of the recent increase in deceased donor organs in the United States resulted from organ donation following death because of drug intoxication (often associated with an increased risk of infection for recipients). In 2018, 17,555 organ donors enabled 36,529 transplants. 10,722 were deceased donors—1,401 of whom had died from drug intoxication, up from 230 in 2006—and 6,833 were living donors (slightly above the number of living donors in 2006 and almost as many as in 2004 and in 2005).[6] Despite these significant increases, and the shrinkage of organ transplant waiting lists, the gap between supply and need remains large, as close to 114,000 patients were awaiting a transplant at the end of 2018.

Proposals for laws, policies, and social practices have variably emphasized first-person consent to postmortem organ donation, on the one hand, or familial decisions to donate after an individual's death, on the other hand. According to Donate America, by the end of 2016, 136 million individuals had registered as organ donors in state registries. In that year, 48% of the donations involving the removal of organs for transplantation were authorized by the decedent through state registries.[7] The other deceased donor organs came from individuals who had indicated in other ways their desire to donate their organs or whose next of kin decided to donate the decedent's organs.

This chapter will focus on what is variously called first-person consent to deceased donation, first-person authorization, or donor designation or declaration by living individuals rather than on familial decisions to donate. This focus does not imply that this is the most effective way to increase the supply of donor organs; both first-person consent or authorization and familial consent or authorization remain important.

In exploring the failure to donate organs and ways to overcome this failure, I will make two assumptions: (1) we need to increase the supply of organs in order to save the lives and to enhance the quality of life of persons with organ failure, and (2) our societal efforts to increase the supply of transplantable organs should respect certain ethical boundaries. Each of these assumptions is somewhat controversial: the first, because of challenges to organ transplantation as an overvalued enterprise relative to its benefits and its costs; the second, because of uncertainties and disputes about the appropriate ethical boundaries, both their specific nature and implications and their strength. I will ignore controversies about the first assumption and only address the second through efforts to clarify and defend important ethical constraints on societal efforts to increase the number of transplantable organs.

Following are several ethical criteria that are relevant to an assessment of current and proposed public policies to address the persistent organ shortage:

1. Effectiveness and efficiency in increasing the supply of organs
2. The acceptability of appeals to various motives—not only altruism—for organ donation
3. Respect for human dignity and moral worth
4. Respect for each individual's right to control the postmortem disposition of his or her bodies and parts, including whether to donate organs
5. Respect for families' wishes and feelings
6. Respect for human remains
7. Fairness in the distribution of burdens and benefits, with particular attention to impacts on disadvantaged groups

These are very similar (though slightly different in formulation) to the "perspectives and principles" proposed by an Institute of Medicine (IOM) Committee on Increasing the Rates of Organ Donation, which I chaired.[8] In seeking to identify standards "commonly found in the United States," as its charge required, the committee "examined current practices, policies, laws, opinion surveys, and cultural and religious traditions as interpreted by the spokespeople for relevant organizations and other experts (e.g., philosophers, theologians, anthropologists, and sociologists)."

While encountering diverse views, the committee also found "a surprising degree of consensus around several fundamental propositions." Many of the disputes it found centered on the meaning or entailments of those standards, rather than on their "existence or validity." Nevertheless, the committee's task was not merely descriptive. It was also "inescapably interpretive" because some standards represent a "latent understanding that provides a commonly accepted foundation for existing policy and practice or a constraint on the range of acceptable solutions for improving the present system." Still, the committee found several standards that represent "a genuine consensus" and provide "a solid framework" for analyzing and assessing actual and proposed policies.

The IOM Committee viewed its versions of Principles 3–6 as specifications of a complex principle of respect for persons. In the context of obtaining cadaveric organs for transplantation, these specifications set "limiting conditions deeply rooted in the cultural, religious, and legal traditions of the

United States." Principles 4 and 5 may come into conflict on occasion, and the IOM Committee rightly assigned priority to the decedent's previously expressed choices over the next of kin's preferences.

Employing these and other standards to assess actual and proposed policies to increase the supply of transplantable organs is not easy. Deceased organ transfer is fraught with meaning and value—the dead human body evokes a variety of beliefs, symbols, sentiments, and emotions, and dying/death involves several rituals and social practices. A proposed policy to increase the supply of transplantable organs may appear to be quite defensible from a rationalistic standpoint, but then turn out to be ineffective and even counterproductive because of these rich and complex contexts of beliefs, values, and practices surrounding the dead body. Excessively rationalistic policies neglect or override deep convictions, symbols, sentiments, and emotions, as well as associated rituals and practices, and, as a result, often fail to accomplish their goals. In addition, policies are often too individualistic (they pay inadequate attention to individuals' relational contexts) and too legalistic and formalistic (they focus too much on laws, such as opt-out versus opt-in legislation, and forms, without adequate attention to social practices, and the like).

A Case of Deceased Organ Donation

The following case can help us identify different frameworks of moral discourse that shape our evaluations of individual and familial decisions to donate or not to donate. These frameworks focus on those particular decisions, rather than on possible public policies, targeted by the above principles. Of course, these frameworks have implications for analyzing and assessing possible public policies.

In early June 1995 a popular, athletic Texan in his twenties, who was undecided about what he wanted to be and do, died unexpectedly from an aneurysm. "In death," as the sports section of a newspaper noted, "he gave half a dozen people their futures, among them a truck driver, a farm manager, a backwoods-resort operator and an American legend named Mickey Mantle."[9] All six operations occurred at about the same time at the Baylor University Medical Center in Dallas.

Newspaper reporters later managed to identify the source of the organs, but, at the family's request, they refrained from disclosing his identity in their reports or to the recipients. His mother explained the family's decision to donate: "Once his soul and spirit is gone, nothing is left. His body is of use to somebody else only in this way. It never even crossed my mind not to donate. To me, it's the decent thing to do. It's the thing we should do." "We thought," she continued, "we might as well make something good come out of our tragedy." Hence, as soon as the doctors asked her, she responded, "Yes, definitely." She made this decision even though her son had never discussed organ donation with her. Even though his Texas driver's license indicated "donor," this fact was not emphasized in reports about the family's decision and may not have been known to the family at the time.[10]

It is instructive to contrast the mother's comment about why she donated her son's organs with various media reports about deceased organ donation. Often with specific reference to this case, the media stress the "sacrifice" of deceased organ donors and praise their "heroic" actions. Others call these actions "extraordinary," a term that could refer to their relative infrequency or to their exceptional normative status—that is, beyond duty and obligation. New Jersey legislation on deceased organ donation a few years ago is cited as the "New Jersey Hero Act."[11]

Before examining the two frameworks of moral discourse implicit in these comments, I will identify several questions raised by this case. First, what criteria must be met before we can appropriately refer to someone as an organ "donor"? As obvious as this question sounds, the answer is far from obvious. The term "donor" sometimes refers to the *decision-maker* about donation— that is, the one who decides to donate organs—and sometimes to the deceased *source* of the organs, whoever made the decision to donate. Obviously, these may be the same. But the decision-maker may not be the source of the organs, and the source may never have been competent to make a decision about donation—perhaps an anencephalic newborn, a child, or a cognitively impaired person—or, if competent, may never have made a decision to donate. For instance, a dead child may be the source of organs, but cannot be the "donor," that is, the one who makes the donation. Furthermore, someone who sells his or her organs is not a "donor," but a vendor or seller. I have long protested the promiscuous use of the terms "donor," "donation," "giver," and "gift." This loose usage creates a false moral aura around activities that are not appropriately called giving or donating.

Second, who was the donor in this case? From the brief report in the newspapers, it appears that the mother viewed herself as the donor, that is, the decision-maker, and her son as the source of the organs. "It never even crossed my mind not to donate," she said. However, in view of the fact that the young man had checked "donor" on his driver's license, he could have legitimately been viewed as the decision-maker about donation. By selecting "donor" status, he became the decision-maker about as well as the source of the transplanted organs. From that standpoint, his mother (if she was aware of his driver's license) merely conveyed or expressed his wishes, in effect, implementing his prior decision to donate.

Even if the young man had never indicated his decision to donate, his mother still could have plausibly held that this is what he would have wanted, because of his fundamental values and commitments. Indeed, his dramatic actions the week before his death expressed those values and commitments: a former lifeguard, he was at a lake when a swimmer attempting to reach an island started to go under and he swam out a long distance and pulled the struggling swimmer safely to shore.[12] His mother could have constructed his willingness to donate from the way he lived—she could have taken his recent heroic actions as indicative of the moral character of a person who would seek to save others, even at some risk, and who would want to have his organs used to benefit others after his death.

Third, it is not surprising that the mother and newspaper reports viewed her as the actual "donor," that is, the decision-maker about the donation of her dead son's organs, in view of the laws and social practices prevalent in the United States at the time. The legal structure for organ donation appears in state versions of the Uniform Anatomical Gift Act, as formulated in the late 1960s and then rapidly adopted by all fifty states and the District of Columbia.[13] Within that "gift" framework, competent individuals can determine what will be done with their organs after their deaths. In the absence of a valid expression of the decedent's prior wishes, the family can decide whether to donate his or her organs.

As a matter of social practice, the default mechanism of the family became the primary mechanism—not many individuals signed donor cards, organ procurement teams frequently did not find them, and, in occasional cases of conflict between the decedent's expressed wish to donate and the family's opposition, procurement teams generally (until more recently) yielded to the family for mistaken legal reasons but understandable ethical reasons. The legal concerns were misplaced because the Uniform Anatomical Gift Act (UAGA), as implemented by the states, provided broad immunity from criminal and civil liability for good faith actions on the basis of a signed document of gift. (Further changes in the UAGA, to be discussed later, strengthened the priority of first-person consent or donor designation.) The moral concerns focus on harm to the grieving family and on risks to practices of deceased organ donation as a result of the bad publicity generated by fighting a family that vigorously objects to the decedent's prior decision to donate.

While the law is, and has been, primarily individualistic, social practice has been heavily communitarian in approaching the deceased person as part of the social network of the family. One ethical and practical challenge is bringing the individualistic and communitarian perspectives together for educational and other purposes. Public education needs to target individuals as potential decision-makers for themselves but also as members of families who may be the default decision-makers.

In the context of these laws and social practices, the moral and practical importance of not blocking deceased donations is evident. Even if the individual while alive does not explicitly make a decision to donate, it is important that he or she not block familial donation by saying "no." Checking "no" on the donor card or driver's license or entering "no" in a registry effectively blocks any subsequent action by the family. In practice, now changing, procurement teams often allowed the family to block the decedent's "yes," but the decedent's "no," where known, has been determinative. Not blocking donation can itself express passive benevolence or altruism—the individual refrains from asserting or acting on his or her legal and social right not to donate.

Similarly, when an individual has expressly indicated his/her wish to donate, it is morally important that the family not take advantage of social practice and block the donative transfer. There are good reasons to affirm in law, as the amended UAGA (2006) proposed and many states now do, the primacy of the individual decedent's decision to donate over familial dissent, even though practical difficulties may limit enforcement.[14] Despite several anecdotes, it is not clear how often families have actually objected to a decedent's valid document of gift. In any event, it is not likely that we will see major gains in deceased organ donation by enforcing the primacy of first-person consent.[15] Nevertheless, that enforcement is essential in order to implement the individual's preferences for postmortem disposition of his or her body. In a survey in June 2012, 80% of the fifty-eight Organ Procurement Organizations (OPOs) in the United States reported honoring first-person authorizations for organ donation over family objections.[16]

Frameworks of Moral Discourse about Organ Donation

Two frameworks of moral discourse appear in discussions of the Texas mother's act of donation as well as in other such cases: morality of aspiration and morality of duty; supererogation and obligation; ideal and right; praise-worthiness and blameworthiness.[17] These paired categories are not totally separate, and the lines between them are not always clear. Not surprisingly, we move back and forth between them. The mother's framework, which stressed that her action was "the decent thing to do . . . the thing we should do," appears to be one of obligation, duty, and right action. By contrast, commentators often use the language of aspiration, supererogation, ideals, and good actions to describe and praise acts of deceased organ donation. These two frameworks of moral discourse produce different descriptions of and responses to nondonation.[18]

Within a morality of aspiration or supererogation, nondonation does not produce guilt—it might produce shame if an agent has committed himself/herself to living up to an ideal that would entail donation. Others should not be indignant or complain about the agent's nondonation. Instead, praise and gratitude are appropriate responses to acts of organ donation. By contrast, within a morality of duty or obligation, nondonation represents a moral failure and should produce a feeling of guilt; and others may be indignant and complain. Praise and gratitude are inappropriate responses to donation—after all, the donor just did his or her duty.

Both patterns of moral discourse play significant roles in our social-moral practices related to deceased organ donation. One important question is whether and on what grounds we could establish an obligation of benefi-cence, or obligatory beneficence, that extends to deceased organ donation. In various editions of *Principles of Biomedical Ethics*, Tom Beauchamp and I describe a continuum between obligation and supererogation, without bright lines to separate them, noting that it is extremely difficult to pinpoint obligations of beneficence. "We bounce back and forth between viewing actions as charitable and as obligatory; and we sometimes feel guilty for not doing more, at the same time doubting that we are obligated to do more."[19] "Strongly recommended" is plausible intermediate language. A framework of obligation may include both general beneficence and specific beneficence, and specific beneficence may include a duty to rescue that is independent of roles, as well as role-related beneficence. If deceased organ donation is oblig-atory, it largely falls under the duty to rescue.

It is plausible to argue from liberal, secular premises for a (moral) duty of easy rescue: Apart from special moral relationships, such as contracts, a person D has a determinate obligation of beneficence toward person R, a specific duty to rescue R, if and only if each of the following conditions is satisfied (assuming that D is aware of the relevant factors).[20] (D stands for potential donor, while R stands for potential recipient.)

(1) R is at risk of significant loss of or damage to life, health, or some other basic interest;

(2) D's action is needed (singly or in concert with others) to prevent this loss or damage;

(3) D's action (singly or in concert with others) will probably prevent this loss or damage;

(4) D's action would not present significant risks, costs, or burdens to D (or to others);

(5) The benefit that R can be expected to gain outweighs any harms, costs, or burdens that D is likely to incur (or that others are likely to incur as a result).

We could increase the weight or strength of D's obligation by increasing the probable benefit to R, that is, by increasing the probability and magnitude of a positive outcome for R (conditions 1–3), with an obvious impact on the fifth condition. We could also decrease the risk, cost, or burden to D (condition 4), again with an impact on the fifth condition. Even when D does not know the specific R or Rs at risk, the fact that several Rs are in need and that D's action could help them is sufficient to extend this specific obligation of beneficent action. In short, deceased organ donation appears to satisfy these conditions for obligatory specific beneficence, a duty to rescue, independent of particular roles.

Converging with a duty to rescue in liberal, secular morality, a strong duty of deceased organ donation also emerges in Judaism (because of the priority of saving human life) and in Christianity (because of neighbor-love), among other religious traditions. However, this "overlapping consensus" does not provide a warrant for the society to adopt an enforceable *legal* obligation to donate. From the standpoint of the law, deceased organ donation should remain supererogatory and praiseworthy. Even if both moral frameworks—(1) deceased organ donation as obligatory, and (2) deceased organ donation as supererogatory and praiseworthy—are appropriate and important in societal discourses, the legal framework should not impose an enforceable obligation. This does not rule out the possibility of various measures, including nudges, to promote organ donation.

In general, the society's organ donation policies should primarily *express* community rather than *impose* community.[21] Even if these policies articulate communal norms, such as a moral obligation to donate organs in order to save lives, it would be more justifiable and effective to express communal solidarity than to try to impose those norms. The society should make it easier and safer for individuals to act beneficently. So-called Good Samaritan laws often work this way in the United States. A few jurisdictions do impose a legal obligation to act to rescue someone in trouble—usually a failure to try to do so is a misdemeanor punishable by a modest fine. However, most Good Samaritan laws in the United States facilitate rather than obligate beneficent actions. And they do so mainly by reducing risks or perceived risks to potential Good Samaritans, for example, by protecting Good Samaritans from legal liability for good faith actions. Such laws also suggest a direction for society's interventions to increase deceased organ donation.

Facilitating Deceased Organ Donation by Changing the Individual's Risk/Cost-Benefit Calculation

There are several possible ways to facilitate deceased organ donation by making it more reasonable for individuals and/or families to donate. Four are particularly relevant to first-person consent to postmortem donation. The first two focus on the relative value of *cadaveric organs* to initial rights-holders and to potential recipients; the second two focus on the risks and benefits of *acts* of donation. These may be combined in various ways.

First, we could try to *increase* the perceived *value of donated organs* by stressing their benefits to potential recipients and to the society. In principle this approach could be useful in both obligation and supererogation models, and it has been widely used, particularly through media attention to the needs of potential transplant recipients and to the successful outcomes of transplantation. A 2012 survey found that among those who wanted to donate their organs, the "single biggest reason," checked by 73.8%, was "to save the life or be of help to others in need."[22] In combining the frameworks we noted earlier, 5.5% indicated that it was what they wanted to do, the right thing to do, a good thing to do. Among those who were not willing to donate their organs, close to 50% indicated that nothing could change their minds, but 20.9% indicated that the "one thing" that could change their minds was "to save a life or be of help to others in need."[23] Although information about the benefits of donated organs to others is important, merely attempting to increase the perceived value of donated organs fails to address what is crucial in many individual (and familial) decisions to donate, viz., the perceived risks, costs, and burdens of *acts* of donation, which we will consider in what follows.

Second, we could try to *reduce* the perceived *value of organs* to decedents (and families). The mother who donated her dead son's organs in Texas insisted that they had no value, except insofar as they could be useful to others. This perspective views organs as "spare parts" that will go to "waste" if not used in transplantation.[24] The 2012 survey found that only 5.5% of those who wanted to donate their organs identified the sentiment "I won't need them any longer" or "why not?" as their "single biggest reason."[25] In view of this small percentage, it is doubtful that societal policies or educational efforts to devalue organs for rights-holders, even in death, apart from their donation to others are appropriate or potentially effective, in part because of the complex beliefs, sentiments, and rituals surrounding the dead body in various communities.

Third, we could attempt to *reduce* the perceived risks, costs, and burdens of *acts of donation*. These risks, costs, and burdens apparently lead some to conclude that deceased organ donation is heroic or sacrificial, perhaps even too heroic or too sacrificial, thus providing a warrant for not donating organs. After all, some level of risks, costs, and burdens can defeat obligations of beneficence—for instance, rescue efforts may appear to be dauntingly unreasonable because of the risk they involve.

Surveys indicate that individuals have a variety of reasons for not registering as organ donors. These include a lack of thought about organ donation or reluctance to contemplate death. But also important for many individuals is a perception of excessive risk, for instance, of being declared dead prematurely or having life-sustaining procedures stopped prematurely if one is a registered organ donor.[26] In this context, the widespread and deep-seated misunderstandings about "brain death" are significant obstacles. Such misunderstandings help to create and sustain mistrust because some people fear that being on record as an organ donor may lead the medical team to declare a patient dead prematurely. Polls suggest that some of these fears may have diminished.[27] But even among families deciding to donate a loved one's organs, there are "complaints about the lack of information on brain death."[28] The previous chapter in this volume discussed the scientific, medical, and philosophical uncertainties and difficulties in determining death in different contexts of organ donation, all of which may be relevant for prospective donors but may also generate distrust.

More generally, we need to reduce background mistrust, in part through expressions of community toward, and solidarity with, individuals and families. Organ donation presupposes well-founded trust in the overall system within which it occurs. For instance, the public's willingness to donate organs appears to depend in part on its confidence in the fairness of the system of organ distribution. We only need to recall the numerous cynical comments about how quickly celebrities such as Mickey Mantle receive a transplant. There is no evidence that Mantle's transplant was out of line, but some transplant centers would not have listed him in view of his overall condition. It is important to assure the public that donated organs will be used in fair as well as effective ways, without priority to patients who are rich, powerful, or famous. (See chapter 9 in this volume.)

In addition, as the federal Task Force on Organ Transplantation argued about thirty years ago, there are several good reasons—including its possible impact on the public's willingness to donate organs—to eliminate ability to pay as a criterion for access to most transplants.[29] Inability to pay is now rarely a problem for kidney transplantation because of the End-Stage Renal Disease Program of Medicare (but the limited coverage for post-transplant immunosuppressive medications does create problems of access and lead to the loss of transplants). Inability to pay remains a major roadblock for patients needing other expensive transplants. The Task Force argued that it is unfair and even exploitative for the society to ask people, rich and poor alike, to donate organs if poor people would not have an opportunity to get on waiting lists if they needed a transplant. Hence, it is important to include all citizens as potential donors in the community of potential recipients through specific or broad healthcare coverage—this is one way to increase the general background trust essential for deceased organ donation. Yet one study determined that in 2003 only 0.8% of transplant recipients lacked health insurance while 16.9% of organ donors were uninsured: "Many uninsured Americans donate organs, but they rarely receive them."[30]

Fourth, we could try to *increase* the perceived benefits of *acts of donation* to donors, as well as to potential recipients and the society. Familial donors report many positive effects, along with some negative effects, of their acts of donation.[31] In the Texas case, the mother said, "I just can't believe people don't donate more. This was the best thing we could have ever done. Whoever the people are that got the organs, we're just grateful to them to keep part of him alive in this way. We're grateful they are living." It is more difficult to identify plausible benefits to living individuals who are trying to decide whether to donate, but there are some possibilities.

One obstacle to increasing the perceived benefits to organ donors from their acts of donation may be somewhat surprising. It is the interpretation of deceased organ donation as almost exclusively altruistic in the United States. Postmortem donations of organs are deemed to be purely other-directed. For example, in his excellent book, *The Most Useful Gift*, Jeffrey Prottas says, "the voluntary decision to donate must be based on altruistic motives; otherwise, it is not permitted."[32] That is an overstatement—in deceased organ donation (in contrast to living organ donation), an inquiry into motives is highly unusual, in the absence of suspicions that financial compensation is involved. Familial donors may have mixed motives—ranging from altruism, which is often central, to a sense of obligation, to a desire to find redemptive meaning in a tragic set of circumstances, to a hope that their loved one can live on in others, to a desire for praise, honor, fame, and so forth. Stated reasons also vary for individuals' prior consent to postmortem organ donation, but they are largely other-directed reasons.[33] The question is whether additional motives can be generated for those whose altruism or sense of obligation is not strong enough to motivate donation. According to the IOM Committee on Increasing Rates of Organ donation,

> organ donation has been praised as a highly disinterested, sacrificial, and heroic act that may appear to be out of the ordinary person's reach because it is so demanding. The act of donation is voluntary, in the sense that others cannot claim it as a right. This does not mean, however, that altruism is the only possible or acceptable motivation or that donation policies should appeal only to altruism.[34]

Once we recognize that the system for obtaining organs does not require pure altruism as the donor's sole motivation and that motives are often mixed, then we can begin to consider not only how the society could *remove disincentives* to donation (e.g., by eliminating costs or other burdens associated with deceased organ donation) but also how it might *provide incentives*—that is, additional motivating reasons—to supplement a sense of altruism or of moral obligation when that sense is not strong enough to motivate a donor declaration. Honoring the act of donation and the donor/source of the organs has certainly been one way—for example, through letters from the US Surgeon General or the President or through public ceremonies that recognize and praise deceased organ donors and their families.

Can we find more meaningful and powerful incentives, perhaps even financial ones, within acceptable moral limits? I will not here examine arguments for buying and selling organs, an arrangement I have opposed elsewhere not as intrinsically wrong but as ethically unacceptable in our context as well as politically impracticable, at least in the short-run, because of the difficulties of overturning the National Organ Transplant Act's ban on the transfer of organs in exchange for valuable consideration.[35]

We need to start, as the earlier analysis suggests, by distinguishing *systems* for the transfer of organs (donation/gift versus sales/purchases) from the *motivations* of participants in organ transfers. Within each system individuals engaged in postmortem organ transfer may be acting on a variety of motives. There is no reason to suppose that altruism is the only motivation for making donations or gifts—as our ordinary experiences of gift exchanges suggest. And there is no reason to suppose that altruism—for example, toward one's family—is absent from sales.

No doubt, some proposals to provide financial incentives for organ donation are really ways to purchase organs. However, short of actually buying and selling organs, it may be possible to use financial incentives as tools to increase deceased organ donations without blurring the line between donations and sales.

The label "rewarded gifting" is often used to demarcate some financial (and other) incentives from sales/purchases of organs. Let's start with Thomas Peters's early proposal of a pilot program to test the effects of providing a death benefit of $1,000 for recoverable donated organs.[36] His proposal would have provided death benefits not for acts of donation but for donated organs actually recovered. This appears to be close to a sale/purchase. If the reward is provided only when the gift of the organ has actually been delivered, then, as William F. May argues, "the transaction differs very little from an outright sale" (with all its attendant problems).[37]

Some possible modifications might be more compatible with sociomoral practices of donation. For instance, we could provide the death benefit as a tangible societal expression of gratitude for *acts of donation* by eligible donors, rather than for recoverable organs. As a regular practice, for example, the society could cover the organ "donor's" funeral expenses up to a certain level (say, $1,000) in order to express, quite concretely and tangibly, its gratitude for the act of donation, whether by the individual while alive or by the family at the time of death, and to share in the disposition of the final remains following the removal of any usable donated organs. Such a practice of conveying gratitude would express communal solidarity with the deceased and the bereaved who decide to donate or, at least, do not block donation.[38] Along similar lines, the Nuffield Council on Bioethics in the United Kingdom recommends a pilot program "to test the public response to the idea of offering to meet funeral expenses for those who sign the Organ Donation Register and subsequently die in circumstances where they could become organ donors."[39]

Still another possible policy would involve a double gift: organ donation and financial donation to a charitable organization. An individual while alive (or the next of kin after his/her death) could select a registered charitable organization to receive a financial donation that would be provided by the government upon the donor's death and the retrieval of his/her organs. Proponents of this policy stress that it could provide positive incentives to potential donors while retaining and emphasizing altruism and generosity. It avoids concerns about commercialization and commodification "because there is no financial or material benefit conferred to the donor or the donor's family."[40]

In principle, any of these approaches could be developed in ways that would avoid sales/purchases with their attendant ethical problems. Whether they would in fact be effective is a separate question, and focus groups and pilot studies may be necessary to generate the evidence necessary to change policies. Surveys in the United States have indicated increased receptivity to the possibility of financial incentives, such as assistance in paying for funeral expenses, an award of cash to the donor's estate, or a contribution to a selected charity. In a 2012 poll, 25.4% indicated that a financial incentive would increase the likelihood of their organ donation, a significant increase over the 16.7% who indicated this in a 2005 poll. Nevertheless, a majority of the population (63.6%) still indicated that a financial incentive would not make any difference in their decision. About 9.5% indicated they would be less likely to donate if financial incentives were offered. Their primary reason (34.2%) was that the transfer of organs should remain a donation or a gift and not be a profitable bargaining tool. This reason neglects the distinction we are drawing here between a *system*, such as a gift or donation system, and the *motives* for actions within that system. Some respondents also worried about possible abuses (12.9%), and others deemed the practice to be against their religion (9.0%). (I do not here discuss the possibility of creating a non-financial incentive for registered organ donors of preferential access to organ transplants if needed, because, in my judgment, it creates practically insurmountable problems for a fair scheme of organ allocation.[41])

Nudging the Individual's Organ Donation Declaration

In *Nudge: Improving Decisions about Health, Wealth, and Happiness*, Richard Thaler and Cass Sunstein define a nudge "as any aspect of the choice architecture that alters people's behavior in a predictable way without forbidding any options or significantly changing their economic incentives."[42] Contexts of decision-making embody a "choice architecture," whether or not we are aware of it. Hence, it is essential to attend to the "choice architecture" of the context in which people make decisions and the impact of that structure on those decisions. Choice architecture includes nudges, and any public policy regarding organ donation will inevitably nudge choices in one direction or the other. For example, defaults are unavoidable in any legal or policy structure for organ donation, and where they are set can nudge potential organ donors to donate or not to donate, even though potential donors remain free to decide one way or the other.

Nudges and defaults have been widely discussed over the last several years as options when rational persuasion is not sufficient to accomplish the ends that are sought, such as improving public health or promoting deceased organ donation. They have often been touted because they leave the final choice to the individual and thus are arguably compatible with respecting autonomy. As a result, their proponents generally fail adequately to probe the ethical presuppositions and implications of nudges, except perhaps for their ends and effectiveness. This is a mistake, and I will offer further ethical analysis and assessment with regard to selected nudges in the context of organ transfer and procurement.

Public policies that nudge individuals to make certain decisions deemed to be in the society's (or the individual's) best interests may try to shift the individual's risk- or cost-benefit ratio as discussed earlier. The proposal for modest financial incentives for organ donation fits within the Thaler-Sunstein category of a nudge because it does not "significantly" change economic incentives the way a market would. Having already discussed this nudge, I will consider two major types of nudge—mandated choice or required response and opt-out policies based on tacit/silent/presumed consent to donation. Together these nudges target first-person consent or donor declaration, designation, and registration, rather than familial decisions.

Mandated Choice, Required Response

Mandated choice or *required response* has been proposed as an ethical and effective way to nudge individuals to sign donor cards, complete other documents of gift, or enroll in donor registries.[43] In conjunction with some other state-mandated task, such as obtaining or renewing a driver's license or filing income tax forms, these policies would promote individuals' decision-making about deceased organ donation while, at the same time, nudging their decision toward consent to donation. They thus differ from routine or mandatory inquiries about or requests for organ donation directed at the next-of-kin after an individual's death.

Questions about the effectiveness and the degree of compatibility of these policies with respect for individual autonomy focus on several possible features, including the range of possible choices or responses, the penalties, if any, for no choice or no response, and a registry for nondonors or objectors to donation. Mandated choice requires the individual to make a choice, often but not necessarily binary, about organ donation. In required response policies, the range of possible responses is usually larger than a choice for or against organ donation. Still weaker versions involve "prompted choice" or even inquiries about individuals' preferences. I will focus mainly on mandated choice. Required response and prompted choice are softer nudges that do not constrain autonomous choices as much as mandated choice does, but they may also provide less definitive guidance than a forced choice.

Proponents contend that a policy of mandated choice would be both right and effective—it would both respect personal autonomy (because individuals may choose whether or not to register as postmortem organ donors) and increase the supply of transplantable organs from deceased donors. If mandated choice would not effectively increase organ donation rates, there would be little reason to adopt it. Merely clarifying what individuals want to happen to their organs after death would probably not be a sufficient reason.

There is little empirical evidence to support the claim that mandated choice will actually increase rates of deceased organ donation. A report of the American Medical Association (AMA) Council on Ethical and Judicial Affairs appealed to "empirical evidence that mandated choice would be acceptable to the public and therefore effective in increasing the organ supply."[44] It found some evidence in a survey in which 90% of the respondents indicated that they would support a program of mandated choice. However, the Council's inference confuses the public's acceptance of and even support for a *program* of mandated choice with their willingness as *individuals* to say "yes" if they were forced to make a choice.

According to the Council, under mandated choice, individuals who are reluctant to contemplate their own deaths and the disposition of their bodies after their deaths would have to confront these possibilities. This would presumably remove some current obstacles to deceased organ donation. However, merely requiring a choice, without other major changes—including extensive and adequate public education, engendering public trust, and so forth—would probably be ineffective and possibly even counterproductive. Some factors that currently dissuade individuals from donating would also apply under mandated choice, and they would probably prevent such a policy from substantially increasing rates of organ donation. If forced to choose in the current context, some individuals would probably check "no," not because they actually oppose the donation of their organs after their deaths, but for other reasons, such as a fear of being on record as postmortem donors of organs as well a deep distrust of governmental involvement in such matters. In saying "no," they would block their family's possible decision to donate after their deaths. And this could actually decrease the supply of transplantable organs.

One proposal to address this problem structures the mandated choice or response to inquire about the individual's willingness to be listed on the registry for deceased organ donation. The individual could indicate "yes," in which case his or her name would be included on the organ donor registry, or "no," in which case his or her name would not be recorded on a nondonor registry. In contrast to some earlier unsuccessful state programs—for example, in Texas and Virginia[45]—successful programs, such as the one in Illinois, now inquire about individuals' willingness to donate and enter positive responses in the registry, without creating a registry of nondonors or objectors to donation. This avoids the blockage of possible familial decisions to donate. For instance, in California, the applicant for renewal of a driver's license can check "Yes, add my name to the donor registry" or "I do not wish to register at this time." The latter response is not recorded anywhere and thus leaves the door open for familial decisions to donate organs after the individual's death. This system generates a registry of first-person declarations or designations as organ donors, but it does not produce a registry of nondonors or objectors to donation.

This nudge in the direction of donation comes at a serious ethical cost. I concur with the Nuffield Council on Bioethics that "any system set up to document people's wishes that mandates a response to a question about organ donation should also include the option of expressing objection."[46] Otherwise the nudge becomes a push or a shove, violates the commitment apparently embedded in the law to respect the individual's wishes, and risks misleading many applicants about the effect of the choice or response they are making.

Concerns also focus on the putative coerciveness of a required choice or response policy. Tony Calland, Chair of the Ethics Committee of the British Medical Association, which supports a policy of presumed consent, stresses, "We would not support the kind of coercion involved in mandated choice."[47] However, a mandated-choice policy is not inevitably coercive or, if coercive, not necessarily unjustifiably so. Even though, under such a policy, the individual would face a directive to indicate his/her choice about deceased organ donation, the policy's conditions will determine whether it is actually coercive. Of course, a mandated-choice policy would be coercive if it imposed penalties for a decision either for or against organ donation, and it would be coercive if it imposed certain penalties for not making and indicating a decision. For instance, it would be deemed coercive if donation were the default for a refusal to make a decision or if the individual declining to respond could not receive, say, a driver's license, as some proposed policies dictate. Then the question becomes whether such coercion can be justified to promote the important objective of increasing the rates of organ donation. Furthermore, at least in the United States, this level of governmental intrusion in the context of other state-mandated tasks is likely to be sharply opposed and even counterproductive. It is not defensible to think about a nudge in general or abstract terms that neglect the specifics of the interaction, the nature of the decision, and the like. The "prompted choice" model, if it is more than a mere euphemism for mandated choice or required response, may be a promising, softer way to influence choices toward organ donation without penalties.

Proponents of mandated choice often assume a very individualistic, rationalistic, legalistic, and formalistic version of autonomous choices. They fail to see that people might exercise their autonomy in various ways—for example, by informally delegating the donation decision to their family or by not blocking their family's subsequent decision, each of which can be an exercise of autonomy as well as altruistic in motivation. Indeed, one possible way to increase the probable effectiveness of mandated choice or required response—or, for that matter, the current opt-in system without either required choice or required response—would be to allow individuals to designate a surrogate to make a decision about organ donation after their deaths. This would have the advantage of increasing the individual's sense of security by placing the postmortem decision in trusted hands.[48] Such a delegation is already common in advance directives about care at the end of life.

In short, ethical, social, and political concerns about governmental intrusions and interventions in mandated choice are worrisome. Moreover, psychological and behavioral studies that support nudges do not necessarily support forced choices. At any rate, uncertainty about the potential effectiveness of mandated choice, as well as lingering concerns about governmental intrusion and coercion, led the IOM Committee on Increasing the Rates of Organ Donation to hold, "*At this time*, states should not enact legislation requiring people to choose whether or not to be an organ donor (mandated choice)"[49] (italics added). The committee recognized that extensive public education would be essential for an effective mandated choice, but also that if public education is intensified, such a policy may not be necessary.

Opt-Out Policies

In opt-in systems of deceased organ donation, operative in the United States and several other countries, the default—in the absence of explicit consent to donation—is nondonation. By contrast, several European countries have adopted laws, policies, and practices that set the default at donation when a deceased individual has not explicitly stated his or her wishes. Opt-out systems thus allow the decedent's organs to be removed for transplantation unless he or she previously objected or, in some models, unless the family now objects.

There are at least two distinct moral foundations of opt-out laws. One is the society's ownership of or dispositional authority over cadaveric organs.

An opt-out law with this foundation is often labeled *routine removal* or *routine salvaging*. Even when the society claims ownership or dispositional authority over the organs of deceased persons, it may still grant individuals and/or families legal rights to opt out, largely because of consequentialist concerns, such as avoiding social conflict, instead of individuals' and/or families' moral rights. Such a system need not adopt vigorous public educational campaigns, easy opt-out procedures, and the like, but it may choose to do so for practical and other reasons.

A second moral basis—and the only basis compatible with the framework of values in the United States at this time—is individual ownership or dispositional authority over dead bodies and their parts (with the family as the default decision-maker). The transfer of organs from a deceased person to recipients is effectuated through *silent* or *tacit consent* or *presumed consent*; that is, the individual's lack of dissent is construed as consent. Within this framework, such consent is ethically valid only if there is adequate understanding of the options and clear, easy, reliable, and nonburdensome ways for individuals to opt out. These are preconditions for an ethically acceptable opt-out system based on the individual's primary right to control what happens to his or her bodily parts after death.[50]

Laws that construe the individual's lack of objection as valid consent may assign different roles to the next-of-kin. In a *strong* or *hard* opt-out model, there is no obligation to consult the decedent's family; by contrast, a *weak* or *soft* opt-out model recognizes such an obligation.[51] In the latter model, it is not always clear why familial consultation is required or allowed. If it is a way to ensure that the decedent's lack of declared objection reflected his/her willingness or desire to donate organs, it functions as an ethical safety check. It is a precaution in case an individual changed his or her mind but failed to register that change. If, however, family consultation is considered a way to solicit and honor the family's wishes, rather than the decedent's prior wishes, this undermines the rationale for the opt-out model. The decedent's nonobjection to donation simply provides, at most, a basis for asking the next-of-kin for permission.

A study of twenty-five countries with opt-out legislation determined that health professionals in all those countries inform the next-of-kin of their intention to remove the decedent's organs for transplantation. Twenty-one of these countries allow the next-of-kin to oppose and thwart a donation that is based on the decedent's nonobjection alone or on his or her registered decision to donate; in the other four countries health professionals will let the next-of-kin stop a donation that is based only on the decedent's nonobjection, but will not do so if the decedent actually registered his or her wish to donate.[52] This study further concluded that whether the legal structure is opt-in or opt-out, express donation or presumed donation, procurement teams still generally consult family members.[53] Debates persist about whether these practices of familial consultation and nonobjection reflect moral wisdom— for instance, in not wanting to harm a grieving family—or professional bias and whether they should be maintained or changed.

The main argument for adopting an opt-out system is that it is potentially more effective than opt-in systems of organ procurement and does not violate anyone's autonomy rights. Claims about the effectiveness of opt-out systems rest in part on evidence from behavioral research about the place and effects of defaults. For example, setting defaults creates options that require little or no effort and thus partly rely on inertia, and the defaults represent the status quo so that changes involve trade-offs.[54] Defaults can also signal that some actions, such as the donation of organs, are supported by social norms and by policy-makers. Furthermore, different default policies may shape the meaning people assign to the act of postmortem organ donation. Studies suggest that participants under opt-in conditions tend to view donation as a more substantial and weighty action while participants under opt-out conditions tend to view nondonation as a more significant breach of responsibility.[55] Such differences in meaning may influence individuals' decisions.

The following ethical tension can arise in opt-out systems: On the one hand, defaults can be effective nudges if individuals view pursuing the alternative, such as nondonation, as requiring some effort. On the other hand, for an ethically valid silent, tacit or presumed consent to organ donation, individuals should have clear, easy, reliable, and nonburdensome ways to register their objection.

The empirical evidence most commonly invoked in support of an opt-out system is that countries with that system generally have higher rates of deceased organ donation than opt-in countries.[56] If we rank countries according to the rates of deceased donors per million population, those with the highest rates, led by Spain, tend to have opt-out systems. In 2004, the United States with its opt-in system was an aberration because it ranked second only to Spain: Spain had 34.6 deceased donors per million population while the United States was a distant second with 24.1; most of the countries closest to the United States also had opt-out systems.[57] More recently, a few other countries with opt-out systems have surpassed the United States, at least in some years—for instance, Portugal and Belgium in 2009 and Portugal and Croatia in 2014.[58]

Nevertheless, there is vigorous debate about whether the higher rates of deceased organ donation in countries with opt-out legislation result mainly from their laws or from associated policies, infrastructure, organization, and the like, as well as from broader social and cultural factors.[59] For instance, according to one systematic review,

> Presumed consent alone is unlikely to explain the variation in organ donation rates between countries. Legislation, availability of donors, organisation and infrastructure of the transplantation service, wealth and investment in health care, and public attitudes to and awareness of organ donation may all play a part, but their relative importance is unclear.[60]

As a result, it is far from clear that the introduction of an opt-out policy can be counted on to improve the rates of deceased organ donation.

Frequently overlooked in these debates is the possible interaction in opt-out systems between deceased and living organ donation, particularly of kidneys. One study concluded that opt-out policies are associated with lower rates of living kidney donation. Even though a causal relationship cannot be established, countries considering opt-out legislation in their effort to increase deceased kidney donation should also "carefully consider and reduce any negative effect on rates of living donation."[61] This is particularly relevant in the United States, where in 2018 just over 39% of the acts of kidney donation were by living donors and just over 30% of the kidneys transplanted came from living donors.[62] In 2013 the United States had the world's highest rate of organ donation per million population when both living donors (for kidneys and portions of livers) and deceased donors are combined.[63]

Other concerns surround proposals to adopt opt-out laws and policies. Even if we could assume that the introduction of such laws and policies would increase the supply of transplantable organs, it is not clear that they would be more cost effective in the United States than improving and enhancing the current opt-in system. After all, it would be costly to establish the conditions for ethically valid silent, tacit, or presumed consent, including ensuring public understanding and establishing clear, easy, reliable, and nonburdensome ways for objectors to opt out. With a similar infusion of funds, the current opt-in system could conceivably be made more effective than it is and perhaps as effective as an opt-out system if the latter could even be adopted.

Another argument focuses on the distribution of the burdens of decision-making and action. Some argue that an opt-out system would enable the majority more easily to realize its will. According to opinion polls in the United States, the donation default is more likely to be correct than the current nondonation default.[64] However, such numbers alone cannot determine the fairness of the default. One question is whether it is fairer to burden those who want to donate or those who do not want to donate, and the answer may depend on whether there is a moral (though not legal) obligation of deceased organ donation. The nature of the burden is also relevant. Defenders argue that the burden of opting out, in an ethically valid system, would be minimal. However, the burden would be greater for vulnerable populations, given their lower socioeconomic status, educational limitations, language barriers, and so forth.

Another consideration of fairness also focuses on these vulnerable populations, many of whom in the United States would be uninsured or underinsured and would be unlikely to have access to expensive extra-renal transplants if needed because these transplants are not covered by the federal End-Stage Renal Disease (ESRD) Program. As we noted earlier, the uninsured often give but rarely receive organs. Furthermore, because of the limited coverage of immunosuppressive medications under the ESRD Program, problems of access still arise in the context of kidney transplantation in the United States.

Others argue that an opt-out system would relieve the decedent's family of the burden of receiving requests for organ donation and making decisions under very difficult circumstances following their loved one's death. Nevertheless, in a weak or soft policy, procurement teams would have an obligation to consult the family, and, even in a strong or hard policy, as we have seen, procurement teams usually still involve the family in some way. However, it is not persuasive to argue against an opt-out system on the grounds that it would deprive the family of an opportunity to make a meaningful and perhaps therapeutic decision in tragic circumstances.

Nor is it persuasive to argue against an opt-out system on the grounds that it would reduce opportunities for altruism and generosity. Nothing about an opt-out system necessarily precludes the possibility of express organ donation based on altruism or generosity. And, as previously noted, these motivations and virtues can be expressed in passive ways—for instance, in declining to opt out—as well as in active ways. Not standing on or exercising one's right to opt out can itself embody and display generosity and altruism. It is a mistake to assume that only explicit consent in an opt-in system can express altruism and generosity.

There is nothing objectionable in principle about relying on tacit or silent consent in certain contexts, including organ donation. It can be real consent in carefully defined social practices and circumstances.[65] Nevertheless, it is still appropriate to use such labels as "presumed consent to donation" or "presumed donation" or "presumed lack of objection to donation" because we cannot be sure that a particular individual understood and voluntarily consented through his or her silence. This consent is not presumed on the basis of a theory of human goods or obligations. Even if we hold, as I have argued, that there is a beneficence-based obligation of deceased organ donation, and not merely an ideal of supererogatory donation, not all moral obligations are or should be legally enforced. Nor do they always provide a basis for presuming consent to their fulfillment in the absence of explicit consent.[66]

My conclusion is similar to the one we adopted on the IOM Committee on Increasing the Rates of Organ Donation: Even though opt-out legislation is ethically justifiable in some contexts, it is not ethically justifiable in the United States at this time. It would probably be ineffective and possibly counterproductive. Hence, even if it could be adopted in most or all states—which is highly unlikely from a political standpoint—and even if we could establish all the conditions for ethically valid silent, tacit, or presumed consent, the system would probably reduce rather than increase the supply of transplantable organs and, on those grounds, would not be ethically justifiable.

According to the best available—though limited—evidence, many persons would opt out and this would thereby block familial decisions, further reducing the supply of organs for transplantation. Results from a 2005 National Survey of Organ Donation suggested that approximately 30% in the US population would opt out under an opt-out law, while another 5.9% indicated that they did not know whether they would opt out. If 28% to 36% or so opted out, their decisions would preclude familial donations and possibly or probably would reduce the overall number of organs available for transplantation.[67] In the 2012 National Survey of Organ Donation fewer (23.4%) indicated they would opt out under a system of presumed consent; however, the report of the survey fails to indicate how many selected "don't know." Still, a significant number said they would opt out, and opting out would block subsequent familial decisions. The reasons that many now give for not signing documents of gift or entering donor registries in the current opt-in system in the United States would also operate in an opt-out system and, in all likelihood, would lead many individuals to opt out in order to avoid being on record as organ donors, even if they are not opposed to their organs being donated.

In view of all these considerations, the IOM committee's report concluded:

> *At this time*, states should not replace the existing legal framework, which requires explicit consent for organ donation, with a framework under which people are presumed to have consented to donate their organs after death unless they have declared otherwise. (italics added)

It would not be feasible for some states in the United States to experiment with an opt-out system while others retain the current opt-in system, because of the need for (relative) uniformity across the states. However, the Committee went on to stress,

> it would be appropriate for all interested parties to seek to create over time the social and cultural conditions that would be essential for the adoption of an effective and ethical system of presumed consent.[68]

Part of the debate about the available evidence centers on a "chicken-egg" problem: Is a strong, viable consensus needed for effective opt-out laws and policies or do those laws and policies help to create such a consensus? A strong case can be made that, as Jennifer Bard stresses, presumed consent laws "must be built on a foundation of public support; they cannot create it."[69] She points to the example of Wales, which adopted presumed consent legislation effective December 1, 2015—the first UK country to adopt presumed consent. Wales already had one of the higher rates of deceased organ donation in Europe. Furthermore, officials in Spain, with the world's highest rates of deceased organ donation per million population, recommend that countries seeking to increase their rates of organ donation devote vigorous efforts to improving their organization of the whole process of organ procurement and transplantation. This, in their judgment, will lead to increased organ donation. Accordingly, and in contrast to many, they recommend against spending too much time and energy on changing the legal system (e.g., to opt out), on public campaigns, and on donor cards.[70]

Combined Systems

Many of the legal and policy options we have examined are not mutually exclusive but can be combined in potentially fruitful and ethically valuable ways. As noted, in 2015 Wales became the first country in the United Kingdom to introduce what it calls a "soft opt-out" system for organ and tissue donation.[71] Nine out of ten people in the country support organ donation but only three out of ten register as donors. This revised system, which applies to everyone over the age of eighteen who lives and dies in Wales, combines several of the options in this chapter. It retains an opt-in option for those who wish to donate their organs—they may do so by completing a form that takes only two minutes to complete. Others may opt out if they do not want to be organ donors. What is new is that individuals who "do nothing" are "deemed" to have no objection to postmortem organ donation and thus are "deemed" to have consented to it. Individuals may also avoid making a decision about organ donation by selecting a representative to do so after their deaths.

The family—or representative—will be involved in all cases in order to provide medical and lifestyle information for helping to determine the safety and quality of the decedent's organs. No organ donation will proceed without such involvement. Even where there is "deemed consent," families may still object on behalf of the decedent if they know that he or she did not want to become a donor. But they may not override the decedent's decision to opt in or opt out. Of course, if the decedent previously appointed a representative, he or she is the decision-maker on behalf of the decedent.

It is too early to know whether this combination system will be effective. After close to eight months, 52% of the Welsh population had not yet shared their organ donation decision. In addition, historically, the family has objected 43% of the time based on lack of knowledge about the decedent's wishes; hence participants are urged to discuss their wishes with their families. Nevertheless, this combination system avoids most ethical pitfalls.

The Welsh system shares elements with the German National Ethics Council's 2007 report *Increasing the Number of Organ Donations: A Pressing Issue for Transplant Medicine in Germany*.[72] This proposal, which is one of the most rigorous and fully developed proposals available, combines elements of opt-in and opt-out systems, retaining declared consent and adding presumed consent. This "two-tier model" includes systematically asking individuals to make personal declarations and informing them that their organs may be removed in the absence of a declaration unless their relatives object. The language for approaching individuals (e.g., "inviting," "calling upon," and "appealing to") appears to be softer than mandated choice or required response. This combination proposal also avoids most ethical problems, but it has not been implemented.

Conclusion

Drawing together several themes, I would characterize my approach as firmly individualistic but also communitarian. A possible label would be "liberal communitarian." As a liberal approach, it starts from and continues to affirm the emphasis on individuals' rights to make their own decisions about deceased organ donation. And it favors laws to prevent the family from overriding the decedent's prior express wish to donate (parallel to what already occurs in regard to the decedent's prior decision against donation).

My approach is communitarian in its recognition of the individual's prima facie moral obligation to rescue others through deceased organ donation. However, that moral obligation does not authorize the state, society, or others to claim dead bodies and their parts against the decedent's prior objections (or against the family's current objections unless the decedent made a valid donation). Despite emphasizing a prima facie ethical obligation of deceased organ donation, my approach still appreciates the relevance for various purposes, including legislation, of a model of supererogation. We cannot demand organ donation.

Thus, instead of *imposing* community through sanctions for failures to donate in accord with ethical norms, we should *express* community. The society can and should make it easier and more reasonable for individuals (and families) to discharge an obligation (or to live up to an ideal) of deceased organ donation in part by reducing actual and perceived risks, costs, and burdens of acts of donation and by modestly increasing the benefits of those acts to donors. In addition, through certain nudges and defaults, such as opt-out policies, it can represent communal norms, again without imposing them and without infringing or violating the individual's autonomous choices.

My approach recognizes that individuals' (and families') willingness to donate generally presupposes their trust in medicine and the society, for example, in the criteria and procedures for determining death and for distributing donated organs, subjects of two other chapters. Also important is the society's expression of communal solidarity in individual and familial suffering, in part through the provision of healthcare. Indeed, it is morally problematic to request organ donation from residents who have difficulty obtaining basic healthcare, much less expensive procedures such as organ transplants. The expression of community in these several ways is indispensable.

My approach remains "liberal" in that it recognizes and prioritizes individuals' legal and social rights to decide whether to donate or withhold their own organs after death. Under certain conditions, tacit, silent, presumed, or deemed consent can be ethically valid, even if express consent remains a normative ideal and provides greater certitude about the validity of the consent to postmortem organ donation. A combination system, versions of which have been adopted in different places, is more promising ethically and more likely to be successful.

However, we need to be realistic about the prospects for various proposed policies to increase first-person consent to deceased organ donation in the United States. There are no "magic bullets" to accomplish this goal, especially in light of the complex beliefs, values, and practices surrounding the dead body. Over the years, many promising proposals have not been adopted, and the ones that have been adopted have usually had only limited success—hence, the stagnation that I stressed at the outset.

In addition to being realistic, we need to be cautious about interventions into a system that works relatively well. Not only do we need evidence that new laws and policies would probably be more effective than what we already have but also we need to avoid a possible reduction of the current rates of first-person (and familial) organ donation through misguided interventions.

Notes

1. This chapter has been developed over several years in lectures, seminars, and public policy deliberations as well in published articles. An earlier version, which appeared under the same title in the *Kennedy Institute of Ethics Journal* 11, No. 1 (March 2001): 1–16, originated in the André Helleger's Memorial Lecture at Georgetown University in 1995 and in the Alloway Lecture at the University of Toronto and the Canadian Bioethics Association in 1997. Subsequent versions have also been delivered or discussed in seminars at several other institutions, most recently in a seminar at the Centre for the Advanced Study of Bioethics at the University of Münster in Münster, Germany, in 2016 and at the Virginia Military Institute and the University

of Minnesota School of Medicine (The John Najarian Lecture) in 2018. I am indebted to a number of individuals in those settings for perceptive criticisms and helpful suggestions. In addition, I am grateful to the suggestions and criticisms of colleagues on the Institute of Medicine Committee on Increasing the Rates of Organ Donation, which I chaired and which issued its report *Organ Donation: Opportunities for Action* in 2006 (publication information appears in note 8). I have drawn some ideas and formulations from the draft chapter I prepared on presumed consent for that committee's deliberations, and I have drawn some ideas and formulations from the publication of the original version (especially for the sections "A Case of Deceased Organ Donation" and "Facilitating Deceased Organ Donation by Changing the Individual's Risk/Cost-Benefit Calculation").

2. See the data from the Organ Procurement and Transplantation Network (OPTN), available at https://optn.transplant.hrsa.gov/data/view-data-reports/national-data/# (last accessed March 14, 2019).

3. See ibid.

4. Mike M. Ahlers and Jeanne Meserve, "Traffic Fatalities Fall to their Lowest Level since 1949," *CNN U.S.*, April 1, 2011, available at http://www.cnn.com/2011/US/04/01/traffic.fatalities/ (last accessed March 14, 2019).

5. Katharine Q. Seelye, "As Drug Deaths Soar, a Silver Lining for Transplant Patients," *New York Times*, October 6, 2016.

6. See https://optn.transplant.hrsa.gov/data/view-data-reports/national-data/# (last accessed March 14, 2019). See also Christine M. Durand, Mary G. Bowring, Alvin G. Thomas, et al., "The Drug Overdose Epidemic and Deceased-Donor Transplantation in the United States: A National Registry Study," *Annals of Internal Medicine* 168 (May 15, 2018): 702–711; and Camille Nelson Kotton, "Every Cloud Has a Silver Lining: Overdose-Death Donor in Organ Transplantation," Editorial, *Annals of Internal Medicine* 168 (May 15, 2018): 739–740.

7. Donate Life America, 2017 Annual Report, including the 2017 National Donor Designation Report Card, https://www.donatelife.net/wp-content/uploads/2016/06/2017_AnnualUpdate_singlepages_small.pdf (last accessed March 14, 2019).

8. See James F. Childress and Catharyn T. Liverman, eds., *Organ Donation: Opportunities for Action* (Washington, DC: The National Academies Press, 2006), chap. 3.

9. "A Hero in Death: Mantle Organ Donor Helped Save Six Lives," from *Dallas Morning News*, reprinted in *The Atlanta Constitution*, August 7, 1995, 6C.

10. Ibid.

11. See http://www.njleg.state.nj.us/2008/Bills/PL08/48_.PDF.

12. "A Hero in Death: Mantle Organ Donor Helped Save Six Lives."

13. National Conference of Commissioners on Uniform State Laws, *Uniform Anatomical Gift Act* (Chicago, IL: National Conference of Commissioners, 1968).

14. National Conference of Commissioners on Uniform State Laws, now known as the Uniform Law Commission, *Revised Uniform Anatomical Gift Act* (Chicago, IL: National Conference of Commissioners, 2006, last amended in 2009). Another version developed in 1987 was not widely adopted, and the 2006 version was in part an effort to secure uniformity across states. However, as of late 2018, a few states

(Florida, New York, Pennsylvania) had not yet adopted the 2006 version. See https://www.uniformlaws.org/committees/community-home?CommunityKey=015e18ad-4806-4dff-b011-8e1ebc0d1d0f (last accessed March 14, 2019).

15. Childress and Liverman, eds., *Organ Donation: Opportunities for Action*, especially pp. 68–69.

16. W. J. Chon, M. A. Josephson, E. J. Gordon, et al., "When the Living and the Deceased Cannot Agree on Organ Donation: A Survey of US Organ Procurement Organizations (OPOs)," *American Journal of Transplantation* 14 (2014): 172–177.

17. Versions of these distinctions appear in a number of sources, such as Lon Fuller's *The Morality of Law*, revised edition (New Haven, CT: Yale University Press, 1969).

18. My use of the term "failure" rather than "nondonation" deliberately highlights the connection to these moral frameworks.

19. Tom L. Beauchamp and James F. Childress, *Principles of Biomedical Ethics*, 4th edition (New York: Oxford University Press, 1994), p. 268.

20. These conditions are drawn, with modifications, from Beauchamp and Childress, *Principles of Biomedical Ethics*, 7th edition (New York: Oxford University Press, 2013), p. 207.

21. See Childress, "Contact Tracing: A Liberal-Communitarian Approach," *The Responsive Community: Rights and Responsibilities* 1, No. 1 (Winter 1990–1991): 69–77.

22. *2012 National Survey of Organ Donation Attitudes and Behaviors* (U.S. Department of Health and Human Services, Health Resources & Services Administration, Healthcare Systems Bureau, Division of Transplantation, September 2013), p. 32, available at http://organdonor.gov/dtcp/nationalsurveyorgandonation.pdf (last accessed August 10, 2014).

23. Ibid., p. 30.

24. See the critique of the language of "spare parts" in Renée C. Fox and Judith P. Swazey, *Spare Parts: Organ Replacement in American Society* (New York: Oxford University Press, 1992).

25. *2012 National Survey of Organ Donation Attitudes and Behaviors*, p. 32.

26. See the summary in James F. Childress, *Practical Reasoning in Bioethics* (Bloomington: Indiana University Press, 1997), chap.14. Surveys have often reported that individuals are more willing to donate a deceased family member's organs than their own.

27. See *2012 National Survey of Organ Donation Attitudes and Behaviors*.

28. See, e.g., Laura Siminoff, Robert M. Arnold, Arthur L. Caplan, et al., "Public Policy Governing Organ and Tissue Procurement in the United States," *Annals of Internal Medicine* 123 (1995): 10–17.

29. Task Force on Organ Transplantation, *Organ Transplantation: Issues and Recommendations* (Rockville, MD: Office of Organ Transplantation, Health Resources and Services Administration, U.S. DHHS, April, 1986).

30. A. A. Herring, S. Woolhandler, D. U. Himmelstein, "Insurance Status of U.S. Organ Donors and Transplant Recipients: The Uninsured Give, but Rarely Receive," *International Journal of Health Services* 38, No. 4 (2008): 641–652

31. See, e.g., Siminoff, Arnold, Caplan, et al. "Public Policy Governing Organ and Tissue Procurement in the United States," p.16.

32. Prottas, *The Most Useful Gift: Altruism and the Public Policy of Organ Transplants,* A Twentieth Century Fund Book (San Francisco: Jossey-Bass Publishers, 1994), p. 50.

33. *2012 National Survey of Organ Donation Attitudes and Behaviors,* p. 32.

34. See Childress and Liverman, eds., *Organ Donation: Opportunities for Action,* p. 85.

35. See Childress, *Practical Reasoning in Bioethics,* chap. 15.

36. Thomas G. Peters, "Life or Death: The Issue of Payment in Cadaveric Organ Donation," *Journal of the American Medical Association* 265 (1991): 1302–1305.

37. William F. May, *The Patient's Ordeal* (Bloomington: Indiana University Press, 1991), p. 181.

38. Pennsylvania never implemented the legislation it passed that allowed the provision of $300.00 to funeral homes to help organ donor families cover the costs of funeral expenses, in part because of uncertainty about whether it would violate the National Organ Transplant Act's ban on providing organs for valuable consideration. See Sheryl Gay Stolberg, "Pennsylvania Set to Break Taboo on Reward for Organ Donations," *New York Times,* May 9, 1999.

39. Nuffield Council on Bioethics, *Human Bodies: Donation for Medicine and Research* (London: Nuffield Council, October, 2011), 6.46. http://nuffieldbioethics.org/wp-content/uploads/2014/07/Donation_full_report.pdf (last accessed March 14, 2019). See also Nuffield Council on Bioethics, "Ethics Body Suggests NHS Pays for Funerals of Organ Donors," Press Release October 10, 2011. Available at http://www.nuffieldbioethics.org/news/ethics-body-suggests-nhs-pays-funerals-organ-donors (last accessed March 14, 2019).

40. See Stephen Jan, Kristen Howard, and Alan Cass, "A Proposal to Increase Deceased Organ Donation through an Altruistic Incentive," *BMJ* 340 (2010): c2182.

41. See the discussion in Childress and Liverman, eds., *Organ Donation: Opportunities for Action,* esp. pp. 253–259. A relatively recent Israeli law gives priority status to candidates for organ transplants who have been registered as organ donors for at least three years prior to entering the waiting list as a candidate for an organ. Two analysts hold that "although needing some modifications, the new Israeli law is based on [a] sound ethical approach that seems to begin already to bear fruit." See Jacob Lavee and Dan W. Brock, "Prioritizing registered donors in organ allocation: an ethical appraisal of the Israeli organ transplant law," *Critical Care* 18, No. 6 (December 2012): 707–711.

42. Richard H. Thaler and Cass R. Sunstein, *Nudge: Improving Decisions about Health, Wealth, and Happiness* (New Haven, CT: Yale University Press, 2008), p. 6.

43. See Aaron Spital, "Mandated Choice for Organ Donation: Time to Give It a Try," *Annals of Internal Medicine* 125, No. 1 (1996): 66–69, among his other works. Richard Thaler and Cass Sunstein prefer a policy of presumed consent but they support mandated choice because it appears to be an easier sell politically even if less effective. See *Nudge,* p. 180. Robert Veatch has been a vigorous and long-time proponent of required response of competent persons. See his *Death, Dying, and the Biological Revolution,* revised edition (New Haven, CT: Yale University Press, 1989); *Transplantation Ethics* (Washington, DC: Georgetown University Press, 2000), chap.

10; and Veatch and Lainie Ross, *Transplantation Ethics*, 2nd edition (Washington, DC: Georgetown University Press, 2015).

44. American Medical Association Council on Ethical and Judicial Affairs, "Strategies for Cadaveric Organ Procurement: Mandated Choice and Presumed Consent," *Journal of the American Medical Association* 272 (1994): 809–812. This opinion was replaced in 2005 by "Presumed Consent and Mandated Choice for Organs from Deceased Donors," a more cautious opinion. See *Code of Medical Ethics of the American Medical Association*, 2010–2011 edition (Chicago: American Medical Association, 2010), pp. 75–77.

45. See the discussion of the problems in Texas and Virginia in Childress and Liverman, eds., *Organ Donation: Opportunities for Action*, pp. 177–179.

46. Nuffield Council on Bioethics, *Human Bodies: Donation for Medicine and Research* (London: Nuffield Council on Bioethics, 2011), 6:55. Contrast Richard H. Thaler and Cass R. Sunstein, "How Required Choice for Organ Donation Actually Works in Practice," Nudge Blog, October 10, 2010, http://nudges.org/2010/10/10/how-required-choice-for-organ-donation-actually-works-in-practice/ (last accessed March 14, 2019).

47. Quoted in Jeremy Laurance, "Change Law on Organ Donation, Doctors Say," *The Independent*, November 2, 2009.

48. See Judith Areen, "A Scarcity of Organs," *Journal of Legal Education* 38 (1988): 555–565. She says, "If people were given the option of using such a durable power of attorney for organ donation instead of a donor card, efforts to educate the public about the need for organs might produce more organs." Parallel to durable powers of attorney for treatment/nontreatment decisions, "an individual who prepares a durable power of attorney that transfers power to authorize organ donation will be able to inform the surrogate in advance as to his own wishes on the subject and relieve the surrogate of the burden of trying to ascertain what the donor might have wanted. At the same time, the donor will have the comfort of knowing that organs cannot be retrieved without the approval of the surrogate" (pp. 563–564). See also John Saunders, "Bodies, Organs and Saving Lives: The Alternatives," *Clinical Medicine: Journal of the Royal College of Physicians* 10 (2010): 26–29, at 28.

49. See the summary in Childress and Liverman, eds., *Organ Donation: Opportunities for Action*, pp. 177–179.

50. David Orentlicher has argued—mistakenly, in my judgment—that we have already had an experiment in presumed consent legislation in the United States. He focuses on the laws in several states that authorized medical examiners or coroners to remove corneas for transplantation from bodies under their auspices without notification to or explicit consent or permission from either the decedent while alive or the next of kin, even if the relatives were readily available. See his "Presumed Consent to Organ Donation: Its Rise and Fall in the United States," *Rutgers Law Review* 61 (2008–2009): 295–331. In fact, these laws involved routine removal or salvaging with the possibility of opting out but they were not presumed consent laws. To be "presumed consent" laws—much less ethically acceptable presumed consent laws—more efforts to educate the public and to establish clear, easy, nonburdensome, and reliable

mechanisms for opting out would have been necessary. This "little known experiment," as Orentlicher labels it, can hardly be called an experiment in "presumed consent to donation," because it is not plausible to presume that silence or nondissent is consent when so few people in a state are even aware of the law.

51. See Arthur L. Caplan, "Ethical and Policy Issues in the Procurement of Cadaver Organs for Transplantation," *New England Journal of Medicine* 314 (1984): 981–983.

52. Amanda M. Rosenblum, Lucy D. Horvat, Laura A. Siminoff, et al., "The Authority of Next-of-Kin in Explicit and Presumed Consent Systems for Deceased Organ Donation: An Analysis of 54 Countries," *Nephrology, Dialysis, Transplantation* 27 (2012): 2533–2546.

53. Ibid. The similarity of practices of organ procurement, whether in an opt-in or an opt-out system, was observed years ago and still persists. See Prottas, *The Most Useful Gift*, from 1994.

54. E. J. Johnson and D. G. Goldstein, "Do Defaults Save Lives?" *Science* 302 (2003): 1338–1339.

55. Shai Davidai, Thomas Gilovich, and Lee D. Ross, "The Meaning of Default Options for Potential Organ Donors," *Proceedings of the National Academy of Sciences* 108, No. 38 (September 18, 2012): 15201–15205.

56. Among the many studies that argue for the greater effectiveness of PC laws, see Alberto Abadie and Sebastien Gay, "The Impact of Presumed Consent Legislation on Cadaveric Organ Donation: A Cross-Country Study," *Journal of Health Economics* 25 (2006): 599–620.

57. See Council of Europe, "International Figures on Organ Donation and Transplantation," *Transplant Newsletter* 10, No. 1 (2005): 5–22; and Childress and Liverman, eds., *Organ Donation: Opportunities for Action*, p. 28.

58. C. Rudge, R. Matesanz, F. L. Delmonico, and J. Chapman, "International Practices of Organ Donation," *British Journal of Anaesthesia* 108 (2012): 148–55. Rates of deceased organ donation will vary somewhat depending on whether "dead" donors include only those who "brain dead" (i.e., who are declared dead by neurological standards) or also those who are "non-heart-beating donors" (i.e., those who are declared dead by cardiopulmonary standards). See the previous chapter.

59. See Firat Bilgel, "The Impact of Presumed Consent Laws and Institutions on Deceased Organ Donation," *European Journal of Health Economics* 13 (2012): 27–38.

60. Amber Rithalia, Catriona McDaid, Sara Suekarran, Lindsey Myers, and Amanda Sowden, "Impact of Presumed Consent for Organ Donation on Donation Rates: A Systematic Review," *BMJ* 338 (2009): a3162. Chris J. Rudge and Elizabeth Buggins write, "The impact of opting-out legislation remains controversial, and difficult to assess, but perhaps a truer measure of the possible benefits would be a demonstration that consent rates are higher in countries with such legislation. European data on the refusal rate are limited, but there does not seem to be a clear association between the legislative framework and the reported refusal rate. . . . An effective donation structure, based on local responsibility for maximizing donation, seems to be the key to success." Rudge and Buggins, "How to Increase Organ Donation: Does Opting Out Have a Role?" *Transplantation* 93, No. 2 (January 27, 2012): 141–144, at p. 144.

61. Lucy D. Horvat, Meaghan S. Cuerden, S. Joseph Kim, et al., "Informing the Debate: Rates of Kidney Transplantation in Nations with Presumed Consent," *Annals of Internal Medicine* 153, No. 10 (November 16, 2010): 641–649.

62. For these data on recovered kidney donors and kidneys transplanted in 2018, see https://optn.transplant.hrsa.gov/data/view-data-reports/national-data/# (last accessed March 19, 2019).

63. "Life after Death: Ideas for Increasing the Rates of Organ Donations Are Controversial," *The Economist*, February 18, 2012.

64. See the discussion in Childress and Liverman, eds., *Organ Donation: Opportunities for Action*, pp. 218–219.

65. Childress, *Practical Reasoning in Bioethics*, chap. 14, explicating and developing A. John Simmons, "Tacit Consent and Political Obligation," *Philosophy & Public Affairs* 5, No. 3 (1976): 274–291.

66. Contrast Micah Hester, "Opting-Out: The Relationships between Moral Arguments and Public Policies in Organ Procurement," *Cambridge Quarterly of Healthcare Ethics* 18 (2009): 159–165.

67. J. A. Wells, *National Survey of Organ Donation: 2005 Preliminary Results*, Presentation at the Institute of Medicine Workshop on Increasing Rates of Organ Donation (Washington, DC: Institute of Medicine Committee on Increasing Rates of Organ Donation, June 20, 2005); summarized in Childress and Liverman, eds., *Organ Donation: Opportunities for Action*, pp. 215–216.

68. Childress and Liverman, eds., *Organ Donation: Opportunities for Action*, p. 227.

69. Jennifer S. Bard, "Lack of Political Will and Public Trust Dooms Presumed Consent," *American Journal of Bioethics* 12, No. 2 (2012): 44–46.

70. Eurotransplant, *Organ Donation: Towards a Mutual Understanding* (Leiden: Eurotransplant Information Exchange Program, July 2010), p. 24. See also John Fabre, Paul Murphy, and Rafael Matesanz, "Presumed Consent: A Distraction in the Quest for Increasing Rates of Organ Donation," *BMJ* 341 (2010): c4973.

71. For the information that follows, see the official website *Organ Donation Wales* at http://organdonationwales.org/?lang=en (last accessed November 10, 2016).

72. German National Ethics Council (Nationaler Ethikrat), *Increasing the Number of Organ Donations: A Pressing Issue for Transplant Medicine in Germany* (Berlin, 2007), http://www.ethikrat.org/files/Opinion_Increasing_the_number_of_organ_donations.pdf.

9

Putting Patients First in Organ Allocation

An Ethical Analysis of Policy Debates in the United States

Introduction

Organ allocation policy involves a mixture of ethical, scientific, medical, legal, and political factors, among others. It is thus hard, and perhaps even impossible, to identify and fully separate ethical considerations from all these other factors. Yet I will focus primarily on the ethical considerations embedded in debates in the United States about organ allocation policy. I will argue that it is important to put patients first—in the language of the title of one of the major public hearings[1]—but even then significant ethical questions will remain about exactly how to put patients first.

I would not characterize the current organ-allocation system in the United States as fundamentally unfair or unjust, in part because there are debates about various criteria of fairness and justice and in part because the United Network for Organ Sharing (UNOS), operating the national Organ Procurement and Transplantation Network (OPTN) under a contract with the federal government's Department of Health and Human Services (DHHS), has made substantial progress over time and continues to seek improvements in fair or equitable access. However, I do believe that organ allocation policy can be further improved—largely by putting patients across the nation first, apart from particular professional and institutional interests—and that the 1998 DHHS final rule points in the right direction, as indicated in what follows. Nevertheless, I cannot endorse the DHHS rule in toto largely because it does not adequately attend to the probability of successful outcomes among transplant candidates for particular organs. In my judgment, this criterion needs more attention, both on its own terms and in relation to medical urgency, than the DHHS regulations suppose.

Debates about the Community of Ownership
of Donated Organs

I had the good fortune to serve as vice-chair of the federal Task Force on Organ Transplantation, which in April 1986 issued its report *Organ Transplantation: Issues and Recommendations*.[2] One of this task force's major responsibilities, as mandated by the National Organ Transplant Act, was to make "recommendations for assuring equitable access by patients to organ transplantation and for assuring the equitable allocation of donated organs among transplant centers and among patients medically qualified for an organ transplant." It took me some time to discern that our debates about "equitable access" and "equitable allocation" were, in part, debates about who "owns" donated organs.

Apart from special cases of directed donation to named recipients, donated organs belong to the community, the public, and not to procurement and transplant teams. This fundamental conviction undergirded the Task Force's deliberations about and recommendations for equitable organ allocation: Donated organs should be viewed as scarce public resources to be used for the welfare of the community. Organ procurement and transplant teams receive these donated organs as "trustees" and "stewards" on behalf of the whole community. Thus, they should not have unlimited dispositional authority over donated organs.

Over the years since the Task Force's report, the term "community" has been widely but variously used.[3] Unfortunately, it has often been excessively narrowed. In the current debate, it frequently means the "transplant community,"[4] which is sometimes limited to transplant surgeons, professionals, and their institutions, though it sometimes includes organ donors, organ recipients, transplant candidates, and their families. But even the latter interpretation of "community" is still too narrow because it fails to include the larger community, which comprises not only all these parties but also all of us as potential donors and potential recipients (and relatives of potential donors and potential recipients).

Policies of organ allocation should be designed for the public as a whole. This view of community ownership of and dispositional authority over donated organs provides strong support for wide and diverse public participation in setting the criteria for allocating donated organs. Calls for public participation stem in part from the nature of organ procurement in the United States—it depends on voluntary, public gifts; that is, gifts by individuals and their families to the community. Indeed, there are important moral connections between policies of organ procurement and policies of organ allocation. On the one hand, the success of policies of organ procurement may reduce scarcity and hence obviate some of the difficulties in organ allocation. On the other hand, distrust is a major reason for the public's reluctance to donate organs, and policies of procurement may be ineffective if the public perceives the policies of organ allocation as unfair and thus untrustworthy.[5] In short, public participation—for example, in the OPTN—is very important and even indispensable to ensure actual and perceived fairness. "Organ allocation falls into the region of public decision-making," as Jeffrey Prottas insists, "not medical ethics and much less medical tradition."[6] Thus, policies of organ allocation should be designed, in part, by the public.

Two additional points about community ownership of donated organs and public participation in setting organ allocation criteria merit attention. First, while observing that prior to 1986 organs donated for transplantation had effectively belonged to the surgeons who removed them, Prottas contends that the fundamental philosophical shift to community ownership effected by the Task Force report both changed matters and left them the same. On the one hand, professional dominance remains, in part because of technical expertise and medical gatekeeping. On the other hand, professional dominance is now more circumscribed and publicly accountable. With organ allocation now in the public domain, in part because transplant professionals had sought governmental assistance for transplantation, there are now more participants, particularly public participants, and the terms of the debate have changed:

> Alternative allocation systems are now defended in public debate, and equity as well as efficiency must be considered and defined. Physicians dominate the debate, through knowledge as well as power, but they must justify their actions now as trustees of the public. The organs are no longer theirs.[7]

Second, some ambiguities about community ownership persist in debates in the OPTN and elsewhere about policies of organ allocation: Do donated organs belong to the national community or to regional, state, or local communities? Different answers to this question may or may not lead to different policies, but they certainly create different presumptions and pose different problems. Nevertheless, from either starting point, various arguments may support using organs on one geographical level rather than another. If we start from local (or state or regional) "ownership" of donated organs, then organs would be allocated first in the local community, perhaps subject to some requirements to "share" organs (e.g., a zero-antigen mismatch in kidney transplantation). If, however, the relevant community for organ distribution is the national community, as I believe it is, then that community has the right and the responsibility to allocate the organs to patients anywhere in the country according to acceptable standards and logistical constraints. Nevertheless, it may and often should allow organs to be used at the local level, if, for instance, transporting those organs would jeopardize their viability for transplantation. Such logistical problems remain especially important for heart and lung transplantation, somewhat important for liver transplantation (where the situation has improved), but only modestly important for kidney transplantation.

Although logistical problems thus remain variably important, there is nothing more than anecdotal evidence, to the best of my knowledge, to warrant the additional common claim that local allocation provides a substantial incentive for organ donation that would be lost under a national system. A truly national approach should reduce the relevance of "accidents of geography" in organ allocation and allow such geographical factors to enter only when and where they are clearly relevant for transplantation outcomes.

In short, it is now time to return to the Task Force's conception of the national community as the relevant community of dispositional authority in organ allocation and to take steps to minimize "accidents of geography"— accidents regarding where transplant candidates live or are listed—in organ allocation to the greatest extent possible with the use of the best available technologies for each type of organ. The moral point is not that the local community should "share" some organs it obtains with the larger, national community—the language of "sharing" suggests that the local community "owns" the donated organs. Rather, donated organs belong to the national community, and the "trustees" and "stewards" of those organs should allocate them according to criteria that minimize "accidents of geography" in putting patients first.

Principles of Just, Fair, and Equitable Allocation

Justice and Morally Relevant and Irrelevant Characteristics

To state the last point differently, it is, in my judgment, generally unjust to use "accidents of geography" in organ allocation because they are not morally relevant to who should receive donated organs (unless, again, local or regional priority is required because transporting the organs would be impossible or would adversely affect their viability for transplantation). But what exactly is justice, and how should principles of justice function in organ allocation?

Justice, which may be defined as rendering to each person his or her due, includes both formal and material criteria. The formal criterion of justice involves similar treatment for similar cases or equal treatment for equals. Various material criteria of justice specify relevant similarities and dissimilarities among parties and thus determine how particular benefits and burdens will be distributed.[8] There is debate about the moral relevance and moral weight of different material criteria, such as need, merit, societal contribution, status, and ability to pay. Different theories of justice tend to stress different material criteria. However, some material criteria may be acceptable in some areas of life, such as employment, but not in others, such as the allocation of scarce life-saving organ transplants.

Even though principles of justice permit rationing under conditions of scarcity, they rule out allocation criteria that are based on morally irrelevant characteristics, such as race or gender. However, it is much easier to agree on what is unjust, such as distribution by gender or race, than on what is just. A fundamental question concerns which material criteria satisfy the requirements of justice and are justifiable for organ allocation. As I have argued, public participation is one way—but only one way and by no means sufficient—to reduce possible biases from particular professional or institutional interests in the public process of determining which material criteria are relevant to organ allocation. In short, public participation is one way to put patients first.

Just Material Criteria in Organ Allocation: Patient Need, Probability of Success, and Time on the Waiting List

There is general agreement that three material criteria are relevant, just, and justifiable in organ allocation—patient need, probability of a successful outcome, and time on the waiting list. These are recognized in UNOS policies, which attempt to balance them but which then allow local priority to produce "accidents of geography." They are also evident in the DHHS regulations, which, however, pay insufficient attention to the probability of a successful outcome, particularly in relation to the other two criteria.

The first two material criteria—patient need and probability of a successful outcome—appear at two major stages in organ allocation: (1) forming a waiting list by determining the pool of transplant candidates, and (2) allocating available organs to patients on the waiting list. The third material criterion—time on the waiting list—obviously applies only at the second stage of allocation. The difficult ethical and practical questions at each stage involve specifying the criteria—what exactly do they mean, how can we measure them, and so forth?—and weighting them in case they conflict—should one take priority over the others, should allocation policies attempt to balance them, and so forth? Even though there is little dispute about the general relevance of these three criteria, and much of that dispute focuses on waiting time rather than the other two criteria, vigorous and widespread debate occurs about how to specify and weight all three criteria.

Setting Criteria for Admission to Waiting Lists

There is general agreement that the waiting list of transplant candidates should be formed according to the medical criteria of need for and probability of benefiting from an organ transplant. However, consensus breaks down at the point of specification that requires determining whether to define these medical criteria broadly or narrowly, where to set the standards for need or for minimal efficacy, and which factors are relevant in determining both need and probable benefit. It also breaks down in determining which of these criteria should have priority in case of conflict.

Vigorous efforts have been undertaken, particularly through UNOS, to develop fair policies of allocating organs to patients on waiting lists, but it has been more difficult to ensure equitable access to waiting lists, perhaps in part because of transplant-center discretion. And yet, decisions about who will be admitted to the waiting list appear to constitute a primary source of unequal access to organ transplants. In the absence of minimum criteria for admission to the waiting lists for organ transplants, transplant teams have had the sole authority to decide whether and when to register a patient. According to one report, "a patient can be registered at any time before the transplant is urgently needed and can electively turn down available organs while accumulating waiting time that may misrepresent the patient's medical condition."[9]

It is thus essential to avoid the inappropriate, unnecessary, unfair, and premature listing of transplant candidates. DHHS rightly proposes a performance goal for the OPTN of defining "objective and measurable medical criteria to be used by all transplant centers in determining whether a patient is appropriate to be listed for a transplant."[10] These criteria should establish minimum medical need, as DHHS indicates, but they should also attend to probability of success, which DHHS doesn't adequately address or stress (even though it is mentioned more or less in passing).

Point Systems for Allocating Organs

It is obviously necessary to have point systems for allocating organs across the national community. Such systems appear to provide objective, public, and impartial ways to allocate organs by reducing institutional and professional discretion and possible bias. They thereby assure the public that all patients will be treated as equals according to the standards reflected in the point system.

With the exception of time on the waiting list, the material criteria explicitly used in different point systems for organ allocation are largely medical in that they involve medical techniques used by medical personnel and arguably influence the transplant's likely success or failure. They are not, however, value free.[11] Selecting different factors and then assigning to them various weights (points) reflects various values. The vigorous debate about how much weight each criterion should have is only partly technical and scientific (e.g., the impact of human leukocyte antigen (HLA) matching in kidney transplantation); it is to a great extent ethical. Let me take one example: In kidney transplantation, such factors as quality of antigen match and logistical score focus on the chance of a successful outcome; both medical urgency and panel-reactive antibody in different ways focus on patient need; and time on the waiting list introduces a nonmedical factor, even though it may overlap with panel-reactive antibody because sensitized patients tend to wait longer for transplants.

The points assigned to these various factors thus reflect value judgments about the relative importance of patient need, probability of success, and waiting time. Similar observations apply to other organ transplants.

Specifying and Balancing Patients' Needs and Probable Benefits

Both patient need for a transplant and the probability of a successful transplant are ethically relevant in selecting patients for the waiting list and in selecting patients to receive a particular organ. I would argue that both the urgency of medical need and the probability of successful outcome should be used to determine which candidate should receive a particular organ, after the pool of transplant candidates has been established by the same criteria. Obviously, a patient's risk of imminent death is a strong reason for allocating an organ to that patient. But a major reason for also considering the probability of a successful outcome is to avoid wasting the gift of life. Organs are donated for effective use, and providing an organ to a patient who has only a very limited chance of success increases the probability that he or she will then need another transplant for survival, further reducing the chances for others as well as for his or her own successful transplantation.

It is important to specify as completely as possible both criteria. The DHHS regulations quite rightly require further specification of medical need, according to status categories that adequately differentiate patient needs.[12] One important reason is that medical urgency is a manipulable category, which has reportedly been abused at times by physicians eager to protect their own patients by declaring them medically urgent to increase their chances for a transplant.[13] However, the DHHS regulations, in my judgment, do not adequately attend to the probability of success, which is also morally relevant.

To be sure, after concentrating on medical urgency as the primary criterion, the DHHS preamble and regulations often add a proviso to the effect that the application of the criterion of medical urgency is limited by medical judgment about not wasting an organ through a transplant that would be futile. For instance, the standard of equalizing waiting times within the medically urgent status emphasizes "that the sickest categories of patients should receive as much benefit as feasible under this standard, in accordance with sound medical judgment."[14] And among the "key constraints on organ allocation" that DHHS would require the OPTN to take into account is a limited version of the probability of a successful outcome: "There are patients with urgent need for whom transplantation is futile. Organs cannot be used without an assessment of the immune system and other physical conditions of patients."[15]

This DHHS proviso is important, but it is also necessary to try to build this ethical criterion of probability of success into the publicly formulated criteria of allocation rather than leaving it to medical discretion. This will be very difficult to accomplish—for instance, what counts as a success when we consider length of graft survival, length of patient survival, quality of life, rehabilitation?—and it may even be ultimately impossible. However, with both medical and public input in an open process conducted over time, we should be able to determine whether we can specify this criterion, along with status categories having to do with urgency of need. At the very least, through this process, it might be possible to set certain minimum thresholds of probable benefit.

One reason further specification is needed is that even judgments of "futility" are subject to considerable debate. For instance, as used in the medical literature, "medical futility" may mean (1) a procedure cannot be performed because of a patient's biological condition, (2) a procedure will not produce the intended physiological effect, (3) a procedure cannot be expected to produce the benefit that is sought, and (4) the anticipated benefits of a procedure will be outweighed by its burdens, harms, and costs. Given that the last is really a judgment of utility, rather than futility, only the first three should count, but even they are not objective and value free. For instance, some clinicians hold that a treatment is futile only if there is no chance it will be effective, whereas others label a treatment as futile if its chance of success is 13% or lower.[16] Clearly, a public process is needed to provide greater specification of "sound medical judgment" in this regard.

Such a public process will also need to consider how to balance these two morally relevant criteria of patient need and probable success. Tensions between medical urgency and probability of success may vary greatly depending on the organ in question. For instance, the category of medical urgency will probably not be as important when an artificial organ can be used as a backup (for example, dialysis for end-stage renal failure). In liver transplantation, to take another example, the dominant practice has been to give the sickest patient the highest priority (within the local area), but "medical utility" (and some would include cost-effectiveness) would often dictate placing the liver in a fitter patient to realize the greatest medical benefit (at the lowest cost). Another reason for some attention to those with a higher probability of benefit is that "as time goes on . . . the fitter patients become increasingly ill, their survivability on the waiting list declines, and their operative risk soars."[17] It is not possible to determine generally, apart from different types of organ transplants, what weights to assign to urgency of patient need and probability of success; what is needed is a public process to consider and determine their respective weights for organ-specific allocation policies.

The Moral Relevance of Time on the Waiting List and of Seeking to Equalize Waiting Times

It is fair to allocate organs according to both medical need and probability of success, but when there are no substantial differences in degree of medical need and probable benefit among various transplant candidates, it is fair to use their time on the waiting list (or queuing or first-come, first-served) to break the tie.

Indeed, if two or more patients are equally good candidates for a particular organ according to the medical criteria of need and probability of success, using their different times on the waiting list may be the fairest way to make the final selection. Such an approach presupposes that there is a firm (and morally acceptable) consensus on what constitutes substantial differences in medical need and probability of success, as well as on criteria for admission to the waiting list.

Some critics charge that time on the waiting list is morally irrelevant or even morally pernicious. For example, Olga Jonasson argues that "length of time on the waiting list is the least fair, most easily manipulated, and most mindless of all methods of organ allocation."[18] She is right if this criterion is used by itself without regard to the other important criteria of urgency of need and probability of success or if it is viewed as the primary criterion. But the use of waiting time in patient selection, when medical need and probability of success are roughly equal, can be justified by various principles and values, such as fair equality of opportunity. Nevertheless, ethical and practical problems do arise in its application. For instance, when does the transplant candidate's waiting time start—when the patient seeks medical treatment for the condition that leads to end-stage organ failure or when the patient is registered with the OPTN, to take just two possibilities? The latter has been used, but, as critics note, it is easy to manipulate, for example, by putting patients on the list as early as possible and well before their condition really merits such placement. Hence, DHHS is rightly requiring that the OPTN set minimum standards across transplant centers for admission to the waiting list.

Also, the fairness of using time on the waiting list as a criterion depends in part on background conditions. For example, some people may not seek care early because they lack insurance; others may receive inadequate medical advice about how early to seek transplantation; and so forth. It will help, in line with the DHHS regulations, to establish not only firm standards for admission to the waiting list but also firm status categories and then to count only the time within a particular status: "The relevant 'tie-breaker' will no longer be total waiting time, perhaps years, but will become waiting time within a group of patients with equal medical urgency."[19] Such a development will facilitate the fair use of waiting time as a criterion of allocation.

If it is ethically acceptable, as I have argued, to use different times on the waiting list to break ties among transplant candidates, based on medical need and probability of success, is it also ethically important to try to reduce unequal waiting times among patients in particular status categories and across geographical boundaries? The DHHS performance goal is to make average waiting times as equal as possible among patients with similar degrees of need (here I would go beyond the DHHS regulations and include probability of success too, at least above a certain threshold). The goal is to equalize average waiting times within similar categories of transplant candidates. Inequalities, such as a fivefold difference in waiting times for liver transplants, should serve as triggers to inquire into ways to reduce the inequalities. It is a legitimate public goal to try to equalize, as much as possible, times on the waiting list, given that those times have some bearing on suffering, on urgency of need, and on probability of success, in addition to being independently significant. Increasing equality, through reducing arbitrary differences in time on the waiting list among otherwise similar transplant candidates, is required by formal justice.

Conclusions

Organ allocation poses a "tragic choice."[20] Short of adequately increasing the supply of transplantable organs, we cannot fully realize all our values at the same time. Hence, it is morally imperative to seek the best possible balance of the whole range of relevant values, which are reflected in the material criteria of patient need, probability of success, and waiting time.

First, we need to defuse the moral rhetoric about various organ-allocation systems. Several organ-allocation systems appear to fall within the range of ethically acceptable or relatively just and fair systems, but all of them require moral fine-tuning in the name of justice and fairness. And various participants in the debate appear to be acting in good faith, even when they seriously disagree.

Second, society should seek to further specify, to weight, and to balance patient need, probable success, and waiting time through a process that involves the fullest possible and most diverse public participation. Obviously, ethically acceptable allocation criteria cannot be formulated without the substantial input of transplant surgeons and other physicians, as well as other healthcare professionals and scientists. Nevertheless, donated organs belong to the whole community, and procurement and transplant teams receive those organs on behalf of the whole community, for which they serve as "trustees" and "stewards."

It is time to put patients first and to devise procedural and substantive criteria to protect current and future patients' rights and welfare. By putting patients first, we should be able to find common ground or reach an overlapping consensus. One way to do so is to ask, along the lines of the Golden Rule or the Rawlsian social contract, behind the veil of ignorance, which set of criteria we would find acceptable for allocating organs to ourselves or to our families, without knowing our own or our families' precise circumstances. This is a fair way to reflect on possible material criteria for just organ allocation.

Third, the morally relevant community of ownership of, or dispositional authority over, donated organs is the national community, subject to logistical constraints that must be met in order to provide viable organs for transplantation. Thus, the allocation system should focus on patients across the country and should minimize, as much as possible, "accidents of geography." This is the main point at which I would criticize the OPTN's current system—the procedural assignment of priority to the local community in allocation, even in combination with other substantive criteria (such as medical urgency in liver allocation), results in an unacceptable patchwork of allocation and produces various inequalities across the country. The alternative is not a single, national list that ignores the potential impact, for instance, of shipping organs great distances on the probable success of the transplant. What is required is a shift in orientation—to thinking about donated organs as belonging to the national community and then to specifying and balancing allocation criteria in part according to logistical realities.

The failure to take a national perspective has now resulted in further fragmentation, as some states have adopted laws that require organs donated within their boundaries to be used for patients within their boundaries and to be shared with other states only if no patient within their states could benefit from the organ. Such a result should have been anticipated by various participants in this debate over the last few years. Medical and political boundaries may not coincide. (Obviously, it is also important to consider the limitations of national boundaries, but I cannot do so here.[21])

Fourth, several of DHHS's proposed regulations should move organ allocation in even more equitable directions. In particular, I have argued that it is essential to set minimum criteria for access to waiting lists for various organ transplants and also to set uniform status categories, such as medical urgency. With these changes, which the OPTN is already pursuing, at least to some extent, it may be possible to use differences in waiting time more fairly as a criterion of allocation, when medical urgency and probability of success are roughly equal among transplant candidates. Furthermore, with these changes, it should be possible to begin to reduce inequalities of waiting time, in part because patients will be admitted to the waiting list in a more consistent way and because their status will be clearer. It is ethically desirable to reduce inequalities of waiting time, both because equality is an important value and because longer waiting times often correlate with longer suffering, further deterioration, and lower chances of successful outcomes.

This point may not come through as clearly as it might in the Institute of Medicine (IOM) report *Organ Procurement and Transplantation*.[22] This report criticizes certain uses of waiting time as an allocation criterion but, rather than rejecting waiting time altogether, calls for its "appropriate consideration." It properly notes that although "disparities in overall median waiting times for liver transplants have been cited as an indicator of the unfairness of the current system," those disparities do not provide "an appropriate measure of the fairness of the system." Thus, the report recommends discontinuing the use of waiting time as an allocation criterion for liver transplant candidates in certain statuses. Those in statuses 2B (who require continuous medical care and satisfy other conditions) and 3 (who require continuous medical care but do not satisfy the other conditions for 2B) are not as severely ill as those in statuses 1 (whose death from fulminant liver failure is expected in fewer than seven days) or 2A (who are in intensive care for treatment of chronic liver failure and who are expected to die in fewer than seven days). Those in statuses 2B and 3 present such a heterogeneous population in terms of range of severity of illness that waiting time is an inappropriate allocation criterion. The IOM report recommends that "an appropriate medical triage system . . . be developed to ensure equitable allocation of organs to patients in these categories." I concur: waiting time should be a tie-breaker when urgency of medical need and probability of successful treatment are roughly equal.

My biggest problem with the proposed DHHS regulations, which the IOM report generally affirms, is not that they emphasize medical urgency—it is appropriate to emphasize this criterion particularly for liver transplants in contrast to kidney transplants—but that they do so without sufficient attention on the level of policy to probable benefit and to balancing probable benefit with medical urgency. Some process needs to be devised, in the OPTN or elsewhere, with both professional and public participation, to work out a fuller conception of "medical utility," which includes both urgency of need and probability of benefit.

Fifth, it is essential to stress, as the proposed DHHS regulations do, ongoing monitoring and evaluation and appropriate revision of any organ-allocation system for various reasons, including to determine whether a particular point system has discriminatory effects and needs modification, whatever modeling programs might have predicted originally. For instance, in 1995 UNOS determined that it needed to alter its point system for allocating cadaveric kidneys in order to eliminate points previously assigned to some levels of HLA match and to increase the role of time on the waiting list, in part to increase the access and to reduce the waiting time of African Americans seeking cadaveric kidney transplants.[23]

Sixth, the so-called green screen is a major source of unequal access to extra-renal organ transplantation in the United States. At this time, a patient's ability to pay, either directly or through third-party coverage, is an important de facto material criterion for access to extra-renal transplants. The strategies that DHHS has recommended for the Department and for the OPTN in trying to make access more equal may help in small ways, but, in the final analysis, this issue must be addressed by the society as a whole, with the involvement of the federal and state governments.

Many of the arguments for providing funds to ensure equitable access to organ transplantation are similar to arguments for providing funds for other medical procedures. But one argument, used by the Task Force, specifically focuses on the distinctiveness or uniqueness of organ transplantation, particularly because of the social practices of procurement of organs for transplantation. This argument identifies an important moral connection between organ procurement, including organ donation, and organ distribution and allocation. In its efforts to increase the supply of organs, our society requests donations of organs from people of all socioeconomic classes—for example, through public appeals for organ donations or through state "required request" and "routine inquiry" statutes, which mandate that institutions inquire about an individual's or family's willingness to donate, or even request such a donation. However, it is unfair and even exploitative for the society to ask people, rich and poor alike, to donate organs if their own access to donated organs in cases of end-stage organ failure would be determined by their ability to pay rather than by their medical need, probability of success, and time on the waiting list.

This principled argument may be combined with an argument that focuses on the consequences of different policies. There are legitimate worries about the impact of unequal access to organ transplants (based on inability to pay) on the system of organ procurement, which includes gifts of organs from individuals and their families. There is substantial evidence that attitudes of distrust limit organ donation; this distrust appears to be directed at both organ procurement (e.g., the fear the potential donors will be declared dead prematurely) and organ distribution and allocation (e.g., the concern that potential transplant recipients from higher socioeconomic classes will receive priority).[24] Thus, it is not at all surprising that after Oregon decided to stop providing Medicaid funds for most organ transplants "a boycott of organ donations was organized by some low-income people."[25] And cynical comments about how quickly some famous people receive scarce organ transplants reflect public suspicion of organ allocation policies.

Finally, as the previous point suggests, there are important moral connections between organ procurement, including organ donation, on the one hand, and equitable access to organ transplantation and equitable organ allocation, on the other hand. It is obvious that increasing the supply of organs would reduce some problems of organ allocation, but, perhaps less obviously, public trust in the organ allocation system also appears to be important for the public donation of organs. As the Task Force on Organ Transplantation stressed over three decades ago, "there is increasing public demand that the criteria for patient selection be public and fair. This demand stems in part from the nature of the organ procurement system, which depends on voluntary gifts to strangers. Indeed, because of the close connection between organ procurement and the politics of organ distribution, it is essential that the criteria for patient selection are fair and are perceived to be fair. Otherwise, distrust may perpetuate the scarcity of organs."[26] Our fragile system of organ transplantation depends for its very existence on public trust and thus on the public's willingness to entrust their or their relatives' organs to the trustees and stewards who will allocate them on behalf of the national community to which the organs belong.[27]

Notes

1. The Joint Hearing of The House Commerce Committee Subcommittee on Health and Environment and The Senate Labor and Human Resources Committee, *Putting Patients First: Resolving Allocation of Transplant Organs*, June 18, 1998.
2. National Task Force on Organ Transplantation, *Organ Transplantation: Issues and Recommendations*, April 1986.
3. Ann Mongoven, "Federal Hearings on Liver Transplant Allocation and Donation," *BioLaw* (1997): S373–S389.
4. United Network for Organ Sharing, "The UNOS Statement of Principles and Objectives of Equitable Organ Allocation," *UNOS Update*, August 20, 1994.
5. James F. Childress, "Some Moral Connections between Organ Procurement and Organ Distribution," *Journal of Contemporary Health Law and Policy* 3 (1987): 85–110.
6. Jeffrey M. Prottas, "Nonresident Aliens and Access to Organ Transplant," *Transplantation Proceedings* 21 (1989): 3428.
7. Jeffrey M. Prottas, *The Most Useful Gift: Altruism and the Public Policy of Organ Transplants* (San Francisco, CA: Jossey-Bass Publishers, 1994), p. 153.
8. Tom L. Beauchamp and James F. Childress, *Principles of Biomedical Ethics*, 4th edition (New York: Oxford University Press, 1994), chap. 6.

9. United Network of Organ Sharing, US Department of Health and Human Services, *1994 Annual Report of the U.S. Scientific Registry for Transplant Recipients and the Organ Procurement and Transplantation Network, Transplant Data: 1988–1993* (Richmond, VA: UNOS, and Bethesda, MD: Division of Organ Transplantation, Bureau of Health Resources Development, Health Resources and Services Administration, US Department of Health and Human Services, 1994), p. v–3.

10. Department of Health and Human Services, "Organ Procurement and Transplantation Network: Final Rule," 42 CFR Part 121, *Federal Register* 63 (1998): 16296.

11. Dan Brock, "Ethical Issues in Recipient Selection for Organ Transplantation," in Deborah R. Matthieu, ed., *Organ Substitution Technology: Ethical, Legal, and Public Policy Issues* (Boulder, CO: Westview Press, 1988), pp. 86–99.

12. Department of Health and Human Services, "Organ Procurement and Transplantation Network: Final Rule."

13. A. P. Monaco, Comments in Roundtable Discussion, *Transplantation Proceedings* 21 (1989): 3418.

14. Department of Health and Human Services, "Organ Procurement and Transplantation Network: Final Rule," p. 16314.

15. Ibid.

16. See Beauchamp and Childress, *Principles of Biomedical Ethics*, 4th ed., p. 289.

17. Olga Jonasson, "Waiting in Line," *Transplantation Proceedings* 21 (1989): 3391.

18. Ibid., p. 3392.

19. See Department of Health and Human Services, "Organ Procurement and Transplantation Network: Final Rule."

20. Guido Calabresi and Phillip Bobbitt, *Tragic Choices* (New York: Norton, 1978).

21. James F. Childress, *Practical Reasoning in Bioethics* (Bloomington, IN: Indiana University Press, 1997), pp. 230–32.

22. Committee on Organ Procurement and Transplantation Policy, Division of Health Sciences Policy, Institute of Medicine, *Organ Procurement and Transplantation: Assessing Current Policies and the Potential Impact of the DHHS Final Rule* (Washington, DC: National Academy Press, 1999).

23. United Network of Organ Sharing, US Department of Health and Human Services. *1994 Annual Report of the U.S. Scientific Registry for Transplant Recipients and the Organ Procurement and Transplantation Network, Transplant Data: 1988–1993,* pp. v–6-7, passim.

24. Childress, "Some Moral Connections between Organ procurement and Organ Distribution," and *Practical Reasoning in Bioethics*, chaps. 12 & 14.

25. H. G. Welch and E. B. Larson, "Dealing with Limited Resources: The Oregon Decision to Curtail Funding for Organ Transplantation," *New England Journal of Medicine* 319 (1988):171–173.

26. Task Force on Organ Transplantation, *Organ Transplantation: Issues and Recommendations*, pp. 85–86.

27. This paper originated in my testimony before the Joint Hearing of The House
    Commerce Committee Subcommittee on Health and Environment and The Senate
    Labor and Human Resources Committee "Putting Patients First: Resolving Allocation
    of Transplant Organs," June 18, 1998. It benefited from discussions with audiences at
    Yale University and the University of Pittsburgh, spring 1999, before being published
    in the *Cambridge Quarterly of Healthcare Ethics* 10, No. 4 (October 2001): 365–376.
    This chapter, which originated over 20 years ago, has not been updated to address the
    controversies in 2018–2019 about geographical disparities in organ allocation, par-
    ticularly in liver transplantation. The author is currently working on this topic.

PART IV
ETHICS IN PUBLIC
HEALTH POLICY

10
Public Health Ethics
Mapping the Terrain

James F. Childress, Ruth R. Faden, Ruth D. Gaare [Bernheim],
Lawrence O. Gostin, Jeffrey Kahn, Richard J. Bonnie, Nancy E. Kass,
Anna C. Mastroianni, Jonathan D. Moreno, and Phillip Nieburg

Public health ethics, like the field of public health it addresses, traditionally has focused more on practice and particular cases than on theory, with the result that some concepts, methods, and boundaries remain largely undefined. This paper attempts to provide a rough conceptual map of the terrain of public health ethics. We begin by briefly defining public health and identifying general features of the field that are particularly relevant for a discussion of public health ethics.

Public health is primarily concerned with the health of the entire population, rather than the health of individuals. Its features include an emphasis on the promotion of health and the prevention of disease and disability; the collection and use of epidemiological data, population surveillance, and other forms of empirical quantitative assessment; a recognition of the multidimensional nature of the determinants of health; and a focus on the complex interactions of many factors—biological, behavioral, social, and environmental—in developing effective interventions.

How can we distinguish public health from medicine? While medicine focuses on the treatment and cure of individual patients, public health aims to understand and ameliorate the causes of disease and disability in a population. In addition, whereas the physician-patient relationship is at the center of medicine, public health involves interactions and relationships among many professionals and members of the community as well as agencies of government in the development, implementation, and assessment of interventions. From this starting point, we can suggest that public health systems consist of all the people and actions, including laws, policies, practices, and activities, that have the primary purpose of protecting and improving the health of the public.[1] While we need not assume that public health systems are tightly structured or centrally directed, we recognize that they include a wide range of governmental, private and non-profit organizations, as well as professionals from many disciplines, all of which (alone and together) have a stake in and an effect on a community's health. Government has a unique role in public health because of its responsibility, grounded in its police powers, to protect the public's health and welfare, because it alone can undertake certain interventions, such as regulation, taxation, and the expenditure of public funds, and because many, perhaps most, public health programs are public goods that cannot be optimally provided if left to individuals or small groups.

The Institute of Medicine's landmark 1988 definition of public health provides additional insight: "Public health is what we, as a society, do collectively to assure the conditions in which people can be healthy."[2] The words "what we, as a society, do collectively" suggest the need for cooperative behavior and relationships built on overlapping values and trust. The words "to assure the conditions in which people can be healthy" suggest a far-reaching agenda for public health that focuses attention not only on the medical needs of individuals, but on fundamental social conditions that affect population levels of morbidity and mortality. From an ethical standpoint, public health activities are generally understood to be teleological (end-oriented) and consequentialist— the health of the public is the primary end that is sought and the primary outcome for measuring success.[3] Defining and measuring "health" is not easy, as we will emphasize below, but, in addition, "public" is a complex concept with at least three dimensions that are important for our discussion of ethics.

First, public can be used to mean the "numerical public," i.e., the target population. In view of public health's goal of producing net health benefits for the population, this meaning of public is very important. In measurement and analysis, the "numerical public" reflects the utilitarian view that each individual counts as one and only one. In this context, ethical analysis focuses on issues in measurement, many of which raise considerations of justice. For example, how should we define a population, how should we compare gains in life expectancy with gains in health-related quality of life, and whose values should be used in making those judgments?

Second, public is what we collectively do through government and public agency—we can call this "political public." Government provides much of the funding for a vast array of public health functions, and public health professionals in governmental roles are the focal point of much collective activity. In the United States, as Lawrence Gostin notes, government "is compelled by its role as the elected representative of the community to act affirmatively to promote the health of the people," even though it "cannot unduly invade individuals' rights in the name of the communal good."[4] The government is a central player in public health because of the collective responsibility it must assume and implement. The state's use of its police powers for public health raises important ethical questions, particularly about the justification and limits of governmental coercion and about its duty to treat all citizens equally in exercising these powers. In a liberal, pluralistic democracy, the justification of coercive policies, as well as other policies, must rest on moral reasons that the public in whose name the policies are carried out could reasonably be expected to accept.[5]

Third, public, defined as what we do collectively in a broad sense, includes all forms of social and community action affecting public health—we can call this "communal public." Ethical analysis on this level extends beyond the political public. People collectively, outside of government and with private funds, often have greater freedom to undertake public health interventions since they do not have to justify their actions to the political public. However, their actions are still subject to various moral requirements, including, for instance, respect for individual autonomy, liberty, privacy and confidentiality, and transparency in disclosure of conflicts of interest.

General Moral Considerations

In providing a map of the terrain of public health ethics, we do not suggest that there is a consensus about the methods and content of public health ethics.[6] Controversies persist about theory and method in other areas of applied or practical ethics, and it should not be surprising that variety also prevails in public health ethics.[7] The terrain of public health ethics includes a loose set of general moral considerations—clusters of moral concepts and norms that are variously called values, principles, or rules—that are arguably relevant to public health. Public health ethics, in part, involves ongoing efforts to specify and to assign weights to these general moral considerations in the context of particular policies, practices, and actions, in order to provide concrete moral guidance.

Recognizing general moral considerations in public health ethics does not entail a commitment to any particular theory or method. What we describe and propose is compatible with several approaches. To take one major example, casuistical reasoning (examining the relevant similarities and differences between cases) is not only compatible with, but indispensable to our conception of public health ethics. Not only do—or should—public health agents examine new situations they confront in light of general moral considerations, but they should also focus on a new situation's relevant similarities to and differences from paradigm or precedent cases—cases that have gained a relatively settled moral consensus. Whether a relatively settled moral consensus is articulated first in a general moral consideration or in precedent cases does not constitute a fundamental issue—both are relevant. Furthermore, some of the precedents may concern how general moral considerations are interpreted, specified, and balanced in some public health activity, especially where conflicts emerge.

Conceptions of morality usually recognize a formal requirement of universalizability in addition to a substantive requirement of attention to human welfare. Whatever language is used, this formal feature requires that we treat similar cases in a similar way. This requirement undergirds casuistical reasoning in morality as well as in law. In public health ethics, for example, any recommendations for an HIV screening policy must take into account both past precedents in screening for other infectious diseases and the precedents the new policy will create for, say, screening for genetic conditions. Much of the moral argument will hinge on which similarities and differences between cases are morally relevant, and that argument will often, though not always, appeal to general moral considerations.[8] We can establish the relevance of a set of these considerations in part by looking at the kinds of moral appeals that public health agents make in deliberating about and justifying their actions as well as at debates about moral issues in public health. The relevant general moral considerations include:

- producing benefits;
- avoiding, preventing, and removing harms;
- producing the maximal balance of benefits over harms and other costs (often called utility);

- distributing benefits and burdens fairly (distributive justice) and ensuring public participation, including the participation of affected parties (procedural justice);
- respecting autonomous choices and actions, including liberty of action;
- protecting privacy and confidentiality;
- keeping promises and commitments;
- disclosing information as well as speaking honestly and truthfully (often grouped under transparency); and
- building and maintaining trust.

Several of these general moral considerations—especially benefiting others, preventing and removing harms, and utility—provide a prima facie warrant for many activities in pursuit of the goal of public health. It is sufficient for our purposes to note that public health activities have their grounding in general moral considerations, and that public health identifies one major broad benefit that societies and governments ought to pursue. The relation of public health to the whole set of general moral considerations is complex. Some general moral considerations support this pursuit; institutionalizing several others may be a condition for or means to public health (we address this point later when we discuss human rights and public health); and yet, in particular cases, some of the same general moral considerations may limit or constrain what may be done in pursuit of public health. Hence, conflicts may occur among these general moral considerations.

The content of these various general moral considerations can be divided and arranged in several ways—for instance, some theories may locate one or more of these concepts under others. But, whatever theory one embraces, the whole set of general moral considerations roughly captures the moral content of public health ethics. It then becomes necessary to address several practical questions. First, how can we make these general moral considerations more specific and concrete in order to guide action? Second, how can we resolve conflicts among them? Some of the conflicts will concern how much weight and significance to assign to the ends and effects of protecting and promoting public health relative to the other considerations that limit and constrain ways to pursue such outcomes. While each general moral consideration may limit and constrain public health activities in some circumstances, for our purposes, justice or fairness, respect for autonomy and liberty, and privacy and confidentiality are particularly noteworthy in this regard.

Specifying and Weighting General Moral Considerations

We do not present a universal public health ethic. Although arguably these general moral considerations find support in various societies and cultures, an analysis of the role of cultural context in public health ethics is beyond the scope of this paper. Instead, we focus here on public health ethics in the particular setting of the United States, with its traditions, practices, and legal and constitutional requirements, all of which set directions for and circumscribe public health ethics. (Below we will indicate how this conception of public health ethics relates to human rights.)

General moral considerations have two major dimensions. One is their meaning and range or scope; the other is their weight or strength. The first determines the extent of conflict among them—if their range or scope is interpreted in certain ways, conflicts may be increased or reduced. The second dimension determines when different considerations yield to others in cases of conflict.

Specifying the meaning and range or scope of general moral considerations—the first dimension—provides increasingly concrete guidance in public health ethics. A common example is specifying respect for autonomy by rules of voluntary, informed consent. However, it would be a mistake to suppose that respect for autonomy requires consent in all contexts of public health or to assume that consent alone sufficiently specifies the duty to respect autonomy in public health settings. Indeed, specifying the meaning and scope of general moral considerations entails difficult moral work. Nowhere is this more evident in public health ethics than with regard to considerations of justice. Explicating the demands of justice in allocating public health resources and in setting priorities for public health policies, or in determining whom they should target, remains among the most daunting challenges in public health ethics.

The various general moral considerations are not absolute. Each may conflict with another and each may have to yield in some circumstances. At most, then, these general moral considerations identify features of actions, practices, and policies that make them prima facie or presumptively right or wrong, i.e., right or wrong, all other things being equal. But since any particular action, practice, or policy for the public's health may also have features that infringe one or more of these general moral considerations, it will be necessary to determine which of them has priority. Some argue for a lexical or serial ordering, in which one general moral consideration, while not generally absolute, has priority over another. For instance, one theory might hold that protecting or promoting public health always has priority over privacy, while another might hold that individual liberty always has priority over protecting or promoting public health. Neither of these priority rules is plausible, and any priority rule that is plausible will probably involve tight or narrow specifications of the relevant general moral considerations to reduce conflicts. From our standpoint, it is better to recognize the need to balance general moral considerations in particular circumstances when conflicts arise. We cannot determine their weights in advance, only in particular contexts that may affect their weights—for instance, promises may not have the same moral weights in different contexts.

Resolving Conflicts among General Moral Considerations

We do not believe it is possible to develop an algorithm to resolve all conflicts among general moral considerations. Such conflicts can arise in multiple ways. For example, it is common in public health practice and policy for conflicts to emerge between privacy and justice (for instance, the state collects and records private information in disease registries about individuals in order to allocate and provide access to resources for appropriate prevention and treatment services), or between different conceptions of justice (for instance, a government with a finite public health budget must decide whether to dedicate resources to vaccination or to treatment of conditions when they arise). In this paper, however, we focus on one particular permutation of conflicts among general moral considerations that has received the most attention in commentary and in law. This is the conflict between the general moral considerations that are generally taken to instantiate the goal of public health—producing benefits, preventing harms, and maximizing utility—and those that express other moral commitments. For conflicts that assume this structure, we propose five "justificatory conditions": effectiveness, proportionality, necessity, least infringement, and public justification. These conditions are intended to help determine whether promoting public health warrants overriding such values as individual liberty or justice in particular cases.

Effectiveness: It is essential to show that infringing one or more general moral considerations will probably protect public health. For instance, a policy that infringes one or more general moral considerations in the name of public health but has little chance of realizing its goal is ethically unjustified.

Proportionality: It is essential to show that the probable public health benefits outweigh the infringed general moral considerations—this condition is sometimes called proportionality. For instance, the policy may breach autonomy or privacy and have undesirable consequences. All of the positive features and benefits must be balanced against the negative features and effects.

Necessity: Not all effective and proportionate policies are necessary to realize the public health goal that is sought. The fact that a policy will infringe a general moral consideration provides a strong moral reason to seek an alternative strategy that is less morally troubling. This is the logic of a prima facie or presumptive general moral consideration. For instance, all other things being equal, a policy that provides incentives for persons with tuberculosis to complete their treatment until cured will have priority over a policy that forcibly detains such persons in order to ensure the completion of treatment. Proponents of the forcible strategy have the burden of moral proof. This means that the proponents must have a good faith belief, for which they can give supportable reasons, that a coercive approach is necessary. In many contexts, this condition does not require that proponents provide empirical evidence by actually trying the alternative measures and demonstrating their failure.[9]

Least infringement: Even when a proposed policy satisfies the first three justificatory conditions—that is, it is effective, proportionate, and essential in realizing the goal of public health—public health agents should seek to minimize the infringement of general moral considerations. For instance, when a policy infringes autonomy, public health agents should seek the least restrictive alternative; when it infringes privacy, they should seek the least intrusive alternative; and when it infringes confidentiality, they should disclose only the amount and kind of information needed, and only to those necessary, to realize the goal.[10] The justificatory condition of least infringement could plausibly be interpreted as a corollary of necessity—for instance, a proposed coercive measure must be necessary in degree as well as in kind.

Public justification: When public health agents believe that one of their actions, practices, or policies infringes one or more general moral considerations, they also have a responsibility, in our judgment, to explain and justify that infringement, whenever possible, to the relevant parties, including those affected by the infringement. In the context of what we called "political

Degree of Voluntariness

		Voluntary	Mandatory
Extent of Screening	Universal	1	2
	Selective	3	4

Figure 10.1 Features of Public Health Screening Programs

public," public health agents should offer public justification for policies in terms that fit the overall social contract in a liberal, pluralistic democracy. This transparency stems in part from the requirement to treat citizens as equals and with respect by offering moral reasons, which in principle they could find acceptable, for policies that infringe general moral considerations. Transparency is also essential to creating and maintaining public trust; and it is crucial to establishing accountability. (Below we elaborate a process-oriented approach to public accountability that goes beyond public justification to include, as an expression of justice and fairness, input from the relevant affected parties in the formulation of policy.)

Screening Program Example

An extended example may illustrate how these moral justificatory conditions function in public health ethics. Let us suppose that public health agents are considering whether to implement a screening program for HIV infection, tuberculosis, another infectious or contagious disease, or a genetic condition (see Figure 10.1 for some morally relevant features of screening programs).

The relevant justificatory conditions will require public health agents to consider whether any proposed program will be likely to realize the public health goal that is sought (effectiveness), whether its probable benefits will outweigh the infringed general moral considerations (proportionality), whether the policy is essential to realize the end (necessity), whether it involves the least infringement possible consistent with realizing the goal that is sought (least infringement), and whether it can be publicly justified. These conditions will give priority to selective programs over universal ones if the selective programs will realize the goal (as we note below, questions may arise about universality within selected categories, such as pregnant women), and to voluntary programs over mandatory ones if the voluntary programs will realize the goal.[11]

Different screening programs may fail close scrutiny in light of one or more of these conditions. For instance, neither mandatory nor voluntary universal screening for HIV infection can meet these conditions in the society as a whole. Some voluntary and some mandatory selective screening programs for HIV infection can be justified, while others cannot. Mandatory screening of donated blood, organs, sperm, and ova is easily justified, and screening of individuals may also be justified in some settings where they can expose others to bodily fluids and potential victims cannot protect themselves. The question of whether and under what conditions screening of pregnant women for HIV infection should be instituted has been particularly controversial. Even before the advent of effective treatment for HIV infection and the identification of zidovudine (AZT) as effective in reducing the rate of perinatal transmission, there were calls for mandatory screening of pregnant women, especially in "high risk" communities. These calls were defeated by sound arguments that such policies entailed unjustifiable violations of autonomy, privacy, and justice.[12] In effect, the recommended policies failed to satisfy any of the justificatory conditions we have proposed here.

However, once it was established that zidovudine could interrupt maternal-fetal transmission of HIV, the weight of the argument shifted in the direction of instituting screening programs of some type. The focus of the debate became the tensions between the public health interests in utility and efficiency, which argued for mandatory, selective screening in high-risk communities, and considerations of liberty, privacy, and justice, which argued for voluntary, universal screening.[13]

In many situations, the most defensible public health policy for screening and testing expresses community rather than imposes it. Imposing community involves mandating or compelling testing through coercive measures. By contrast, expressing community involves taking steps to express solidarity with individuals, to protect their interests, and to gain their trust. Expressing community may include, for example, providing communal support, disclosing adequate information, protecting privacy and confidentiality, and encouraging certain choices. This approach seeks to make testing a reasonable, and perhaps moral, choice for individuals, especially by engendering public trust, rather than making it compulsory. Several diseases that might be subjected to screening for public health reasons involve stigma, and breaches of privacy and confidentiality may put individuals' employment and insurance at risk. Expressing community is often an appropriate strategy for public health, and, ceteris paribus, it has priority over imposing community through coercive policies.

Processes of Public Accountability

Our discussion of the fifth justificatory condition—public justification—focused on providing public reasons for policies that infringe general moral considerations; this condition is particularly applicable in the political context. While public accountability includes public justification, it is broader—it is prospective as well as retrospective. It involves soliciting input from the relevant publics (the numerical, political, and communal publics) in the process of formulating public health policies, practices, and actions, as well as justifying to the relevant publics what is being undertaken. This is especially, but not only, important when one of the other prima facie general moral considerations is infringed, as with coercive protective measures to prevent epidemics. At a minimum, public accountability involves transparency in openly seeking information from those affected and in honestly disclosing relevant information to the public; it is indispensable for engendering and sustaining public trust, as well as for expressing justice.[14]

Public accountability regarding health promotion or priority-setting for public health funding additionally might involve a more developed fair process. Noting that in a pluralistic society we are likely to find disagreement about which principles should govern issues such as priority-setting in health care, Norman Daniels calls for a fair process that includes the following elements: transparency and publicity about the reasons for a decision; appeals to rationales and evidence that fair-minded parties would agree are relevant; and procedures for appealing and revising decisions in light of challenges by various stakeholders. He explains why this process can facilitate social learning: "Since we may not be able to construct principles that yield fair decisions ahead of time, we need a process that allows us to develop those reasons over time as we face real cases."[15]

Public accountability also involves acknowledging the more complex relationship between public health and the public, one that addresses fundamental issues such as those involving characterization of risk and scientific uncertainty. Because public health depends for its success on the satisfaction of deeply personal health goals of individuals and groups in the population, concepts such as "health" and "risk" cannot be understood or acted upon on the basis of a priori, formal definitions or scientific analysis. Public account-ability recognizes that the fundamental conceptualization of these terms is a critical part of the basic formulation of public health goals and problems to be addressed. This means that the public, along with scientific experts, plays an important role in the analysis of public health issues, as well as in the development and assessment of appropriate strategies for addressing them.

Risk characterization provides a helpful example. A National Research Council report, *Understanding Risk: Informing Decisions in a Democratic Society*, concluded that risk characterization is not properly understood if defined only as a summary of scientific information; rather, it is the out-come of a complex analytic-deliberative process—"a decision-driven ac-tivity, directed toward informing choices and solving problems."[16] The report explains that scientific analysis, which uses rigorous, replicable methods, brings new information into the process, and that deliberation helps to frame analysis by posing new questions and new ways of formulating problems, with the result that risk characterization is the output of a recursive process, not a linear one, and is a decision-driven activity.

Assessment of the health risks of dioxin illustrates this process. While sci-entific analysis provides information about the dose-response relationship between dioxin exposure and possible human health effects, public health focuses on the placement of waste incinerators and community issues in which dioxin is only one of many hazardous chemicals involved and cancer only one of many outcomes of concern. The critical point is that good risk characterization results from a process that "not only gets the science right," but also "gets the right science."[17]

Public health accountability addresses the responsibility of public health agents to work with the public and scientific experts to identify, define, and understand at a fundamental level the threats to public health, and the risks and benefits of ways to address them. The appropriate level of public involve-ment in the analytic-deliberative process depends on the particular public health problem.

Public accountability requires an openness to public deliberation and imposes an obligation on decision-makers to provide honest information and justifications for their decisions. No ethical principle can eliminate the fact that individual interests must sometimes yield to collective needs. Public accountability, however, ensures that such trade-offs will be made openly, with an explicit acknowledgment that individuals' fundamental well-being and values are at stake and that reasons, grounded in ethics, will be

		Adverse Effects of Individuals' Actions	
		Self-regarding	Other-regarding
Voluntariness of Individuals' Actions	Voluntary	1	2
	Non-voluntary	3	4

Figure 10.2 Types of Individual Action

provided to those affected by the decisions.[18] It provides a basis for public trust, even when policies infringe or appear to infringe some general moral considerations.

Public Health Interventions vs. Paternalistic Interventions

An important empirical, conceptual, and normative issue in public health ethics is the relationship between protecting and promoting the health of individuals and protecting and promoting public health. Although public health is directed to the health of populations, the indices of population health, of course, include an aggregation of the health of individuals. But suppose the primary reason for some restrictions on the liberties of individuals is to prevent harm to those whose actions are substantially voluntary and do not affect others adversely. The ethical question then is, when can paternalistic interventions (defined as interventions designed to protect or benefit individuals themselves against their express wishes) be ethically justified if they infringe general moral considerations such as respect for autonomy, including liberty of action?

Consider the chart in Figure 10.2: An individual's actions may be substantially voluntary (competent, adequately informed, and free of controlling influences) or non-voluntary (incompetent, inadequately informed, or subject to controlling influences). In addition, those actions may be self-regarding (the adverse effects of the actions fall primarily on the individual himself or herself) or other-regarding (the adverse effects of the actions fall primarily on others).

Paternalism in a morally interesting and problematic sense arises in the first quadrant (marked by the number "1" in Figure 10.2)—where the individual's actions are both voluntary and self-regarding. According to John Stuart Mill, whose *On Liberty* has inspired this chart, other-regarding conduct not only affects others adversely, but also affects them directly and without "their free, voluntary, and undeceived consent and participation."[19] If others, in the maturity of their faculties, consent to an agent's imposition of risk, then the agent's actions are not other-regarding in Mill's sense.

Whether an agent's other-regarding conduct is voluntary or non-voluntary, the society may justifiably intervene in various ways, including the use of coercion, to reduce or prevent the imposition of serious risk on others. Societal intervention in non-voluntary self-regarding conduct is considered weak (or soft) paternalism, if it is paternalistic at all, and it is easily justified. By contrast, societal interference in voluntary self-regarding conduct would be strong (or hard) paternalism. Coercive intervention in the name of strong paternalism would be insulting and disrespectful to individuals because it would override their voluntary actions for their own benefit, even though their actions do not harm others. Such interventions are thus very difficult to justify in a liberal, pluralistic democracy.

Because of this difficulty, proponents of public health sometimes contend that the first quadrant is really a small class of cases because individuals' risky actions are, in most cases, other-regarding or non-voluntary, or both. Thus, they insist, even if we assume that strong or hard paternalism cannot be ethically justified, the real question is whether most public health interventions in personal life plans and risk budgets are paternalistic at all, at least in the morally problematic sense.

To a great extent, the question is where we draw the boundaries of the self and its actions; that is, whether various influences on agents so determine their actions that they are not voluntary, and whether the adverse effects of those actions extend beyond the agents themselves. Such boundary drawing involves empirical, conceptual, and normative questions that demand attention in public health ethics. On the one hand, it is not sufficient to show that social-cultural factors influence an individual's actions; it is necessary to show that those influences render that individual's actions substantially non-voluntary and warrant societal interventions to protect him or her. Controversies about the strong influence of food marketing on diet and weight (and, as a result, on the risk of disease and death) illustrate the debates about this condition.

On the other hand, it is not sufficient to show that an individual's actions have some adverse effects on others; it is necessary to show that those adverse effects on others are significant enough to warrant overriding the individual's liberty. Controversies about whether the state should require motorcyclists to wear helmets illustrate the debates about this condition. These controversies also show how the inclusion of the financial costs to society and the emotional costs to, say, observers and rescue squads can appear to make virtually any intervention non-paternalistic. But even if these adverse financial and emotional effects on others are morally relevant as a matter of social utility, it would still be necessary to show that they are significant enough to justify the intervention.

Either kind of attempt to reduce the sphere of autonomous, self-regarding actions, in order to warrant interventions in the name of public health, or, more broadly, social utility, can sometimes be justified, but either attempt must be subjected to careful scrutiny. Sometimes both may represent rationalization and bad faith as public health agents seek to evade the stringent demands of the general moral consideration of respect for autonomy. Requiring consistency across an array of cases may provide a safeguard against rationalization and bad faith, particularly when motives for intervention may be mixed.

Much of this debate reflects different views about whether and when strong paternalistic interventions can be ethically justified. In view of the justificatory conditions identified earlier, relevant factors will include the nature of the intervention, the degree to which it infringes an individual's fundamental values, the magnitude of the risk to the individual apart from the intervention (either in terms of harm or lost benefit), and so forth. For example, even though the authors of this paper would disagree about some cases, we agree that strong paternalistic interventions that do not threaten individuals' core values and that will probably protect them against serious risks are more easily justifiable than strong paternalistic interventions that threaten individuals' core values and that will reduce only minor risks. Of course, evaluating actual and proposed policies that infringe general moral considerations becomes very complicated when both paternalistic and public health reasons exist for, and are intertwined in, those policies.

Social Justice, Human Rights, and Health

We have noted potential and actual conflicts between promoting the good of public health and other general moral considerations. But it is important not to exaggerate these conflicts. Indeed, the societal institutionalization of other general moral considerations in legal rights and social-cultural practices generally contributes to public health. Social injustices expressed in poverty, racism, and sexism have long been implicated in conditions of poor health. In recent years, some evidence suggests that societies that embody more egalitarian conceptions of socioeconomic justice have higher levels of health than ones that do not.[20] Public health activity has traditionally encompassed much more than medicine and health care. Indeed, historically much of the focus of public health has been on the poor and on the impact of squalor and sanitation on health. The focus today on the social determinants of health is in keeping with this tradition. The data about social determinants are impressive even though not wholly uncontroversial. At any rate, they are strong enough to warrant close attention to the ways conditions of social justice contribute to the public's health.

Apart from social justice, some in public health argue that embodying several other general moral considerations, especially as articulated in human rights, is consistent with and may even contribute to public health. For example, Jonathan Mann contended that public health officials now have two fundamental responsibilities—protecting and promoting public health and protecting and promoting human rights. Sometimes public health programs burden human rights, but human rights violations "have adverse effects on physical, mental, and social well-being" and "promoting and protecting human rights is inextricably linked with promoting and protecting health."[21] Mann noted, and we concur, that, ultimately, "ethics and human rights derive from a set of quite similar, if not identical, core values," several of which we believe are captured in our loose set of general moral considerations.[22] Often, as we have suggested, the most effective ways to protect public health respect general moral considerations rather than violate them, employ voluntary measures rather than coercive ones, protect privacy and confidentiality, and, more generally, express rather than impose community. Recognizing that promoting health and respecting other general moral considerations or human rights may be mutually supportive can enable us to create policies that avoid or at least reduce conflicts.

While more often than not public health and human rights—or general moral considerations not expressed in human rights—do not conflict and may even be synergistic, conflicts do sometimes arise and require resolution.[23] Sometimes, in particular cases, a society cannot simultaneously realize its commitments to public health and to certain other general moral considerations, such as liberty, privacy, and confidentiality. We have tried to provide elements of a framework for thinking through and resolving such conflicts. This process needs to be transparent in order to engender and sustain public trust.

Acknowledgments

This work was supported by a grant from The Greenwall Foundation. Other project participants were John D. Arras and Paul A. Lombardo, both of the University of Virginia, and Donna T. Chen of the National Institute of Mental Health and Department of Bioethics, National Institutes of Health.

Notes

1. Our definition builds on the definition of health systems offered by the World Health Organization: Health systems include "all the activities whose primary purpose is to promote, restore, or maintain health." See *World Health Report 2000 Health Systems: Improving Performance* (Geneva: World Health Organization, 2000), p. 5.
2. Committee for the Study of the Future of Public Health, Division of Health Care Services, Institute of Medicine, *The Future of Public Health* (Washington, D.C.: National Academy Press, 1988), p. 1.
3. We recognize that there are different views about the ultimate moral justification for the social institution of public health. For example, some communitarians appear to support public health as an instrumental goal to achieve community. Others may take the view that the state has a duty to ensure the public's health as a matter of social justice. Although these different interpretations and others are very important for some purposes, they do not seriously affect the conception of public health ethics that we are developing, as long as public health agents identify and inform others of their various goals.
4. L.O. Gostin, *Public Health Law: Power, Duty, Restraint* (Berkeley: University of California Press; New York: The Milbank Memorial Fund, 2000), p. 20.
5. T. Nagel, "Moral Epistemology," in R.E. Bulger, E.M. Bobby, and H.V. Fineberg, eds., Committee on the Social and Ethical Impacts of Developments in Biomedicine, Division of Health Sciences Policy, Institute of Medicine, *Society's Choices: Social and Ethical Decision Making in Biomedicine* (Washington, D.C.: National Academy Press, 1995), pp. 201–14.
6. For some other approaches, see P. Nieburg, R. Gaare-Bernheim, and R. Bonnie, "Ethics and the Practice of Public Health," in R.A. Goodman et al., eds., *Law in Public Health Practice* (New York: Oxford University Press, 2003), and N.E. Kass, "An Ethics Framework for Public Health," *American Journal of Public Health* 91 (2001): 1776–82.
7. We do not explore here the overlaps among public health ethics, medical ethics, research ethics, and public policy ethics, although some areas of overlap and difference will be evident throughout the discussion. Further work is needed to address some public health activities that fall within overlapping areas—for instance, surveillance, outbreak investigations, and community-based interventions may sometimes raise issues in the ethics of research involving human subjects.

8. Recognizing universalizability by attending to past precedents and possible future precedents does not preclude a variety of experiments, for instance, to determine the best ways to protect the public's health. Thus, it is not inappropriate for different states, in our federalist system, to try different approaches, as long as each of them is morally acceptable.

9. This justificatory condition is probably the most controversial. Some of the authors of this paper believe that the language of "necessity" is too strong. Whatever language is used, the point is to avoid a purely utilitarian strategy that accepts only the first two conditions of effectiveness and proportionality and to ensure that the non-utilitarian general moral considerations set some prima facie limits and constraints and establish moral priorities, ceteris paribus.

10. For another version of these justificatory conditions, see T.L. Beauchamp and J.F. Childress, *Principles of Biomedical Ethics*, 5th ed. (New York: Oxford University Press, 2001), pp. 19–21. We observe that some of these justificatory conditions are quite similar to the justificatory conditions that must be met in U.S. constitutional law when there is strict scrutiny because, for instance, a fundamental liberty is at stake. In such cases, the government must demonstrate that it has a "compelling interest," that its methods are strictly necessary to achieve its objectives, and that it has adopted the "least restrictive alternative." See Gostin, supra note 4, at 80–81.

11. Of course, this chart is oversimplified, particularly in identifying only voluntary and mandatory options. For a fuller discussion, see R. Faden, M. Powers, and N. Kass, "Warrants for Screening Programs: Public Health, Legal and Ethical Frameworks," in R. Faden, G. Geller, and M. Powers, eds., *AIDS, Women and the Next Generation* (New York: Oxford University Press, 1991), pp. 3–26.

12. Working Group on HIV Testing of Pregnant Women and Newborns, "HIV Infection, Pregnant Women, and Newborns," *Journal of the American Medical Association* 264, no. 18 (1990): 2416–20.

13. See Faden, Geller, and Powers, supra note 11; Gostin, supra note 4, at 199–201.

14. In rare cases, it may be ethically justifiable to limit the disclosure of some information for a period of time (for example, when there are serious concerns about national security; about the interpretation, certainty, or reliability of public health data; or about the potential negative effects of disclosing the information, such as with suicide clusters).

15. N. Daniels, "Accountability for Reasonableness," *British Medical Journal* 321 (2000): 1300–01, at 1301.

16. P.C. Stern and H.V. Fineberg, eds., Committee on Risk Characterization, Commission on Behavioral and Social Sciences and Education, National Research Council, *Understanding Risk: Informing Decisions in a Democratic Society* (Washington, D.C.: National Academy Press, 1996): at 155.

17. *Ibid.* at 16–17, 156.

18. See, for example, N. Daniels and J. Sabin, "Limits to Health Care: Fair Procedures, Democratic Deliberation, and the Legitimacy Problem for Insurers," *Philosophy and Public Affairs* 26 (Fall 1997): 303–50, at 350.

19. J.S. Mill, *On Liberty*, ed. G. Himmelfarb (Harmondsworth, England: Penguin Books, 1976): at 71. For this chart, see J.F. Childress, *Who Should Decide? Paternalism in Health Care* (New York: Oxford University Press, 1982), p. 193.

20. See, for example, the discussion in I. Kawachi, B.P. Kennedy, and R.G. Wilkinson, eds., *Income Inequality and Health*, vol. 1 of The Society and Population Health Reader (New York: The New Press, 2000).

21. J.M. Mann, "Medicine and Public Health, Ethics and Human Rights," *The Hastings Center Report* 27 (May–June 1997): 6–13, at 11–12. Contrast Gostin, supra note 4, at 21. For a fuller analysis and assessment of Mann's work, see L.O. Gostin, "Public Health, Ethics, and Human Rights: A Tribute to the Late Jonathan Mann," S.P. Marks, "Jonathan Mann's Legacy to the 21st Century: The Human Rights Imperative for Public Health," and L.O. Gostin, "A Vision of Health and Human Rights for the 21st Century: A Continuing Discussion with Stephen P. Marks," *Journal of Law, Medicine, and Ethics* 29, no. 2 (2001): 121–40.

22. Mann, supra note 21, at 10. Mann thought that the language of ethics could guide individual behavior, while the language of human rights could best guide societal-level analysis and response. See Mann, supra note 21, at 8; Marks, supra note 21, at 131–38. We disagree with this separation and instead note the overlap of ethics and human rights, but we endorse the essence of Mann's position on human rights.

23. See Gostin, supra note 4, at 21.

11

Public Health and Civil Liberties

Resolving Conflicts

Introduction

This chapter considers public health ethics in a particular context—a liberal, pluralistic, democratic society that maintains explicit commitments to several basic civil liberties: bodily integrity, privacy, freedom of movement, freedom of association, and freedom of religion and conscience.[1] In addition to functioning as sociocultural norms, these liberties are embedded in legal and, in some cases, constitutional rights. They are also incorporated into international human rights documents and discourse. Beyond these civil liberties, there are several basic economic liberties, including freedom of contract and uses of property, which this chapter does not address. Nor is this the place to offer a theoretical defense of a liberal, pluralistic, democratic society; I assume this as the context for these reflections about public health ethics.

Examinations of the relations between public health and civil liberties are often framed by one of two major perspectives: conflict or concord. These differ according to whether they hold that conflict between public health and civil liberties is more fundamental and prevalent than their harmony. Of course, both perspectives acknowledge that conflicts do arise between public health and civil liberties, but their starting assumptions differ greatly. One views conflicts as common and inevitable, and trade-offs as unavoidable,[2] while the other views conflicts as occasional, even rare, and trade-offs as generally avoidable.[3] The conflict perspective is also captured in the language of "inherent tensions" between public health and civil liberties "across the spectrum of threats to public health."[4] The concord perspective stresses that respect for civil liberties and rights constitutes an important part of public health policy and practice and is essential for voluntary public cooperation with public health authorities. The dominance of conflict or concord perspectives varies in different sociocultural contexts and over time.

PUBLIC HEALTH AND CIVIL LIBERTIES   253

The perspective of this chapter, which its overall argument supports, is that concord is more basic than conflict. However, difficult conflicts do sometimes erupt, and public health officials, invoking the "police power" of the state, sometimes rightly believe they must restrict civil liberties in order to protect or promote public health. In this chapter, I argue that

- When conflicts do emerge, a presumptivist framework is more defensible and helpful than an absolutist or a contextualist one for determining appropriate public health interventions, some of which may infringe civil liberties.
- The presumptivist framework involves specifying public health ends and goals and viewing civil liberties, also specified, as presumptive directions for and constraints on measures to accomplish those ends and goals.
- The presumptivist framework operates with several conditions for rebutting the presumption, in some circumstances, against interventions that infringe civil liberties.
- Often, rebutting the presumption against infringing civil liberties is not necessary because it is possible to obtain voluntary cooperation and compliance. The metaphor of the Intervention Ladder from the Nuffield Council on Bioethics allows us to explore different ways to secure individuals' cooperation and compliance with public health measures without infringing their civil liberties.

I focus my discussion on a few civil liberties—freedom of movement and association and freedom from intrusions on bodily integrity—and I mainly draw examples from vaccinations, directly observed therapy (DOT) for tuberculosis (TB), and quarantine following probable infectious disease exposure.

Frameworks of Ethical Analysis of Conflicts between Civil Liberties and Public Health

If conflicts emerge between public health and civil liberties, how should they be adjudicated? Among three possible frameworks for adjudication, I argue that a presumptivist framework is preferable to either an absolutist or a contextualist framework.[5]

An absolutist framework holds that a certain value has absolute priority over some or all conflicting values. It is not plausible in public health ethics to take an absolutist approach, whether the absolute value is liberty or public health. Only an extreme libertarian position—verging on anarchism—could assign absolute priority to liberty in the face of, say, a major pandemic that threatens a country's survival. Most libertarians recognize warrants for over-riding liberty in such cases—for instance, David Boaz, an influential liber-tarian, concedes that forcible quarantine, exercised with "great caution, and with appropriate safeguards for due process," appeared to be a "necessary" step in response to the outbreak of SARS (severe acquired respiratory syn-drome) which is known to have infected over 8,000 persons worldwide and killed 775 of them in 2002–2003.[6] Similarly, only an extreme communitarian position—verging on totalitarianism—could assign absolute priority to public health. Most communitarians recognize some liberties as communal values, along with public health and other values.

At the other end of the spectrum is a contextualist approach that refrains from assigning advance weights to either public health goals or civil liber-ties. Instead, it considers all of them equally in particular contexts. The dominant metaphors are "weighing" and "balancing." For instance, Amitai Etzioni holds "that individual rights and social responsibilities, liberty and the common good, have equal standing; that neither should be assumed a priori to trump the other; and that we need to seek a carefully crafted balance between these core values."[7]

It is common for governmental officials to describe their reasoning as *bal-ancing* public health and civil liberties. Often, this focuses on public health and liberty as abstract concepts, as though all public health goals are equally significant and all civil liberties are equally important. Attending to partic-ular contexts offers at least a partial corrective, but this approach still fails to provide an adequate structure for moral reasoning and relies too much on bare intuition. Furthermore, it fails to capture a key commitment of liberal societies to assign presumptive priority to means in public health and else-where that respect civil liberties and voluntary choices. It tends to reduce all judgments to proportionality, failing to see that even policies that pass an overall balancing test still need to be necessary, the least restrictive, the least intrusive, and so forth.

A presumptivist approach, by contrast, requires specification of the public health ends or goals that are sought and then assesses the range of potentially useful and available means. In pursuing public health goals, it starts from a presumption in favor of interventions that respect, and against measures that violate, basic civil liberties. To be sure, this presumption can sometimes be rebutted, but this rebuttal process requires a more precise and nuanced analysis than is available to the contextualist.

The presumptivist framework avoids pitfalls that trouble both absolutist and contextualist approaches. It avoids the extreme and implausible absolutist positions—that public health always trumps liberty/ies or that liberty/ies always trump public health. It is closer in spirit to the contextualist approach but provides a needed and helpful structure for moral reasoning about public health interventions. The presumptivist framework assigns presumptions, starting points, and burdens of proof in deliberation about interventions that could be used to realize the goals of public health. The presumption favors those that do not infringe civil liberties.

Goals of Public Health

The first task in justifying interventions is to identify, specify, and justify the assignment of weights to the goals of public health. Too often "public health" is presented as a univocal and sufficient goal even though it is too broad without further specification. Here I focus on six general types of goals offered as justification for public health interventions.

Public health has historically encompassed actions that individuals cannot perform entirely for themselves, for instance, when collective action is required in public sanitation and in preventing the spread of communicable diseases. The major justification for liberty-limiting interventions is the "harm-to-others principle," presented in John Stuart Mill's *On Liberty*.[8] This principle authorizes the society's intervention into individuals' other-regarding actions, that is, actions that harm others or put them at risk of harm. A version of what Mill calls societal "self-protection" appears in the early 20th century U.S. Supreme Court decision, *Jacobson v. Massachusetts* (1905), which upheld a mandatory vaccination law: "Upon the principle of self-defense, of paramount necessity, a community has the right to protect itself against an epidemic of disease which threatens the safety of its members."[9]

A second goal is protecting people who lack the capacity to protect themselves, even from effects of their own actions.[10] In *On Liberty* Mill gives an example of a person about to cross a dangerous bridge and there is "no time to warn him of his danger." In such a case, Mill said, it would be ethically acceptable to "seize him and turn him back, without any real infringement of his liberty" on the assumption that he does not want to fall into the river.[11] Here a person's lack of information or, as we might broaden this, lack of capacity, combined with the risk to him or her, warrants the intervention. This is a form of weak or soft paternalism that is unobjectionable from the standpoint of civil liberties if it is exercised in good faith.[12]

A third possible goal is protecting an individual's health interests even if she is competent, has adequate information, and voluntarily rejects the intervention on her behalf. This is strong or hard paternalism. Mill argued for an absolute prohibition of coercive interventions in an individual's self-regarding actions, i.e., actions with adverse effects that fall only on the autonomous individual herself or also on others with their consent. Such strong or hard paternalism is very difficult to defend as a warrant for breaches of civil liberties.

A fourth possible goal employs an expanded notion of "harm to others." It rejects Mill's sharp distinction between self-regarding and other-regarding conduct and contends that some apparently paternalistic interventions may be primarily, or at least significantly, aimed at protecting others. Such expansionist views of *public* health hold that in the modern welfare state, so different from Mill's context in the mid-19th century, some apparently self-regarding conduct is now other-regarding in its effects if not in its intention.

Consider the following example: Arguments for mandatory motorcycle helmet laws appear paternalistic in nature, having only the goal of protecting motorcyclists themselves from severe head injuries or death. However, some other arguments focus on the increased risks, burdens, and costs to other individuals and to the society. Such an extension of the harm-to-others principle appears in a Massachusetts court decision:

> From the moment of the injury, society picks the person up off the highway; delivers him to a municipal hospital and municipal doctors; provides him with unemployment compensation if, after recovery, he cannot replace his lost job; and if the injury causes permanent disability many assure the responsibility for his and his family's continued sustenance. We do not

understand a state of mind that permits a plaintiff to think that only he himself is concerned.[13]

A fifth possible goal under the rubric of public health is *population health*. A healthy population is a worthy societal goal in and of itself. It also provides human capital for a more productive society, more capable of competing in the global arena and defending itself from external enemies. Even if individuals' health-damaging actions appear to affect only themselves, they are at the same time depriving society of fully capable and productive citizens. This goal also allows the society to target chronic conditions such as diabetes and/or obesity in its public health programs. Its logic is similar, on a larger scale, to the logic of the expanded "harm-to-others" principle. For instance, after arguing for paternalistic regulation of individuals' conduct in order to protect the individuals themselves, Ronald Bayer adds "because such [paternalistic] efforts can have a broad and enormous impact at a population level."[14] This joins a paternalistic rationale with the societal benefit of population health.

A sixth possible goal also attends to population health but from a distributive rather than an aggregative perspective. This goal, resting on egalitarian conceptions of social justice, involves efforts to close the health gaps between the better off and the worse off in the society. Over the last several decades, for example, this goal has been clearly evident in mandatory vaccination laws, tied to school attendance, that seek to "foster the equitable distribution of the benefits of vaccines, especially among children whose life circumstances make them less likely to be fully immunized."[15]

Of course, it is possible—and common—to combine several of these goals as warrants for policies and practices that limit or override civil liberties. Strong (but not necessarily overriding) unmixed goals, when the proposed interventions conflict with civil liberties, are the first, second, and sixth; the third is the most controversial in a liberal society but has its defenders[16]; the fourth and fifth are commonly invoked but require close attention to the actual effects of individuals' actions on others and on the society before they can override civil liberties. Under these six broad goals, under the rubric of public health, we need to formulate and deliberate about specific, concrete goals.

Justificatory Conditions for Liberty-Limiting Public Health Measures

A presumption in favor of interventions that respect civil liberties in the pursuit of public health goals can be rebutted under some conditions, and it is important to delineate these rebuttal conditions. We can call them *rebuttal conditions* because they specify conditions for rebutting the presumption in favor of respecting specific civil liberties, or we can call them *justificatory conditions* because they specify conditions for justifying infringements of specific civil liberties.[17]

The presumption-rebuttal or justification process occurs in particular contexts when measures that limit, infringe, or violate civil liberties are being considered as possible ways to achieve specific public health goals. The process should be directed at all stakeholders.

The first task of this process, as we noted above, is to specify and weight the public health goals, and so the first rebuttal condition focuses on the following question: Is there a legitimate and important public health end or goal? The other justificatory conditions kick in once there is a specific, legitimate, and important public health goal and some of the possible interventions involve limiting liberties. It is not sufficient merely to assert that public health is at stake. As we have seen, some of the general types of goals are weaker than others in justifying infringements of civil liberties.

Second, would the proposed liberty-limiting measure probably be effective in achieving an important public health goal? If there is no reasonable chance that the liberty-limiting measure—such as forcible quarantine—would achieve its goal, then it is both unwise and unethical. A reasonable prospect of success is a condition for rebutting the presumption in favor of civil liberties of movement and association.

Third, is the proposed liberty-limiting measure necessary? We can imagine circumstances in which liberty-limiting measures, such as forcible quarantine or mandatory vaccination, would be effective but nonetheless ethically unjustifiable because they are not necessary to realize the public health goal being sought. It is often, though not always, possible to secure individuals' voluntary adherence to public health measures without coercion or threat of coercion. Moreover, the logic of presumptive principles or values compels us to seek alternatives before we can justifiably override them. A liberty-limiting measure is necessary only if other measures have failed or have been determined to have no reasonable chance. Only then is it a last resort.

Some frameworks do not include necessity as a justificatory condition, holding instead that it is incorporated into the fifth condition of proportionality. However, it serves as a valuable reminder that consequentialist considerations, such as effectiveness and proportionality, which would also include cost-effectiveness and a wide range of consequences, do not exhaust our moral concerns in public health.

Fourth, is the proposed infringement of liberty the least restrictive or least intrusive means available? In some interpretations, this justificatory condition is simply a corollary of the previous one, necessity. If liberty-limiting measures are necessary, the degree of infringement, as well as the kind of infringement, should be necessary. Nevertheless, it is also useful to consider this condition as a specific requirement of the logic of presumptive principles or values—to minimize the restrictiveness, intrusiveness, and invasiveness of justified infringements, such as infringements of freedom of movement and association and protections of bodily integrity, and to narrow their scope as much as possible. If, for example, public health officials have determined that forcible quarantine is necessary to control a SARS outbreak, they should employ the least restrictive, intrusive, and invasive measures and aim at the narrowest range of possible targets of quarantine consistent with achieving the public health goal being pursued. They might, for instance, select quarantine in home rather than in a hospital or in jail; of course, other factors such as cost will enter into these deliberations too.

Fifth, is the proposed liberty-infringing measure proportionate? From one standpoint, if a proposed limiting-infringing measure is effective, necessary, the least intrusive, etc., then it is proportionate in the sense of being appropriate and fitting.[18] In this chapter, proportionality involves the kind and range of balancing featured in contextualist analyses. It considers not only the probable benefits of the proposed measure, weighed against the relevant liberty interests, but also attends to the probable overall balance of good and harmful short- and long-term effects of the proposed liberty-limiting interventions.

Sixth, is the proposed liberty-limiting measure impartially applied? In a seminar on "Confronting Epidemics: Historical and Contemporary Perspectives," which I co-taught several times with a colleague in law and public health, we were initially surprised to see how often liberty-limiting measures were imposed unfairly, based on race, ethnicity, and social class, among other characteristics. Discrimination based on such characteristics is common in epidemics, particularly in singling out some victims for blame.

In the 2003 SARS outbreak in Canada, Asian persons in Toronto experienced stigmatization and discrimination.[19]

There are concerns that presumptions and rebuttal or justificatory conditions, such as those just delineated, too often stand in the way of effective measures for reaching public health goals. Some advocates for public health worry that these presumptions and rebuttal conditions erect barriers to public health by requiring that liberty-limiting measures pass excessively stringent tests.[20] And yet if the commitment to civil liberties in a liberal, pluralistic, democratic society is meaningful, it at least sets a (rebuttable) presumption against infringements of civil liberties. Moreover, such criticisms fail to note that safeguarding civil liberties regularly goes hand in hand with protecting and promoting public health, in part because of the need for public trust and cooperation. Finally, as I have suggested and elaborate in the next section, respect for civil liberties can often be maintained by persuading or nudging individuals voluntarily to accept and act on public health measures, such as vaccination or quarantine or DOT for TB. Hence, the justificatory conditions compel public health officials to seek measures that may elicit voluntary cooperation before resorting to infringements of civil liberties.

The Intervention Ladder

The metaphor of an Intervention Ladder, introduced by the Nuffield Council on Bioethics,[21] helps us think about a range of interventions that may secure the public's cooperation with public health measures without infringing civil liberties. The interventions higher on this ladder are considered to be more intrusive and thus to require a stronger justification. In line with a presumptivist approach, the justificatory burden increases as higher rungs of the ladder, involving infringements of liberty, are reached. Not every rung is available for every public health measure. My primary examples, as earlier, are vaccinations, DOT for TB, and quarantine for infectious diseases.

Intervention Ladder[22]

8. Eliminate choice
7. Restrict choice
6. Guide choice by disincentives
5. Guide choice by incentives

4. Guide choice by changing the default policy
3. Enable choice
2. Provide information
1. Do nothing

This ladder is not complete, there is overlap among the rungs, and each covers several possible kinds of policies and practices. In some contexts, some of the lower rungs may be unjustifiable for reasons other than infringement of civil liberties—indeed, for the most part, the lower rungs do not infringe civil liberties. Doing nothing—or monitoring the situation (#1)—may seem unproblematic, but if, for example, serious illnesses or deaths are occurring while vaccination rates are being monitored, without any interventions, then it too requires solid ethical justification in view of the risks involved.

Providing accurate and truthful information (#2) also appears ethically unproblematic, whether the goal is to ensure informed choices or to convince citizens and residents to act in certain ways, for instance, to accept certain vaccinations. Ethical issues do arise in efforts to motivate individuals through presenting graphic images, appealing to emotions, stigmatizing conduct, shaming failures to comply with social norms, and the like. Most governments have relied mainly on persuasion and motivation through a variety of educational and advertising campaigns to promote needed vaccinations, but they have employed other interventions as well.

A policy or practice of enabling choices (#3) seeks to secure compliance with public health measures by providing resources or otherwise increasing individuals' capacities to act in certain ways. It does not violate civil liberties to enable people to exercise those liberties in particular ways or to choose to waive their liberties. Enabling choices may involve removing financial, logistical, and other disincentives, obstacles, or barriers. These could be as straightforward as providing free fresh fruit for students or constructing lanes for bicyclists.

Consider the following scenario: public health officials may believe that a particular individual who has TB should be in a DOT program until noncontagious or even cured in order to protect others and to reduce the chances of multidrug resistant TB with its serious risks and huge costs to the individual and the society. It may be possible to secure that individual's compliance by providing vouchers for transportation to a center for DOT along with free care. In this case, the individual's failure to comply may not reflect a lack of will but rather a lack of resources for easy and non-burdensome

compliance. Similarly, programs to increase access to vaccinations and to reduce or eliminate parents' out-of-pocket costs for getting their children vaccinated, according to the recommended schedule, have also been effective.[23]
Such programs do not infringe civil liberties and hence are unobjectionable
from that standpoint.

For some public health measures, it may be possible and ethically justifiable to take another step and to guide individuals' choices by altering defaults
(step #4 on the Intervention Ladder) or using other nudges. This is attrac-
tive because it maintains individuals' liberties while gently pushing their
choices in certain directions. As Richard Thaler and Cass Sunstein argue
in *Nudge: Improving Decisions about Health, Wealth, and Happiness*,[24] a
"nudge" is an aspect of a society's "choice architecture" that seeks to change
what people do without prohibiting any of their options and without significantly modifying their economic incentives. A mere nudge must not be difficult or costly to avoid. Changing the default in an organ donation system
from opt in, as is current in the U.S., England, and Australia, to opt out, as is
common in a number of European countries, selects one nudge over another
in an effort to increase the rates of organ donation. Placing fruit, rather than
less healthy foods such as potato chips, at students' eye level in a school cafeteria counts as a nudge, in contrast to banning junk food altogether from the
choices in the cafeteria.[25]

I briefly consider the role of nudges in one part of mass mandatory immunization programs. It is worth noting that immunization programs in
about half of the countries in the European Union do not have any mandatory
vaccinations, only recommended ones, while the other countries include at
least one mandatory vaccination.[26] Many of the countries only recommending
vaccinations have high coverage nonetheless.[27] Immunization programs
generally aim at herd or population immunity, which does not require universal immunization. Governments that mandate vaccinations generally
exempt some individuals from the requirements. On the one hand, some
children and adults have medical conditions that put them at risk from particular vaccinations; all states in the U.S. recognize medical exemptions.
On the other hand, mandatory vaccination programs threaten another
civil liberty, freedom of religion or, more broadly, freedom of conscience.
Freedom of religious/conscientious action is generally more limited than
freedom of belief. However, in 2019 only five states in the U.S. did not allow
exemptions from immunizations to religious objectors, and fifteen states
also allowed exemptions to persons (or to parents or guardians of minors)

with philosophical, personal, moral, or other objections.[28] In the U.S., such non-medical exemptions are not deemed to be constitutionally required, and they may legitimately be overturned in a declared public health emergency or epidemic.

Not only is there a question about whether non-medical exemptions should be allowed, but there are also questions about how to exempt particular objecting individuals. States have had to consider whether to grant these non-medical exemptions upon request or also to require further steps and formal review. This has become an important question because outbreaks of communicable diseases, particularly pertussis (whooping cough) in some states, have resulted in part from the increased numbers of exemptions.[29] Some states have responded by introducing such formal requirements as an annual written request for exemption followed by a review. The available evidence suggests that such nudges can effectively reduce the number of requests for exemptions.[30] The explanation is simple: parents or guardians whose children have fallen behind on their immunization schedules may find it much easier to request an exemption, in the absence of nudges and slight hurdles, than to complete the immunizations. These nudges and slight hurdles may also serve as a limited test of objectors' sincerity. In any event, they represent only minor and justifiable encumbrances of freedom of religion and freedom of conscience without violating those fundamental civil liberties.

Nudges work for several reasons.[31] One factor is the cost of acting against the nudges, for instance, by taking the non-default option, especially when the default option is recommended by public health officials and is considered socially normative. However, to count as a mere nudge, an option's cognitive, psychological, or other costs must be insignificant. If they are significant, then #4 is indistinguishable from #5 and #6, guiding individuals' choices by incentives or by disincentives. To return to our example of ensuring adherence to DOT by a person with TB, providing vouchers for transportation (an instance of #3) may not be sufficient to secure his or her compliance. It may also be possible and desirable to provide incentives, such as additional money, to motivate compliance. A small incentive, such as money for an inexpensive lunch, could count as a nudge whereas a more substantial amount would fall under #5.

What evidence do we have for the effectiveness of incentives? The Community Preventive Services Task Force, a body of independent, non-federal, unpaid experts in prevention and public health, established by the U.S. Department of Health and Human Services, looked at studies from Australia and the United States of the use of several types of positive incentives, which it labels "incentive rewards," for vaccinations: one time payments; child care assistance; lottery prizes (grocery vouchers and monetary prizes); gift cards (for baby products); and food vouchers and baby products.[32] It concludes, based on the solid evidence of effectiveness of such incentive rewards in increasing the vaccination rates of both adults and children, that there is warrant to recommend their use either alone or conjoined with other interventions.[33]

According to some critics, incentives, especially larger and more significant incentives, are potentially coercive. For instance, one such critic objects to paying people to take care of their health: "Cash might coerce some people into changing behavior . . . ."[34] By contrast, I take the view that providing incentives is not coercive because it expands rather than restricts personal options.[35] However, providing incentives still needs ethical scrutiny in order to avoid either exploitation or undue inducement and in order not to stigmatize disadvantaged persons through cash transfers conditional on their behavioral changes.

Some critics point to incentives' deeper potential harms to individuals (and ultimately to public health). Incentives target individuals' conduct, usually in the short run, but may damage their overall motivational structure and character in the long run. Hence, these critics sound a strong cautionary note.[36] Sometimes, however, it is important to achieve short-term public health goals through altering conduct—for instance, using incentives to get individuals to undergo DOT or to receive vaccinations—even if their motivational structure or character is not improved and perhaps even slightly damaged. Claims of character damage through such incentives are difficult if not impossible to substantiate. As a result, we can make judgments about effectiveness and cost-effectiveness, in light of an important public health goal, but judgments of proportionality will be incomplete because of missing information and evidence about possible threats to character.

The final three rungs on the Intervention Ladder introduce more liberty-limiting and coercive policies than the ones below them; they thus stand in greater tension with civil liberties. Policies at rung #6 on the Intervention Ladder significantly shape individuals' choices through the imposition of disincentives, including but not limited to financial disincentives. Substantially increasing taxes on harmful products, such as cigarettes, is one example. Another is fining people who seek to avoid mandatory vaccinations. In *Jacobson v. Massachusetts* (1905), the U.S. Supreme Court upheld Massachusetts' imposition of a fine for failing to accept a vaccination in a smallpox outbreak and imposition of a jail term for failing to pay the fine.[37]

Despite *Jacobson*, vaccination policy in the U.S. has historically relied mainly on persuasion rather than coercion. However, in the late 1960s efforts to eradicate—and not merely to control—infectious disease, in the context of a campaign against measles, more states adopted laws requiring children to be immunized in order to attend school.[38] These laws, which had already been upheld by the U.S. Supreme Court in 1922, represent a significant non-monetary disincentive or sanction to ensure the vaccination of school-age children; they may also have monetary effects if parents have to resort to home schooling. Even so, the assumption was that parents are basically willing to have their children vaccinated but may need this "special stimulus."[39] Moreover, the use of school attendance laws to ensure vaccinations was based in part on the egalitarian value of increasing children's access to conditions for healthy lives. Some supporters viewed these laws "as a kind of societal safety net to catch the children of the 'hard to reach.' "[40] The laws also had the benefit of protecting other children in interactions at school.

More problematic is applying certain monetary disincentives or sanctions when parents or guardians do not adhere to the official public health schedule for children's vaccinations. Particularly troubling is withholding or reducing food vouchers (e.g., providing food vouchers for one month rather than for three months) or other welfare benefits to families, thus potentially damaging children's health by reducing their available nutrition. Even though a few studies indicate that such financial disincentives or sanctions may be somewhat effective in the short term,[41] critics have rightly challenged them as unfair and potentially harmful to children.[42] Even their effectiveness is not clear cut. Based on its review of a range of recent studies, the Community Preventive Services Task Force found "insufficient evidence to determine the effectiveness of monetary sanction policies to increase vaccination rates in children of families on government assistance." [43] The finding of "insufficient evidence" reflects the limited number of studies testing different sanctions and reaching inconsistent results. The Community Preventive Services Task Force also noted the "limited information on potential harms of these policies."[44]

Starting from a baseline of eligibility for food vouchers or other welfare benefits for preschool-aged children and then threatening to stop those benefits in an effort to motivate parental or guardian behavior is arguably un-fair and harmful to the children as well as coercive to the parents or guardians. It may be unreasonable to reject such sanctions altogether, but they should be used, in line with our justificatory conditions, only as a last resort when persuasion, removal of disincentives, provision of positive incentives, and nudges fail to work, and only when children's nutritional status and other health indices can be maintained.

The final two rungs (#7 and #8) of the Intervention Ladder involve restricting choice or eliminating choice. Examples of restricting choice in-clude legal requirements that food producers remove certain unhealthy ingredients from their food products and former New York City Mayor Michael Bloomberg's proposed ban on the sale of sugared drinks over 16 ounces in certain settings. Both would make it more difficult, to different degrees, for consumers to partake of unhealthy foods. Some of what we discussed under #6 related to disincentives and sanctions for vaccinations would also fall here, for instance, not allowing children to attend school if they have not been vaccinated.

Step #8 goes farther to eliminate choice, sometimes even by forcible con-finement. An obvious example is forcibly quarantining individuals who have been exposed to certain communicable diseases, such as SARS, and who do not voluntarily comply with a quarantine order. Another example is forcibly detaining a person with TB who, after efforts to secure his or her cooperation with DOT, still refuses to adhere to the protocol. Among infringements of civil liberties, forcible detention, as a restriction of free movement and asso-ciation, is easier to justify than forcible administration of the required med-ication through an invasion of the uncooperative person's body. Indeed, the Nuffield Council of Bioethics indicates that it is "not aware of any countries that go so far as to force individuals to be vaccinated."[45]

Some public health measures on the final three rungs of the Intervention Ladder are or may be coercive. In general, they need to pass a higher bar of justification because of their threats to civil liberties. But they can sometimes meet our several justificatory conditions and thus rebut the presumption against their use. Often, however, interventions that stop short of coercion can secure individuals' cooperation without violating their liberties. In such cases individuals voluntarily comply with the recommended public health meas-ures, such as quarantine, vaccinations, or DOT, whatever their motivations for doing so as a result of other interventions. These interventions, as we have seen, may not be objectionable from the standpoint of civil liberties themselves, but they may raise other ethical issues that need attention and resolution in particular circumstances.

Conclusion

In conclusion, we should not overlook, but also should not overemphasize, liberty-limiting interventions in the pursuit of effective public health measures. In public health, concord with civil liberties is more basic than conflict. However, conflicts do emerge, and several rebuttal conditions, or justificatory conditions, need to be met to justify liberty-limiting interventions. The presumptive limits set by civil liberties can often direct public health officials to find ethically preferable interventions that do not sacrifice effectiveness in the pursuit of important public health goals. Focusing mainly on examples from vaccination, DOT for TB, and quarantine, this chapter has considered a variety of interventions, stressing possible ways to secure individuals' compliance with important public health measures without breaches of civil liberties. In many contexts, individuals voluntarily choose to appropriately exercise their civil liberties, such as freedom of movement and association, or waive their rights to civil liberties, such as freedom from intrusion on bodily integrity. In those cases, it is not necessary for public health officials to infringe those liberties.

A distinction between *imposing* community and *expressing* community is useful.[46] Certainly, in some cases, it is ethically justifiable to impose community, in the sense of enforcing communal responsibilities and obligations, in order to protect or promote public health. However, public health officials can generally avoid imposing community by using the various non-coercive interventions discussed in this chapter. This outcome is more likely if the society has also expressed community by displaying solidarity with and respect for all its citizens and residents. This expression of community, which includes respecting civil liberties and rights and providing adequate resources, can usually generate trust and voluntary cooperation through such measures, coupled with truthful public communication and active public engagement.

Notes

1. Lawrence O. Gostin, *Public Health Law: Power, Duty, Restraint*, Revised and Expanded Second Edition (Berkeley: University of California Press; New York: The Milbank Memorial Fund, 2008).
2. Lawrence O. Gostin, "Public Health Law in an Age of Terrorism: Rethinking Individual Rights and Common Goods," *Health Affairs* 21, No. 6 (2002): 79–93; Gostin, "When Terrorism Threatens Health: How Far Are Limitations on Personal and Economic Liberties Justified?" *Florida Law Review* 55 (2003): 1105–1170.
3. George J. Annas, "Bioterrorism, Public Health, and Civil Liberties," *The New England Journal of Medicine* 346 (2002): 1337–1342; Annas, "Bioterrorism, Public Health, and Human Rights," *Health Affairs* 21 (2002): 94–97; Annas, "Your Liberty or Your Life: Talking Point on Public Health versus Civil Liberties," *EMBO Reports* 8, No. 12 (2007): 1093–1098.
4. Ronald Bayer, "The Continuing Tensions between Individual Rights and Public Health: Talking Point on Public Health versus Civil Liberties," *EMBO Reports* 8, No. 12 (2007): 1099–1103
5. For a fuller discussion, see James F. Childress and Ruth Gaare Bernheim, "Beyond the Liberal and Communitarian Impasse: A Framework and Vision for Public Health," *Florida Law Review* 55, No. 5 (2003): 1191–1219; Childress and Bernheim, "Public Health Ethics: Public Justification and Public Trust," *Bundesgundheitsblat: Gusundheitsforschung, Gesundheitsschutz* 51, No. 2 (2008): 158–163; Bernheim, Childress, Alan Melnick, and Richard Bonnie, *Essentials of Public Health Ethics* (Boston: Jones and Bartlett Learning, 2014).
6. David Boaz, "SARS and the Bureaucratic Creep of 'Public Health,'" Commentary, Cato. org, June 18, 2003, http://www.cato.org/publications/commentary/sars-bureaucratic-creep-public-health Accessed July 11, 2013.
7. Amitai Etzioni, "Public Health Law: A Communitarian Perspective," *Health Affairs* 21, No. 6 (2002): 102–104.
8. John Stuart Mill, *On Liberty*, ed. David Spitz (New York: W.W. Norton & Company, Inc., 1975).
9. *Jacobson v. Massachusetts*, 197 U.S. 11 (1905).
10. Gostin, *Public Health Law: Power, Duty, Restraint*.
11. Mill, *On Liberty*, p. 89.
12. James F. Childress, "Paternalism in Health Care and Public Policy," In *Principles of Health Care Ethics*, 2nd edn., ed., R.E Ashcroft, A. Dawson, H. Draper and J. McMillan (Chichester, Eng.: John Wiley & Sons, Ltd., 2007), pp. 223–231; Tom L. Beauchamp and James F. Childress, *Principles of Biomedical Ethics*, 7th edition (New York: Oxford University Press, 2013).
13. Bayer, "The Continuing Tensions between Individual Rights and Public Health."
14. Ibid.
15. James Colgrove, "The Coercive Hand, The Beneficent Hand: What the History of Compulsory Vaccination Can Tell Us about HPV Vaccine Mandates," In *Three Shots at Prevention: The HPV Vaccine and the Politics of Medicine's Simple Solutions*, ed.

K. Wailoo, J. Livingston, S. Epstein, and R. Aronowitz (Baltimore, MD: The Johns Hopkins University Press, 2010).

16. Bayer, "The Continuing Tensions between Individual Rights and Public Health."

17. For other versions of these conditions, see James F. Childress, Ruth R. Faden, Ruth D. Gaare, et al., "Public Health Ethics: Mapping the Terrain," *Journal of Law, Medicine & Ethics* 30, No. 2 (2002): 169–177; Childress and Bernheim, "Beyond the Liberal and Communitarian Impasse"; Childress and Bernheim, "Public Health Ethics: Public Justification and Public Trust."

18. Working Group of the University of Toronto Joint Centre for Bioethics, *Ethics and SARS: Learning Lessons from the Toronto Experience* (Toronto, Canada: The University of Toronto Joint Centre for Bioethics, 2003). This report is available at http://www.yorku.ca/igreene/sars.html Accessed July 31, 2007.

19. J. Schram, "Personal Views: How Popular Perceptions of Risk from SARS Are Fermenting Discrimination," *British Medical Journal* 326 (2003): 939.

20. Gostin, "Public Health Law in an Age of Terrorism"; Etzioni, "Public Health Law: A Communitarian Perspective."

21. Nuffield Council on Bioethics, *Public Health: Ethical Issues* (London: Nuffield Council on Bioethics, 2007). Available at: www.nuffieldbioethics.org Accessed January 17, 2013.

22. This figure was derived from the discussion in Nuffield Council on Bioethics, *Public Health: Ethical Issues.*

23. Community Preventive Services Task Force, *Guide to Community Preventive Services: Universally Recommended Vaccinations: Reducing Clients Out-of-Pocket Costs for Vaccinations.* Review completed October 2008. Available at: www.thecommunityguide.org/vaccines/universally/index.html. Accessed: July 12, 2013.

24. Richard H. Thaler and Cass R. Sunstein, *Nudge: Improving Decisions about Health, Wealth, and Happiness* (New Haven, CT: Yale University Press, 2008).

25. Ibid.

26. M. Haverkate, F.D. Ancona, C. Gimabi, et al., "Mandatory and Recommended Vaccination in the EU, Iceland and Norway: Results of the Venice 2012 Survey on the Ways of Implementing National Vaccination Programs," *Eurosurveillance* 17, No. 22 (2012). http://www.eurosurveillance.org/images/dynamic/EE/V17N22/art20183.pdf Accessed July 17, 2013.

27. Ibid. Specifically for the UK, see D.A. Salmon, S.P. Teret, C.R. MacIntyre, et al., "Compulsory Vaccination and Conscientious or Philosophical Exemptions: Past, Present, and Future," *The Lancet* 367 (2006): 436–442.

28. National Conference of State Legislatures, *States with Religious and Philosophical Exemptions from School Immunization Requirements.* December, 2012. http://www.ncsl.org/issues-research/health/school-immunization-exemption-state-laws.aspx Accessed March 22, 2013.

29. S.B. Omer, W.K.Y. Pan, N.A. Halsey, et al., "Nonmedical Exemptions to School Immunization Requirements: Secular Trends and Association of State Policies with Pertussis Incidence," *Journal of the American Medical Association* 296 (2006): 1757–1763

30. D. A. Salmon and A. W. Siegel, "Religious and Philosophical Exemptions from Vaccination Requirements and Lessons Learned from Conscientious Objectors from Conscription," *Public Health Reports* 116 (2001): 289–295; Salmon, Teret, MacIntyre, et al., "Compulsory Vaccination and Conscientious or Philosophical Exemptions: Past, Present, and Future."

31. Thaler and Sunstein, *Nudge*; E.J. Johnson and D. Goldstein, "Do Defaults Save Lives?" *Science* 302, No. 5649 (2003): 1338–1339.

32. Community Preventive Services Task Force (2011a) *The Community Guide: Universally Recommended Vaccinations: Client or Family Incentive Rewards.* Review Completed, April 2011. http://www.thecommunityguide.org/vaccines/universally/clientoutofpocketcosts.html Accessed August 6, 2012.

33. Ibid. For more on the positive effects of incentives on vaccination rates in Australia, see Salmon, Teret, MacIntyre, et al., "Compulsory Vaccination and Conscientious or Philosophical Exemptions."

34. J. Popay, "Should Disadvantaged People Be Paid to Take Care of Their Health? No," *BMJ* 337 (2008): 141.

35. Jennifer S. Hawkins and Ezekiel J. Emanuel, "Clarifying Confusions about Coercion," *Hastings Center Report* 35, No. 5 (2005): 16–19.

36. Ruth W. Grant, *Strings Attached: Untangling the Ethics of Incentives* (New York: Russell Sage Foundation; Princeton, NJ: Princeton University Press, 2012).

37. Michael Willrich, *Pox: An American History* (New York: Penguin Press, 2011).

38. James Colgrove, "The Coercive Hand, The Beneficent Hand"; Colgrove, *State of Immunity: The Politics of Vaccination in Twentieth-Century America* (Berkeley: University of California Press; New York: Milbank Memorial Fund, 2006).

39. Colgrove, "The Coercive Hand, The Beneficent Hand."

40. Ibid., p. 12.

41. E.J. Hoekstra, C.W. LeBaron, Y. Megaloeconomou, et al., "Impact of a Large-Scale Immunization Initiative in the Special Supplemental Nutrition Program for Women, Infants, and Children (WIC)," *Journal of the American Medical Association* 280 (1998): 1143–1147; L.C. Kerpelman, D.B. Connell, and W.J. Gun, "Effect of a Monetary Sanction on Immunization Rates of Recipients of Aids to Families with Dependent Children," *Journal of the American Medical Association* 284 (2000): 53–59.

42. D. Wood and N. Halfon, "Reconfiguring Child Health Services in the Inner City," *Journal of the American Medical Association* 280 (1998): 1182–1183; C.S. Minkovitz and B. Guyer, "Effects and Ethics of Sanctions on Childhood Immunization Rates," *Journal of the American Medical Association* 284 (2000): 2056; M.M. Davis and J.D. Lantos, "Ethical Considerations in the Public Policy Laboratory," *Journal of the American Medical Association* 284 (2008): 85–87.

43. Community Preventive Services Task Force, *The Community Guide: Universally Recommended Vaccinations: Monetary Sanction Policies.* Review Completed, April 2011. http://www.thecommunityguide.org/vaccines/universally/MonetarySanctions.html Accessed August 6, 2012.

44. The Community Preventive Services Task Force, *The Community Guide: Universally Recommended Vaccinations: Client or Family Incentive Rewards*.
45. Nuffield Council on Bioethics, *Public Health: Ethical Issues*.
46. James F. Childress, *Practical Reasoning in Bioethics* (Bloomington, IN: Indiana University Press, 1997).

12

Triage in a Public Health Crisis

The Case of a Bioterrorist Attack

Introduction: Triage and Bioterrorism

In a letter dated August 30, 2001 (and read before the U.S. Senate Committee on Foreign Relations on September 5, 2001), Joshua Lederberg,[1] a Nobel laureate, focused on the threat of biological warfare, that is, the "use of agents of disease for hostile purposes." Noting that up to a dozen countries have developed such a capability, he further observed:

> Considerable harm could be done (on the scale of, say, a thousand casualties) by rank amateurs. Terrorist groups, privately or state-sponsored, with funds up to $1 million, could mount massive attacks of 10 or 100 times that scale. Important to keep in mind: if the ultimate casualty roster is 1,000, there will have been 100,000 or 1,000,000 at risk in the target zone, legitimately demanding prophylactic attention, and in turn a draconian triage. Several exercises have given dramatic testimony to how difficult would be governmental management of such incidents, and the stresses on civil order that would follow from inevitable inequities in that management.[2]

Among the numerous difficult issues that such bioterrorist attacks raise are several ethical ones, particularly those surrounding "draconian triage," in light of the limited surge capacity of the health-care system, including public health and medical care. One question is whether the *inevitable inequalities* in access to medical resources in any system of triage, rationing, or allocation in response to a bioterrorist attack are necessarily, as Lederberg suggests, "*inevitable inequities*," in the sense of unjust and unfair differences. Justice in its formal sense requires that we treat equals equally and similar cases similarly, while fairness at a minimum requires impartial treatment. Unless triage, rationing, and allocation are always unjust and unfair—a claim that is implausible—then the critical ethical question concerns which material criteria of justice are defensible. If formal justice requires treating similar persons in a similar way, it is essential to determine which similarities (and dissimilarities) are morally relevant, and this is the function of material criteria. Different theories of justice in general and in relation to specific problems, such as rationing health care, identify different properties or characteristics as relevant and the allocation that befits those properties or characteristics.[3] In this essay, I will examine some of the ethical issues that surround triage, rationing, or allocation in response to possible bioterrorist attacks.[4]

Two policy analysts note:

Earlier, policymakers spoke of the general problem of allocating scarce medical resources, a formulation that implied hard but generally manageable choices of a largely pragmatic nature. Now the discussion increasingly is of rationing scarce medical resources, a harsher term that connotes emergency—even war-time—circumstances requiring some societal triage mechanism.[5]

This comment focuses on problems of distributing health care in the society at large, but it applies with particular force to distributing various kinds of health care—for example, vaccines, prophylactic measures, therapy, and supportive care—in a public health crisis such as a bioterrorist attack. "Rationing" and "triage" do seem harsher than "allocation" in ordinary discourse. But even a rigorous distributional system, which may seem harsh and "draconian," may not be unjust and unjustified by utilitarian or egalitarian approaches. Some ethicists favor the "more neutral and descriptive language of patient selection."[6] However, I will focus on the model of triage, because it is commonly used, widely discussed, and perhaps the most instructive, but I will also use the language of rationing, allocation, distribution, and selection, as appropriate.

"Triage," a French word meaning sorting, picking, grading, or selecting according to quality, was first applied in English (as early as 1717) to the separation of wool by quality and later to the separation of coffee beans into three classes: "best quality," "middling," and "triage" coffee. The last class, consisting of bad or broken beans, was the lowest grade. The French under Napoleon developed a system of sorting casualties in war, but did not call it "triage" until later. "Triage" in war implied giving the worst off, rather than the best off, priority (within limits). In the U.S. Civil War, treatment was usually provided in turn without regard to wounded soldiers' specific conditions. However, in World War I, the U.S. army adopted the idea of a sorting station from the French and the British armies as well as the term "triage," which, by World War II, was not as widespread as the term "sorting."[7] One statement of U.S. military policy is that triage/sorting

> implies the evaluation and classification of casualties for purposes of treatment and evacuation. *It is based on the principle of accomplishing the greatest good for the greatest number of wounded and injured men in the special circumstances of warfare at a particular time.* The decision which must be made concerns the need for resuscitation, the need for emergency surgery and the futility of surgery because of the intrinsic lethality of the wound. Sorting also involves the establishment of priorities for treatment and evacuation.[8]

Similar formal policies have been adopted for civilian disasters, such as a nuclear disaster and earthquakes. And, as a result of the great increase in the use of emergency rooms, hospitals established triage systems in the early 1960s in order to facilitate the treatment of emergency patients. In such systems, a triage officer quickly assesses patients' needs as "immediate" (posing a threat of death or serious physical impairment if not treated immediately), "urgent" (requiring prompt but not immediate treatment), and "nonurgent," or in a more complex five-category system as "life-threatening," "urgent," "semiurgent," "nonurgent," and "no need for care."[9]

The term "triage" thus largely refers to particular systems of allocation or rationing. It is not equivalent to allocation, rationing, or distribution in general. As a specific system, triage sorts or grades persons according to their needs and the probable outcomes of interventions. In its more formal developments, a system of triage classifies persons according to set categories. Furthermore, medical triage is a form of allocation or rationing under critical or emergency circumstances, where decisions must be made immediately about particular patients because some of them probably have life-threatening conditions and not all of them can be treated at once.

Utilitarian and Egalitarian Approaches to Allocation

Medical and Social Utility

Triage is one way to ration health care when caregivers cannot meet everyone's needs at the same time and to the same degree. Systems of triage, whether informal or formal, all have had an implicit or explicit utilitarian rationale—they have all been designed to produce the greatest good for the greatest number by meeting human needs most effectively and efficiently under conditions of scarcity. They are designed to satisfy the formal criterion of justice—to treat similar cases similarly and equals equally—and their material criteria for distribution, at a minimum, focus on patients' needs and/or probability of successful treatment.

Those who deny that triage has a utilitarian rationale fail to distinguish *medical utility* from *social utility*. And those who recognize but reject utilitarian triage often ignore this distinction too.[10] In addition, critics may fail to see that utility is one important principle alongside several others; that it merits serious consideration at every point; and that, in certain forms, it is compatible with egalitarian approaches. Indeed, there is a prima facie moral duty—though not an absolute one—to produce the greatest good for the greatest number, subject to other moral limits and constraints.

In its simplest formulation, the principle of utility requires that we assess actions, practices, and policies according to whether they produce the greatest good for the greatest number. In *medical utility*, the relevant population includes only those who currently have medical needs or are at risk for such needs. Allocation decisions that seek to maximize the welfare of that population compare the respective needs and probabilities of benefit of different parties in order to do the greatest good for the greatest number.

If triage is understood as the classification of persons in need or at risk in order to satisfy medical utility, then assigning priority to the best off or the worst off or some mix should depend less on principle than on the particular context, including such factors as the available personnel and technologies, and when, if ever, additional resources can be expected. For instance, what can and should be done for persons who have been exposed to or are at risk of exposure to different biological agents will vary from context to context.

Nicki Pesik, Mark Keim, and Kenneth Iserson identify several factors that they believe should and should not be considered in rationing scarce resources in response to a terrorist attack.[11] All of the criteria they propose involve medical utility, but one also involves (narrow) social utility, while the criteria they oppose mainly involve (broad) social utility. Their list is generally sound, but it neglects some important social functions or special responsibilities that may merit attention and priority in the event of a bioterrorist attack.

Should Consider	Should Not Consider
Likelihood of benefit	Age, ethnicity, or gender
Effect on improving quality of life	Talents, abilities, disabilities, or deformities
Duration of benefit	Socioeconomic status, social worth, or political position
Urgency of the patient's condition	
Direct multiplier effect among emergency caregivers	Coexistent conditions that do not affect short-term prognosis
Amount of resources required for successful treatment	Drug or alcohol abuse
	Antisocial or aggressive behaviors

Degree of need and probability of success, particularly the latter, have been featured in triage systems based on medical utility. According to Pesik and colleagues, the relevant and morally justifiable material criteria in the context of a terrorist attack include likelihood of benefit, effect on quality of life, duration of benefit, and urgency of need. They also add another criterion that focuses on the amount of resources required (what others sometimes call the "principle of conservation").[12] Pesik and colleagues indicate that "the likelihood of benefit using minimal resources takes precedence [in order] to maximize the efficient use of scarce medical supplies." In short, "practitioners must prioritize intervention to those who will benefit most from the fewest resources." Their list of criteria and their concentration on probable benefit with the fewest resources are justifiable within a framework of *medical utility* in response to a bioterrorist attack.

More problematic, however, is their claim that this formulation "widens the scope of patients for whom medical intervention is deemed futile." It is a mistake to use the language of "futility" to characterize a judgment made on the basis of "medical utility." Medical interventions should be deemed futile only when they cannot be performed because of the patient's condition, would not produce a physiological effect, or would not produce a benefit.[13] When medical interventions are denied to particular individuals in order to provide them to others who have a higher probability of benefit with the use of fewer resources, that is a matter of utility, not futility. Those interventions would not necessarily be futile for the individuals who do not receive them;

rather they are unjustifiable in the system of utilitarian triage, as long as resources are limited. Describing such a triage system as widening the scope of
futility ignores the harsh reality and invites self-deception.

Another criterion that Pesik and colleagues propose is "direct multiplier
effect among emergency caregivers." Even though this criterion seeks to
maximize medical utility, it is also a criterion of (narrow) social utility, because it assigns priority on the basis of a specific social function. It is important not only to distinguish medical utility and social utility—while
recognizing that they may overlap at points—but also to distinguish two
types of social utilitarian judgments: *narrow social utility* and *broad social
utility.*

Triage has often included social utility, along with medical utility, in military and civilian disaster contexts. Triage seeks to salvage those in need, and
salvageability may reflect both medical and social judgments. For instance,
according to a major text on surgical triage in the military, "traditionally, the
military value of surgery lies in the salvage of battle casualties. This is not
merely a matter of saving life; it is primarily one of returning the wounded
to duty, and the earlier the better."[14] A similar expansion of salvageability in
triage occurs in protocols for civilian disasters, such as plans in San Francisco
to cope with a devastating earthquake or national plans to cope with nuclear
destruction.[15] And, in the debate years ago about triage following a possible
nuclear attack, Thomas O'Donnell, a moral theologian, argued that "those
casualties whose immediate therapy offers most hope for the conservation
of the common good should receive first priority."[16] Furthermore, he continued, "unless the individual is considered as very important to the common
good, and is salvable, it would seem unreasonable for the medical personnel
to expend their efficiency on a few when it could be conserved for the greater
number in more remediable need." This proposal, he noted, was in accord
with national policy regarding a nuclear disaster. Even though the language
of "conservation of the common good" appears to be unduly broad and
vague, triage that reflects such conceptions generally operates with a narrow
formulation of social utility limited to specific functions and roles within a
circumscribed context.

Even the strongest opponents of social utilitarian frameworks of rationing
may recognize exceptions to a more egalitarian approach, such as a lottery or
queuing. For instance, Paul Ramsey generally argued for random allocation

of scarce life-saving medical resources once judgments of medical utility had been made and scarcity remained. His egalitarian reasoning focused the equal work of human lives.[17] In addition, he stressed the difficulty, if not the impossibility, of securing agreement about the relevant social values in an unfocused, pluralistic society, such as our own. Generally, a "society is largely an unfocused meshing of human pursuits."[18] Nevertheless, Ramsey accepted limited social utilitarian exceptions to an egalitarian framework in certain circumscribed or focused contexts—for instance, he justified assigning priority to persons at risk when they can discharge specific functions highly valued by the community in a crisis or emergency, such as an earthquake. These functions would be similar to those performed by sailors on a lifeboat following a shipwreck.[19]

For Ramsey, on the lifeboat analogy, a pluralistic community, with a variety of values and goals, becomes focused in some disasters as a result of a substantial threat to its survival. Its survival becomes an overriding goal, in part because it is a condition for realizing other goals. Ramsey sometimes suggests that a community could justifiably become focused on goals other than survival and then use those goals to identify exceptional social functions for which people should be saved. At any rate, he rejected exceptions based on individuals' broad social worth, their overall social value, in a pluralistic society. He only admitted exceptions based on specific and urgent instrumental social value, judged according to essential social functions, in limited and focused circumstances: "Triage decisions are all a function of the narrowly defined, exceptional purposes to which a community of men may have been reduced. In these terms, comparative social worthiness can be measured."[20] A society, or parts of a society, under bioterrorist attack, would become such a focused community, with its very survival possibly at stake. Hence, judgments of narrow social utility could be justified in such a setting.

In the case of natural or man-made disasters, victims most in need of help—on whom normally we would lavish resources—must simply be set aside, and nothing be done for them. First priority must be given to victims who can quickly be restored to functioning. They are needed to bury the dead to prevent epidemic. They can serve as amateur medics or nurses with a little instruction—as the triage officer directs the community's remaining medical resources to a middle group of the seriously but not-so-seriously injured majority. Even among these, I suppose a physician should first be treated.[21]

Most of the criteria that Pesik and colleagues excluded, as I have suggested, pertain to broad social utility or social value. Nevertheless, in concentrating on medical utility and one criterion that combines medical utility with narrow social utility ("the direct multiplier effect among emergency caregivers"), they fail to see that a bioterrorist attack may threaten the social system as well as the health-care system and that some social functions other than those related to health care may be essential to prevent major social disruption. Hence, in some contexts, "political position," which they excluded, could be essential to communal survival. Later I will return to how we might determine essential specific social functions and roles.

Egalitarian Perspectives

How do these different conceptions of utility in triage systems fit with egalitarian concerns? It is important to stress that they are not all equally problematic from an egalitarian standpoint. First, in contrast to what some egalitarian critics claim, medical utility does not infringe the principle of equal regard for individual persons and their lives. My claim presupposes that counting numbers of lives is compatible with a principle of equal regard for human lives, but this presupposition has been challenged. For example, John Taurek has argued that numbers should not count in deciding whether to distribute a lifesaving drug (a) to save five persons or (b) to save one person when it is not possible to do both (a) and (b).[22] Let's suppose that a drug could save either the five or the one, but not all, because of their respective medical conditions. Taurek proposes the following in response to such a scenario

> Here are six human beings. I can empathize with each of them. I would not like to see any of them die. But I cannot save everyone. Why not give each person an equal chance to survive? Perhaps I would flip a coin. Heads, I give my drug to these five. Tails, I give it to this one. In this way I give each of the six persons a fifty-fifty chance of surviving. Where such an option is open to me it would seem to best express my equal concern and respect for each person.

By contrast, I would argue that numbers should count and that they can count without infringing equal concern or respect for each person. Without considering all of Taurek's arguments, I would contend that it is implausible for him to suggest, as he does, that saving the many over the one is like saving the rich over the poor.[23] Instead, as Derek Parfit argues in criticizing "innumerate ethics," "if we give the rich priority, we do not give equal weight to saving each. Why do we save the larger number? Because we *do* give equal weight to saving each. Each counts for one. That is why more count for more."[24]

Making such a judgment of medical utility may even be morally required in some cases. Even in Taurek's case, in which an individual owner of a drug has to decide how to use it, we can argue that he or she has an obligation to attempt to save more people, if possible, over the one person, absent more stringent, special moral relations, such as contracts. In the context of a bioterrorist attack, citizens would believe that they have as much right to medical care as any other citizens. Taurek would explain this moral intuition by a sense of prior social agreement about the use of a resource, perhaps involving social contributions through taxation.

While medical utility does not infringe the principle of equal regard for individual lives, social utility does. But judgments of social utility are themselves variable, as I have stressed in distinguishing *broad* and *narrow* social utility. Either one infringes the principle of equal regard or respect. Judgments of *broad social utility* recognize the different social value of people's lives, taken as a whole, including their various functions and roles. By contrast, judgments of *narrow social utility* recognize the differential value of specific social functions and roles and assign priority to the individuals discharging certain functions and performing certain roles.

Judgments of broad social utility infringe the principle of equal regard, and it is not justifiable to use them as a basis for rationing in general or in an emergency, such as a bioterrorist attack. Nevertheless, it is possible to justify triage, based on narrow social utility, at least when focused on specific and urgent functions and essential services, in some crises and emergencies such as a bioterrorist attack.

Even if a narrow social utilitarian framework is adopted, along with medical utility, reasons may exist to include other egalitarian considerations and approaches. Egalitarians often favor approaches that, at least within the limits of medical utility, express the transcendence of persons over their social roles and provide rough equality of opportunity. Hence, some egalitarians argue for a mechanism, such as a lottery or queuing, which embodies these values.

One possibility that merits public deliberation is a weighted lottery.[25] From a social utilitarian standpoint, it will be crucial to ensure that *enough* individuals survive who can discharge essential social functions, but it may not be necessary to save *all* individuals who hold essential social roles. Indeed, it may be fair and just to put essential workers and their families at some risk through a weighted lottery, in which individuals in essential social roles would receive additional weights in order to ensure that enough of them will be saved to meet defined social needs, including but not limited to the provision of health care. In this weighted lottery, some persons in essential social roles would not receive treatment. One argument holds that using a lottery or queuing in rationing, rather than social utilitarian allocation, would probably have the result that those in social power who are at risk would take steps to increase the supply of resources in order to reduce their risk of exclusion.

Several considerations support a possible role for a lottery, even if it is heavily weighted, in the context of tragic choices in response to a bioterrorist attack. As Barbara Goodwin observes,

> quite unphilosophical human beings have resorted to the lottery to make tragic choices in the context of natural or man-made disasters for a long time. When a group of people must distribute some unavoidable evil between themselves, they will almost instinctively choose a lottery as the method even if in the early stages of the discussion each is concerned to assert why she herself should not receive the evil allocation.[26]

She goes on to argue that the optimal context for the lottery, if it is to be just and viewed as just, is a "consensual group," particularly one with a common purpose.

However, as we have seen, when a group has a common purpose, when it becomes a "focused community," it may be possible to make some allocative decisions on the basis of (limited) social utilitarian criteria (for example, who is needed for the survival of the "focused community"?). Nevertheless, if the only common purpose is that each individual in the group wants to survive—for example, patients awaiting an organ transplant or patients in the intensive care unit—a lottery or "first come, first served," which Ramsey calls "an ongoing lottery," may embody equal respect, impartial treatment, and fairness in the competition, if medical utility does not determine the outcome. Thus, a lottery would express and symbolize some fundamental values, and it would provide a way around the lack of consensus in an unfocused, pluralistic society about social utilitarian allocation criteria. In some circumstances of tragic choice, people rightly view the lottery as an acceptable way to allocate goods and burdens because of the limits of "mindful" choice, the blindness or impartiality of the lottery, and "the moral judgment that people should be treated as absolutely equal where basic life chances (chances of life or survival) are involved."[27]

In the 1990s, lotteries were used several times to distribute new drugs that were available only in limited supply. Sometimes the candidates for these scarce drugs, such as protease inhibitors to treat AIDS, either proposed or agreed to a lottery, within certain limits set by medical utility. For instance, when Hoffman-LaRoche decided to offer Inviarase to patients with advanced AIDS outside current clinical trials, Dr. Alberto Avendano of the National Association of People With AIDS proposed a lottery, and both the drug manufacturer and the Food and Drug Administration agreed. Sixty percent of the first 2,000 slots were set aside for patients with CD4 counts less than 50. According to Dr. Avendano, "The lottery seemed the closest to the most fair way." Although some argued that patients with AIDS who had participated in clinical trials should have priority, others stressed the symbolic value of the lotteries. As Evan DeRenzo put it, "Lotteries say that after you meet medical criteria, all persons should have an equal shot at the good of society. Lotteries celebrate an understanding that all humans are endowed with equal dignity."[28]

Perhaps the closest society can come to a community of consent is to ensure transparency and public participation in setting the procedures and material criteria for triage in response to a possible bioterrorist attack, and it should do so.

Public Justification: Transparency, Participation, and Cooperation

My arguments in this essay presuppose a context of public justification. Even when the criteria for rationing or triage are set primarily or exclusively by physicians, they operate in a public context. Secrecy is often impossible—as well as ethically problematic—in part because of the public nature of much health care, especially in hospitals. Because a health care team is involved, the criteria must be justifiable to the various participants. Even triage decisions in intensive care units are "public." William Knaus observes, they are made "in the presence of and with the involvement of a wide variety of interested spectators, other physicians and nurses, along with family members and friends"[29]—one might even add administrators, insurers, and regulators. Thus, he calls for "public accountability" to ensure adequate representation of our pluralistic society. In addition to these general reasons for transparency and public accountability in setting triage criteria, some specific reasons apply in the preparation for a possible bioterrorist attack.

The triage that may be required in response to such an attack may look very different from conventional triage in the emergency room and other civilian contexts, in part because of immediate uncertainty and diagnostic challenges. Emergency physicians Pesik, Keim, and Iserson argue that "to address these issues [raised by Weapons of mass-destruction-terrorism—WMD-T] to the maximum benefit of our patients, we must first develop collective forethought and a broad-based consensus that these decisions must reach beyond the hospital emergency department."[30] They continue: "Critical decisions like these should not be made on an individual case-by-case basis. Physicians should never be placed in a position of individually deciding to deny treatment to patients without the guidance of a policy or protocol."[31] Physicians, along with "emergency care providers, personnel, hospital administrators, religious leaders, and medical ethics committees need to engage in bioethical decisionmaking before an acute bioterrorist attack."

This recommendation is too restricted; it needs to be extended to ensure both transparency and public participation, in a context of public justification.[32] Public trust will be essential in a bioterrorist crisis—hence, the public needs to have confidence in the procedures and standards of triage. Some people, perhaps many, will not receive the needed vaccination, prophylaxis, or treatment. As a result, the criteria need to be publicly articulated and defended in advance.

Beyond their public articulation and defense, procedures and standards of triage need to be developed with public participation—here I go beyond the list of participants identified by Pesik and colleagues to include the general public. Public participation rests on several foundations. It is a matter of justice—the right to participate in decisions, especially governmental decisions, that may have a fundamental impact on life chances—and a matter of symbolic values, particularly the equal value of all, as well as a matter of building and maintaining public trust.

Organ allocation in the U.S. is instructive. The criteria for selecting recipients for donated organs from patients on the waiting list are public and they have been developed and modified with public participation, in part because the public's role is so crucial—the public provides the organs and their trust is essential to their willingness to donate.[33] In response to a bioterrorist attack, maintaining the social order as well as the system of health care will depend on public cooperation, while some, perhaps many, individuals suffer and die. For voluntary cooperation, the public must perceive the triage as necessary and the procedures and standards as fair.

Public officials may be reluctant to disclose information to and to invite the participation of the public in preparing for a possible bioterrorist attack because they view members of the public as nonparticipants in and perhaps even as obstacles to effective responses to bioterrorism. By contrast, Glass and Schoch-Spana hold that the public should be viewed as a capable partner and a capable ally.[34] They believe that a "generally effective and adaptive collective action" is possible, and contend that "failure to involve the public as a key partner in the medical and public-health response could hamper effective management of an epidemic and increase the likelihood of social disruption." They propose five useful guidelines for integrating the public into planning responses to bioterrorism: "(1) treat the public as a capable ally in the response to an epidemic, (2) enlist civic organizations in practical public health activities, (3) anticipate the need for home-based patient care and infection control, (4) invest in public outreach and communication strategies, and (5) ensure planning that reflects the values and priorities of affected populations."[35] Whether their proposal of a network of public responders is excessively optimistic, at a minimum, there must be basic public confidence, trust, and cooperation; otherwise social disruption will be a high risk.

Public justification will be all the more difficult—but all the more indispensable—if the criteria of triage are partially social utilitarian, even in the narrow sense. Determining which social functions are essential requires broad societal participation in order to reflect "the values and priorities of affected populations." According to Baker and Strosberg, social utilitarian systems of allocation are inherently unstable and require either non-disclosure and deception or coercion for their maintenance.[36] They contend that individuals in need or at risk in contexts of limited medical resources will consent only to egalitarian criteria. Certainly, a strongly egalitarian approach, such as a lottery or queuing, has widespread and justifiable appeal. However, in asserting their broad claim, Baker and Strosberg fail to distinguish medical utility from social utility and narrow from broad social utility. As a result, they fail to establish that triage based on medical utility along with narrow social utility in an emergency created, for instance, by a bioterrorist attack would not be publicly justifiable and stable, especially if the public has participated in the process of setting the criteria for triage.

Another important issue that requires public attention concerns the families of essential social personnel. The status of families may be particularly important if a bioterrorist attack converts the initial victims into secondary agents, that is, individuals who can infect others—even though this is not true for anthrax, it is true for several other possible biological agents including smallpox and plague. For instance, in May 20–23, 2000, Denver conducted a bioterrorism exercise called Operation Topoff. As this simulated attack unfolded, participants learned that plague aerosol had been covertly released three days earlier at the city's center for the performing arts, with over 2,000 cases of pneumonic plague, many deaths, and hundreds of secondary cases. Richard Hoffman and Jane Norton, both of Colorado Department of Public Health and Environment, note that

> As more cases were identified, an anticipated issue emerged: who should receive antimicrobial prophylaxis? The governor's committee debated whether to limit prophylaxis to close contacts of infectious cases or offer it more widely (e.g., to all health-care workers, first responders, and public safety workers *and their families*) to gain the support and participation of key workers. The committee decided on the latter approach, but not unanimously.[37]

The rationale in providing antimicrobial prophylaxis to the families of key workers, as well as the workers themselves, focused on the need to secure their voluntary cooperation, which will be critically important in a bioterrorist attack. In addition, the public's trust will also be critically important, and that trust will be contingent, in part, on the public's perception that triage is necessary and fair.

This point also emerges from an analysis of the 2001 exercise, "Dark Winter," in which decision makers were presented with a fictional bioterrorist scenario involving smallpox and had "to react to the facts and context of the scenario, establish strategies, and make policy decisions." According to one summary of the lessons of the exercise,

> Dark Winter participants worried that it would not be possible to forcibly impose vaccination or travel restrictions on large groups of the population

without their general cooperation. To gain that cooperation, the President and other leaders in Dark Winter recognized the importance of persuading their constituents that there was fairness in the distribution of vaccine and other scarce resources, that the disease-containment measures were for the general good of society, that all possible measures were being taken to prevent the further spread of the disease, and that the government remained firmly in control despite the expanding epidemic.[38]

Engendering and maintaining the public's trust will be more likely if the public has participated in setting the procedures and material criteria and hence in determining what to emphasize in medical utility, which functions and roles are essential in judgments of narrow social utility, whether to include families as well as individuals whose functions and roles are essential, whether to provide prophylaxis and other treatments to all individuals in certain roles or to have a weighted lottery, and so forth. Such determinations are not clear-cut—as the Denver experience indicated ("The committee decided . . . but not unanimously")—and the public should participate in making them. As already noted, the issues become even more difficult when, in order to contain infectious diseases, quarantine becomes necessary. The observation is sound that "The public will not take the pill if it does not trust the doctor."

When societies confront tragic choices—where fundamental social-cultural values are at stake—they must, as Calabresi and Bobbit stress, "attempt to make allocations in ways that preserve the moral foundations of social collaboration."[39]

Notes

1. Joshua Lederberg, Letter to Hon. Joseph R. Biden, Jr., August 30, 2001, in *The Threat of Bioterrorism and the Spread of Infectious Diseases*, Hearing before the Committee on Foreign Relations, U.S. Senate, One Hundred Seventh Congress, First Session, September 5, 2001 (Washington, DC: U.S. Government Printing Office, 2001), pp. 5–8.
2. Although this letter is very similar to a statement that Lederberg had presented to the same committee on August 24, 2001, some of the language differs. Instead of "draconian triage," Lederberg referred in the earlier letter to "massive triage." And, instead of "the stresses on civil order that would follow from inevitable inequities in that management," he noted "the stresses that control of such incidents would impose on civil order." These formulations reflect a difference in tone if not in substance. See

Lederberg, Testimony before the Committee on Foreign Relations, U.S. Senate, One Hundred Seventh Congress, August 24.
3. Tom L. Beauchamp and James F. Childress, *Principles of Biomedical Ethics*, 5th edn. (New York: Oxford University Press, 2001).
4. I have drawn some ideas about and formulations of these ethical issues, including a few paragraphs, from James F. Childress, *Practical Reasoning in Bioethics* (Bloomington, IN: Indiana University Press, 1997).
5. Richard Rettig and Kathleen Lohr, "Ethical Dimensions of Allocating Scarce Resources in Medicine: A Cross-National Study of End-Stage Renal Disease," Unpublished manuscript, 1981.
6. John Kilner, *Who Lives? Who Dies: Ethical Criteria in Patient Selection* (New Haven, CT: Yale University Press, 1990), p. xi.
7. For discussions of the history of triage, see Gerald R. Winslow, *Triage and Justice: The Ethics of Rationing Life-Saving Medical Resources* (Berkeley, CA: University of California Press, 1982) and Douglas A. Rund and Tondra S. Rausch, *Triage* (St. Louis: C.V. Mosby, 1980), among others.
8. Quoted in Rund and Rausch, *Triage*, p. 9, italics added.
9. Much of the previous two paragraphs derives from Childress, *Practical Reasoning in Bioethics*, pp. 195–196.
10. Robert Baker and Martin Strosberg, "Triage and Equality: An Historical Reassessment of Utilitarian Analyses of Triage," *Kennedy Institute of Ethics Journal* 2 (June 1992): 103–123.
11. Nikki Pesik, Mark E. Keim, Kenneth V. Iserson, "Terrorism and the Ethics of Emergency Medical Care," *Annals of Emergency Medicine* 37, No. 6 (June 2001): 642–646.
12. Winslow, *Triage and Justice*.
13. See Beauchamp and Childress, *Principles of Biomedical Ethics*, 5th edn., pp. 133–35, 161–62).
14. Winslow, *Triage and Justice*, p. 11.
15. Winslow, *Triage and Justice*.
16. Thomas O'Donnell, "The Morality of Triage," *Georgetown Medical Bulletin* 14 (August 1960), p. 70.
17. Paul Ramsey, *Patient as Person* (New Haven, CT: Yale University Press, 1970), p. 255.
18. Ibid., p. 275.
19. Ibid., Chap. 7.
20. Ibid., p. 258.
21. Ibid.
22. John M. Taurek, "Should the Numbers Count?" *Philosophy & Public Affairs* 6 (Summer 1977): 303.
23. Ibid., pp. 315–316.
24. Derek Parfit, "Innumerate Ethics," *Philosophy & Public Affairs* 7 (Summer 1978): 285–301, at 301.
25. Jon Elster, *Solomonic Judgements* (Cambridge: Cambridge University Press, 1989), pp. 47–48, 113–115; Jon Elster, *Local Justice: How Institutions Allocate Scarce Goods and Necessary Burdens* (New York: Russell Sage Foundation, 1992), p. 110.

26. Barbara Goodwin, *Justice by Lottery* (Chicago: University of Chicago Press, 1992).
27. Ibid., p. 178.
28. Diane Naughton, "Drug Lotteries Raise Questions: Some Experts Say System of Distribution May Be Unfair," *Washington Post Health*, September 26, 1995, pp. 14–15.
29. William Knaus, "Criteria for Admission to Intensive Care Units," In *Rationing of Medical Care for the Critically Ill* (Washington, DC: Brookings Institution, 1989), pp. 44–51.
30. Pesik, Keim, and Iserson, "Terrorism and the Ethics of Emergency Medical Care."
31. Ibid., p. 642.
32. We also need to ensure that physicians, public health professionals, and other health care professionals are at the table when government officials formulate policies for possible bioterrorist attacks. One lesson from the Dark Winter exercise is that "After a bioterrorist attack, leaders' decisions would depend on data and expertise from the medical and public health sectors"; another is that "To end a disease outbreak after a bioterrorist attack, decision makers will require ongoing expert advice from senior public health and medical leaders." Tara O'Toole, Michael Mair, and Thomas V. Ingelsby, "Shining Light on 'Dark Winter,'" *Clinical Infectious Diseases* 34 (April 1, 2002): 981–82. But prospective policies should also reflect those data, expertise, and advice.
33. See Childress, *Practical Reasoning in Bioethics*, Chap. 12.
34. Thomas Glass and Monica Schoch-Spana, "Bioterrorism and the People: How to Vaccinate a City against Panic," *Clinical Infectious Diseases* 34 (2002): 217–23.
35. Glass and Schoch-Spana, "Bioterrorism and the People: How to Vaccinate a City against Panic," p. 217.
36. Baker and Strosberg, "Triage and Equality."
37. Richard E. Hoffman and Jane E. Norton, "Lessons Learned from a Full-Scale Bioterrorism Exercise," *Emerging Infectious Diseases* 6, No. 6 (November–December, 2000): 652–653. Italics added.
38. O'Toole, Mair, and Ingelsby, "Shining Light on 'Dark Winter.'"
39. Guido Calabresi, and Philip Bobbitt, *Tragic Choices* (New York: W.W. Norton & Company, 1978), p. 18.

13

John Stuart Mill's Legacy for Public Health Ethics

On Liberty and Beyond

Introduction

The legacy of J.S. Mill's thought for public health ethics—which here stands for the ethical analysis and assessment of public policies directed at the public's health—has been largely shaped by interpretations and applications of *On Liberty*. However, the implications of *On Liberty* for public health ethics are more complex than is often recognized. And Mill's legacy also is unfortunately oversimplified and truncated if it rests only on *On Liberty*, even when that work's complexity is fully appreciated, because there are other resources for public health ethics in his thought, especially in the ethical framework he actually used in addressing a heated controversy in his day about the government's efforts to reduce the transmission of sexually transmitted diseases.

My goal in this essay is to enlarge and illuminate the common portrayal of Mill's legacy for public health ethics through (1) an examination, in light of issues in public health, of respect for liberty, antipaternalism, and the harm-to-others principle, as these are developed in *On Liberty* and *Political Economy*; and (2) an excavation of Mill's ethical framework for public health laws and policies, as this framework appears in his largely neglected critique of the Contagious Diseases Acts. The examination and excavation will consider the implications of Mill's thought in light of selected current concepts and challenges in public health ethics, such as "harm-reduction" strategies.

Respect for Liberty, Antipaternalism, and the Harm-to-Others Principle

In *On Liberty* Mill argued for "respect for liberty," stated variously as a "principle of liberty," "principle of individual liberty," "principle of freedom." (See, for example, OL 91, 95, 96, 101.)[1] Even though it is common to focus on liberty, following Mill's own language, his position is better understood if we keep in mind that he is referring to liberties. For instance, he noted the "liberties" of thought, speaking, and writing as part of the "political morality" of countries with free institutions and policies of toleration. (OL 16)

In justifying his principle of liberty, Mill avoided arguing for liberty as an abstract right, independent of utility, and appeals instead to utility, "the ultimate appeal on all ethical questions," understood in the "largest sense, grounded on the permanent interests of man as a progressive being" (OL, 12). Here and elsewhere Mill took a rule-utilitarian rather than an act-utilitarian approach. And he had a much richer conception of values than his fellow utilitarian Jeremy Bentham, who viewed pleasure or happiness in purely quantitative terms. Given his principle of liberty, Mill held that restraint is always an "evil" and that, in relation to adults, "it partakes, either in a great or in a small degree, of the degradation of slavery."[2] For Mill, the degradation of dignity is particularly evident, as we will see, in paternalistic interferences in voluntary self-regarding acts but it also permeates the Contagious Diseases Acts and their implementation, the subject of the last part of this essay. Mill argued that we need some general principles for determining when liberty or liberties should be respected. Otherwise our judgments are arbitrary and haphazard: "owing to the absence of any recognized general principles, liberty is often granted where it should be withheld, as well as withheld where it should be granted" (OL 96). His "object" in *On Liberty* was, as he stated in its most famous passage,

> to assert one very simple principle, as entitled to govern absolutely the dealings of society with the individual in the way of compulsion and control, whether the means used be physical force in the form of legal penalties, or the moral coercion of public opinion. That principle is, that the sole end for which mankind are warranted, individually or collectively, in interfering with the liberty of action of any of their number, is self-protection. *That the only purpose for which power can be rightfully exercised over any member of a civilized community, against his will is to prevent harm to others. His own*

good, either physical or moral, is not a sufficient warrant. He cannot be rightfully compelled to do or forebear because it will be better for him to do so, because it will make him happier, because, in the opinions of others, to do so would be wise, or even right. These are good reasons for remonstrating with him, or reasoning with him, or persuading him, or entreating him, but not for compelling him, or visiting him with any evil in case he do otherwise. *To justify that, the conduct from which it is desired to deter him must be calculated to produce evil to some one else. The only part of the conduct of any one, for which he is amenable to society, is that which concerns others.* In the part which merely concerns himself, his independence is, of right, absolute. Over himself, over his own body and mind, the individual is sovereign. (OL 11, Italics added)

It turns out that this "very simple principle" is actually complex, and later in *On Liberty* Mill restates it through two maxims. Furthermore, in "specimens of application," he seeks to "illustrate the "meaning" and "limits" of these two maxims, which together "form the entire doctrine of this Essay," and thus "to assist the judgment in holding the balance between them, in cases where it appears doubtful which of them is applicable to the case" (OL 87). Those two maxims are:

(1) that the individual is not accountable to society for his actions, in so far as these concern the interests of no person but himself. Advice, instruction, persuasion, and avoidance by other people, if thought necessary by them for their own good, are the only measures by which society can justifiably express its dislike or disapprobation of his conduct.

(2) Secondly, that for such actions as are prejudicial to the interests of others, the individual is accountable, and may be subjected either to social or to legal punishments, if society is of opinion that the one or the other is requisite for its protection. (OL 87)

If specified, and limited to those in "the maturity of their faculties," the first maxim, often called the antipaternalism principle or maxim, is *absolute*. It sets a firm limit and boundary around societal and governmental interventions. The second maxim, the so-called harm principle, which is a shorthand expression for the harm-to-others principle,[3] establishes a *necessary* condition for governmental interferences with liberty. (In this essay

I will focus mainly on governmental interferences with only passing attention to societal interferences, even though Mill was concerned about the "moral police" as well as the "physical police" [OL 79].)

The first maxim above indicated that such interventions as advice, instruction, and persuasion would be acceptable even when an individual's conduct affects only himself or herself. Mill also extended this point to governmental actions. He distinguished what he called the government's "authoritative interference" from its nonauthoritative interventions.[4] The former involves "issuing a command and enforcing it by penalties," while the latter involves such policies as "giving advice and promulgating information" or establishing parallel agencies or institutions, without banning private ones. According to Mill, the latter is much easier to justify than the former.

The Harm-to-Others Principle: A Necessary but Insufficient Condition for Governmental Interferences

When specified in the context of voluntary self-regarding conduct, respect for liberty is absolute, but when specified in the context of other-regarding conduct, respect for liberty is presumptively, but only presumptively, binding. Mill is clear that even in other-regarding conduct, there is a (rebuttable) presumption against interference in an individual's liberties: "Even in those portions of conduct which do affect the interest of others, the onus of making out a case always lies on the defenders of legal prohibitions."[5] The burden of making the case falls on those who recommend government interference— any departure from the noninterference principle requires justification and "unless required by some great good, is a certain evil."[6]

Mill accepts the general rules for social interaction that are necessary to reduce the time and energy spent in "merely neutralizing one another."[7] These include prohibiting and punishing such clearly injurious conduct as force, fraud, or negligence. But "moral reprobation" attaches to any number of other acts that are injurious to others, and, in "grave cases," may even warrant "moral retribution and punishment" (OL 73).

Acts that cross the threshold from self-regarding conduct into other-regarding conduct fall under society's "jurisdiction." But even when this necessary condition is met, it is still essential to determine whether either societal or governmental interference is actually justifiable (OL 70). The fact that an action is other regarding does not necessarily indicate that it should be subject to societal or governmental interferences. Nevertheless, the harm principle can and does justify moral opprobrium, and even "social stigma," in some cases where it does not justify legal coercion (OL 100).

When considering whether legal coercion that meets the conditions of the Harm Principle is actually justified, it is important to ask first whether the intervention is necessary for protection. Much depends on the nature of the action in question, its effects, and so forth. For instance, harm may occur in socially acceptable ways, such as in competition for positions. Or harm to others "only with their free, voluntary, and undeceived consent and participation" (OL 13). Or it may not rise to the level of severity or seriousness that would merit prevention or punishment.

Among the "good reasons" for not holding an individual accountable for other-regarding actions in particular cases is that doing so would produce greater harms: Sometimes "the attempt to exercise control would produce other evils, greater than those which it would prevent" (OL 13). Another good reason is that the case is of such a kind that generally the individual will still act better "when left to his own discretion, than when controlled in any way in which society have it in their power to control him" (OL 13). Mill recognized that we can harm others by inaction, as well as by action, but stressed that holding individuals accountable for harms caused by inaction requires greater caution and is less often justified (OL 12).

Certain actions that should be viewed as self-regarding and hence protected from moral or physical coercion may be rightly controlled if they are performed publicly and thus constitute offenses to others. Indeed, some conduct that is not even objectionable in itself may be offensive if performed in public (OL 91). Furthermore, Mill recognized the importance of public order as a rationale for governmental interference.

Mill's Critique of Paternal Government: Antipaternalism

From Mill's standpoint, what we call paternalistic actions display at least two features: they aim to protect individuals from harm or injury or the loss of some goods, and they do so by interfering with one or more liberties of those individuals. Paternalism invokes a metaphor of the relationship between father and child, as depicted in the late nineteenth century when the term first emerged in the English language. Even before then, the metaphor functioned in the language of "paternal government" that Mill and others used to criticize governmental policies (OL 94).

Mill's antipaternalism is evident in his famous statement in *On Liberty*: "Each is the proper guardian of his own health, whether bodily, or mental and spiritual" (OL 14). In *On Liberty* and elsewhere, this metaphor of "guardian" is linked with a number of other strong political-legal metaphors over against "paternal government." These include "sovereign" and "final judge," along with the language of "independence" and the division of life into "spheres" and "circles" or "spaces" or "territories," in order effectively to create and defend restriction- or coercion-free zones. And within the circle, sphere, space or territory of self-regarding conduct, the individual is absolute sovereign. The following important passage comes from Mill's *Political Economy*, which is less familiar than *On Liberty* in debates about paternalism:

> there is a circle around every individual human being, which no government, be it that of one, of a few, or of the many, ought to be permitted to overstep: there is a part of the life of every person who has come to years of discretion, within which the individuality of that person ought to reign uncontrolled either by any other individual or by the public collectively. That there is, or ought to be, some space in human existence thus entrenched around, and sacred from authoritative intrusion, no one who professes the smallest regard to human freedom or dignity will call in question: the point to be determined is, where the limit should be placed; how large a province of human life this reserved territory should include. I apprehend that it ought to include all that part which concerns only the life, whether inward or outward, of the individual, and does not affect the interests of others, or affects them only through the moral influence of example. With respect to the domain of the inward consciousness, the thoughts and feelings, and as much of external conduct as is personal only, involving no consequences, none at least of a painful or injurious kind, to other people: I hold that it is allowable in all, and in the more thoughtful and cultivated often a duty, to assert and promulgate, with all the force they are capable of, their opinion of what is good or bad, admirable or contemptible, but not to compel others to conform to that opinion; whether the force used is that of extra-legal coercion, or exerts itself by means of the law.[8]

Weak and Strong Paternalism

In the moral analysis and assessment of paternalistic actions or policies, one of the most prevalent and important distinctions is between *weak* and *strong* paternalism. Mill drew a similar distinction but without these terms, which were formulated by Joel Feinberg in 1971 and subsequently elaborated by many others, along with other distinctions such as soft and hard paternalism.[9]

In weak paternalism, the intended beneficiary is deemed not to be acting voluntarily. He or she may not be in the "maturity of their faculties" in general or in this specific case. One important question is whether weak paternalism—where the intended beneficiary is not acting voluntarily—is even paternalism at all, at least in any morally interesting and significant sense. One of Mill's famous examples is considered to be an instance and even a paradigm of weak paternalistic interventions. In the context of discussing the sale of poisons and the "proper office of public authority to guard against accidents," Mill presented the following case:

> If either a public officer or any one else saw a person attempting to cross a bridge which had been ascertained to be unsafe, and there were not time to warn him of his danger, they might seize him and turn him back, without any real infringement of his liberty; for liberty consists in doing what one desires, and he does not desire to fall into the river. Nevertheless, when there is not a certainty, but only a danger of mischief, no one but the person himself can judge of the sufficiency of the motive which may prompt him to incur the risks: in this case, therefore (unless he is a child, or delirious, or in some state of excitement or absorption incompatible with the full use of the reflecting faculty), he ought, I conceive, to be only warned of the danger; not forcibly prevented from exposing himself to it. (OL 89)

The second part of this passage, focusing on the risk rather than the certainty of harm, excludes individuals who are not competent to make decisions for themselves—an instance of weak paternalism—and then requires disclosure of risks to those who are "in the maturity of their faculties." Throughout Mill is assuming that such adults can form their own preferences and choose and act accordingly and that, indeed, they are the best judges of their own interests. (The first part justifies a temporary, forcible intervention, but then seems to close off the possibility of allowing the person to continue once properly informed of the certainty of the harm, presumably because of an unsupported assumption that no one would rationally desire to fall into the river.)

In *strong* paternalism, the intended beneficiary is deemed to be acting voluntarily but in ways that damage or threaten his or her best interests. For Mill, strong paternalistic governmental policies are absolutely unjustifiable infringements of "respect for liberty" (OL 10–13). In contrast to weak paternalistic interventions of various kinds, strong paternalistic interferences are not justifiable because, as Ronald Dworkin notes in his interpretation of Mill's antipaternalism, they are disrespectful, demeaning, and insulting to the beneficiary.[10] Indeed, to use less common Millian language, they degrade human dignity—they involve "degrading restraint."[11]

In addition to Mill's broad utilitarian grounding of the principle of respect for liberty, he offered other utilitarian reasons for his specific suspicions of "paternal government." He stressed the odds that the paternalist will be mistaken: "[t]he strongest of all the arguments against the interference of the public with purely personal conduct, is that when it does interfere, the odds are that it interferes wrongly, and in the wrong place" (OL 78). Mill's fundamental assumption is also evident here: that adults know their own interests better than anyone else.

Expanding the Scope of Weak Paternalism: Challenges to the Sharp Distinction between Voluntary and Nonvoluntary Actions

Because weak paternalistic governmental policies are considered to be more easily justifiable, Mill's sharp distinction between voluntary and nonvoluntary actions has been challenged in order to weaken the grip of his antipaternalism. One line of attack holds that in modern society various social forces shape individuals' decisions, choices, and actions in ways that render them nonvoluntary—examples include problems of overweight and obesity that result in part from behavioral patterns generated by social forces such as advertising. However, actions can be influenced without being determined and without becoming nonvoluntary or involuntary.

An important challenge comes from so-called libertarian paternalism, based on empirical evidence from psychology and behavioral economics about our bounded rationality and limited self-control.[12] Even if Mill's thought could incorporate such findings, there is still the important question about how much less voluntary our actions are under bounded rationality and limited self-control, whether this degree of "nonvoluntariness" justifies paternalistic "nudges," and whether this degree of "nonvoluntariness" is consistent with the individual's exercise of liberty in making choices in the context of "nudges"—which "libertarian paternalists" want to affirm. More importantly, as Joel Feinberg argues, Mill's antipaternalism "was also meant to apply to almost-but-not-quite fully voluntary choices as well, and probably also even to some substantially non-voluntary ones . . . [but probably not] to choices near the bottom of the scale of voluntariness."[13]

Expanding the Scope of Public Health: Challenges to the Sharp Distinction between Self-Regarding and Other-Regarding Conduct

Many debates about governmental interventions in health-related matters have centered on the nature and scope of public health. Given Mill's sharp distinction between self-regarding and other-regarding conduct, and the justification of authoritative governmental intervention only into the latter, he, not surprisingly, viewed legitimate public health measures as directed only toward other-regarding conduct, under the harm-to-others principle (along with some weak paternalistic interventions). Mill's response to philosopher William Whewell is particularly noteworthy. In arguing for paternal government, Whewell had asked:

> What is the meaning of restraints imposed for the sake of public health, cleanliness and comfort? Why are not individuals left to do what they like with reference to such matters? Plainly because carelessness, indolence, ignorance would prevent their doing what is most for their own interest.[14]

In response, Mill recognized a role for governmental public health interventions, but not for paternalistic ones:

> —Say, rather, would lead them to do what is contrary to the interest of other people. The proper object of sanitary laws is not to compel people to take care of their own health, but to prevent them from endangering the health

of others. To prescribe by law, what they should do for their own health alone, would by most people be regarded as something very like tyranny.[15]

A contemporary challenge to Mill's antipaternalism in health-related policies disputes the line he drew between self-regarding and other-regarding conduct. First of all there is some debate about exactly how Mill drew this line between self-regarding conduct and other-regarding conduct. Properly understood, conduct that is other-regarding affects others and their interests directly, adversely, and without their consent. Even though Mill could talk about the "health of the community," as a utilitarian he attended mainly to the impacts on individuals and their interests and, collectively, the sum of those impacts.

The reinterpretation and expansion of public health in the late twentieth and early twenty-first centuries have incorporated more of what Mill would have considered merely self-regarding acts—overweight and obesity provide a good example. Mill's paradigm was contagious diseases and actions, such as drunken conduct, that directly harm others without their consent or that harm the society.

Certainly Mill recognized that, in some circumstances, conduct that would otherwise be self-regarding, such as drunkenness, can become other-regarding, for instance, when "a person is led to violate a distinct and assignable obligation to any other person or persons" (OL 75). This would constitute a breach of a public duty. However, Mill was suspicious of efforts to convert what appears to be self-regarding conduct into other-regarding conduct by identifying all sorts of adverse effects on others or on the society itself. For example, Mill insisted:

> If grown persons are punished for not taking proper care of themselves,
> I would rather it were for their own sake, than under pretence of preventing
> them from impairing their capacity of rendering to society benefits which
> society does not pretend it has a right to exact. (OL 76)

Mill called for toleration of a variety of sexual activities—even suggesting that future generations would view his own society's mores with amazement—but he also recognized strong moral and legal obligations to nonconsenting persons (i.e., those who are not aware of and thus do not consent to the risks involved) in the context of sexual activities. For instance, as we will discuss later in the context of the Contagious Diseases Acts, he recognized a strong obligation to protect "innocent" persons from sexually transmitted diseases, in particular, the nonconsenting spouse of a person who engages prostitutes and any children he and the spouse might have. Furthermore, Mill emphasized a distinct and weighty parental obligation to children, even arguing that to bring a child into the world without being able to give the child "at least the ordinary chance of a desirable existence" constituted a "crime against that being" (OL 100). Not only is this a "moral crime" against the nonconsenting offspring, it is also a "moral crime" against the society that should have legal consequences (OL 97).

Another possible justification for governmental interference is that some putatively self-regarding harmful acts are in fact "contagious," particularly by setting a bad example—what we might today call "social contagion," which some have suggested is at work in patterns of obesity in certain communities. Mill discussed the claim that a person might be "injurious by his example; and ought to be compelled to control himself, for the sake of those whom the sight or knowledge of his conduct might corrupt or mislead" (OL 75). He conceded that a person's self-regarding "mischief" "may seriously affect, both through their sympathies and their interests, those nearly connected with him and, in a minor degree, society at large." But where the injury is "merely contingent" or "constructive" (i.e., through others' sympathy for the individual, and the like), then it should be tolerated for the sake of freedom. Furthermore, where no one else is harmed, Mill contended, "the example, on the whole, must be more salutary than hurtful. Since, if it displays the misconduct, it displays also the painful or degrading consequences which, if the conduct is justly censured, must be supposed to be in all or most cases attendant on it" (OL 78). Of course, Mill's counterargument does not recognize the complex mechanisms of influence that have been uncovered by modern social science research. An additional question concerns which governmental policies, such as incentives and nudges, he could accept beyond educating the young and providing information and advice.

Finally, policy-makers' intentions and motives are often mixed—for example, they may seek to benefit particular individuals, to protect the public health, to avoid burdens to third parties, and so forth. Rarely are governmental interventions in modern liberal societies defended as purely paternalistic. Most often proponents of such interventions appeal to the protection of other individuals or of the society itself, sometimes because of threats to public resources. In the modern welfare state, in contrast to the mid-nineteenth century when Mill was penning On Liberty, an important justification for governmental interference in what Mill would have considered purely self-regarding conduct may be plausibly based on the excessive and unfair use of public resources.

Mill's Ethical Framework for Analyzing and Assessing Ends and Means in Public Health Policies: The Case of the CDAs

Ethical Considerations and Specific Cases

In examining actual or proposed public health policies, Mill invoked a much wider range of ethical considerations than respect for liberty, the harm-to-others principle, and antipaternalism. As previously noted, these further ethical considerations also display a strongly communitarian and moralistic streak. They enrich but, in my judgment, do not contradict what Mill said in *On Liberty*, given its focus on the *limits* of societal and governmental control over the individual, especially through coercion. These ethical considerations all play roles, in interconnected ways (but without a clear rank order), in Mill's evaluation of public health policies and practices. They are both positive and negative:

- Recognition that "suffering is a great public evil" (CDA 360) and that public health is a legitimate goal of governmental policy (CDA 357)
- Effectiveness in achieving the goal of public health
- Balancing the positive and negative effects of different means to the goal of public health
- Expression of individual and societal benevolence/beneficence, through governmental laws and policies
- Degradation of dignity, often closely connected with violations of "respect for liberty," but not reducible to them
- Equality and impartiality as two precepts of justice,[16] with particular attention to equality between men and women and all those with "equal claims" as well as impartiality, for example, among diseases, especially contagious diseases

- Fairness, for example, in the distribution of the costs of public health measures and as well as in the opportunity to participate in setting public health policy through voting
- The symbolic and communicative significance of public policies, including what we now call "harm-reduction policies" as well as the selection of certain diseases for governmental attention

Following are three examples—two brief and one extensive—of Mill's application of these several ethical considerations, along with the principles in *On Liberty*, to specific public health problems.

While a member of the House of Commons, Mill supported a motion to require the provision of "smoking compartments for each class of passengers" on railway carriages. He viewed smoking and stale smoke on railway carriages as a "positive nuisance." This was not yet perceived as a major public health problem, but it was a major "nuisance" despite some railway companies' own rules. Mill did not oppose giving smokers "permission" to smoke, especially on long journeys, but he thought this should apply only to trains of a certain length and only in "compartments of the hindermost carriages." In response to the suggestion that this policy should be a matter for public opinion, Mill objected that "public opinion in this instance was swayed by a majority of smokers. It was a case of oppression by a majority of a minority."[17]

A second example concerns a bill to regulate the sale of arsenic. In debate about this bill, Mill focused on the degradation of dignity in the unequal treatment of men and women in the bill. As a result of some notorious cases of women using arsenic to commit murder, a clause was added to the original bill to prohibit the sale of less than ten pounds of arsenic to anyone "other than a male person of full age." The degradation of women reflected in this clause outraged Mill: "It singles out women for the purpose of degrading them." With its "insult" to and "disparagement" of women, it puts on women "the stamp of the most degrading inferiority." A paternalistic law that enacted a similar ban for everyone would treat "all mankind . . . as children," but, at least, it would involve equal justice and avoid "insult or disparagement peculiarly to any" (Letter 48/63–65). Degradation of dignity, particularly but not only of women, was also important in Mill's unrelenting opposition to the Contagious Diseases Acts (CDAs), to which we now turn.

Mill's Principled and Consequentialist Objections
to the CDAs

The public health issue that received Mill's most extensive and impassioned attention was the transmission of sexually transmitted diseases by prostitutes to soldiers and sailors, who then transmitted these diseases to their spouses and children. In his vigorous and uncompromising opposition to the CDAs, which were the main measures adopted by the government to reduce this transmission, Mill's arguments deployed the full array of ethical considerations identified earlier, moving well beyond—but not necessarily contradicting—the framework of *On Liberty*.

Deep, widespread concerns emerged in mid-nineteenth-century England about the increasing spread of sexually transmitted diseases among soldiers and sailors with potentially devastating effects on both military preparedness as well as on "innocent" spouses and children. Reportedly one in three cases of illness in the army resulted from sexually transmitted diseases, and close to three hundred out of one thousand hospital admissions for the soldiers were for syphilis or gonorrhea.[18] These alarming numbers had been increasing for decades by 1864 when the first CDA was passed.

For the civilian population, statistics for outpatients indicate that by mid-century half or more of the surgical outpatients—reportedly lower among medical outpatients—had some form of venereal disease. Particularly troubling was the rise of hereditary syphilis, which tended to be particularly lethal during an affected infant's first year of life.[19] While not uncontroversial, such statistics in mid-Victorian society

> convinced medical and military authorities that an epidemic of venereal disease was sweeping the nation. Although alarmed, doctors were confident that this epidemic could be stemmed through the sanitary supervision of prostitutes and that existing therapeutic and diagnostic methods were adequate to carry out the medical provision of such a regulation system.[20]

The CDAs of 1864, 1866, and 1869 together represented a vigorous effort through public policy to reduce the spread of venereal diseases. These acts were passed with little transparency or public attention, and major opposition did not emerge until 1869, when the number of districts subject to the acts grew to eighteen. As noted earlier, these acts were defended as ways to protect enlisted soldiers and sailors in garrison towns and ports and, ultimately, their spouses and offspring from sexually transmitted diseases, particularly syphilis and gonorrhea, for which only ineffective treatments were then available.[21]

In the areas where the acts were in effect, special plainclothes police could identify a woman as a "common prostitute"—a vague and undefined category that left identification up to the discretion of the special police—and ask her to undergo an examination every two weeks. If the woman did not voluntarily consent to the examination, she was taken to the local magistrate and had to show that she did not engage in fornication, whether for money or for pleasure. If the examination indicated that the woman had syphilis or gonorrhea she would be placed for up to nine months in a special "lock hospital" with wards for patients with venereal diseases.[22] Despite a major repeal campaign, the acts remained in effect until 1886.

Mill was in Parliament 1865–1868, and in 1866 he had opposed the only one of these acts passed during his time in the Parliament. But his most vigorous public opposition came later in his testimony before the Royal Commission of 1870 on the Administration and Operation of the Contagious Diseases Acts of 1866 and 1869—he appeared before the commission on May 13, 1871—and in his involvement in opposition groups and in his efforts to persuade others, for instance, in his letters. He stated his overall argument somewhat more systematically in his letters than in his oral testimony before the commission, because he presented that testimony in response to specific questions rather than as a formal statement. My analysis will focus on his testimony and supplement it with his letters and other writings.

Critique of the CDA's Unequal Distribution of Restrictions on Liberties

Based on Mill's very simple principle and its two maxims and on their applications in *On Liberty*, readers might suppose that Mill would have found it justifiable for the harm-to-others principle to, as he put it, "overbear" respect for liberty in these circumstances. After all, there was clear harm to the enlisted soldiers and sailors, who in their roles had a distinct, assignable obligation to the public, and there was clear harm to their "innocent" spouses and children who were infected as a result of their husbands'/fathers' sexual relations with prostitutes. So harm there was. And Mill could and did consider these sexually transmitted diseases and the suffering associated with them to be a "great public evil" (CDA 360). Much of the harm, experienced by many spouses and all children, was unconsented to—hence, they were "innocent" victims. So, at first glance, it might seem odd that Mill did not think that the harm-to-others principle could override respect for liberty in this context, specifically the liberty of "common prostitutes."

However, as Jeremy Waldron rightly emphasizes, Mill did not focus on liberty in the abstract, as an abstract good to be weighed against public health as a good, but rather on the concrete, specific liberties of particular individuals and groups.[23] Mill was thus interested in *whose* and *which* liberties were restricted by any legislation, including the CDAs. It's not the overall amount of liberty but the distribution of specific liberties that is crucially important. In addition, as I will show, Mill invoked the full range of ethical considerations identified earlier in analyzing and assessing the CDAs, in showing how they could possibly be improved, and in arguing, in the final analysis, that, even with such improvements, they would still be ethically unacceptable.

At the hearing's outset both the Royal Commission and Mill stressed that his views would focus on the "principles" of the legislation, because, as he conceded, he lacked "practical knowledge" and "practical experience" of its operation. Unsurprisingly, he focused immediately on "the security of personal liberty."

> I do not consider [the legislation] justifiable on principle, because it appears to me to be opposed to one of the greatest principles of legislation, the security of personal liberty. It appears to me that legislation of this sort takes away that security, almost entirely from a particular class of women intentionally, but incidentally and unintentionally, one may say, from all women whatever, inasmuch as it enables a woman to be apprehended by the police on suspicion and taken before a magistrate, and then by that magistrate she is liable to be confined for a term of imprisonment, which may amount, I believe, to six months, for refusing to sign a declaration consenting to be examined. (CDA 351)[24]

Mill's principled objection to this legislation thus focused at first on its unequal distribution of restrictions on liberties between men and women, what he elsewhere described as "its gross inequality between men & women" (Letter 1519/1688). In his judgment, no reason existed for subjecting women to medical inspection that would not apply with greater force to the men who use their services (Letter 1625/1789). Indeed, it is unjustifiable to restrict women's liberty since they spread disease to nonconsenting persons only through the consenting soldier or sailor.[25] The surveillance, the *espionage*, required to detect "common prostitutes," the women putting soldiers and sailors at risk, could just as easily be used to detect the men engaged in risky conduct. After all, it involved observing women in certain areas, going in and out of buildings suspected to be brothels (Letter 1625/1790).

The medical examination required to carry out the CDAs degrades personal dignity more so for women than for men. In Mill's judgment, this "insulting indignity" is more painful and humiliating for women, even for those who are prostitutes, than for men (Letter 1625/1790). This for Mill is a reason for examining men as well as women *or* instead of women (CDA 356). But he recognized that this was not politically feasible because of men's objections (CDA 355).

Furthermore, from Mill's perspective, a *compulsory* examination is more degrading than a *voluntary* one.[26] Indeed, if a woman voluntarily accepted the medical examination, with the understanding that, if she were determined to have a sexually transmitted disease, she would then be sent to the hospital and detained there until cured, this procedure would not be objectionable "on the score of personal liberty" (CDA 354). Nor would it be objectionable on grounds of inequality between men and women, even though it would still be objectionable on other grounds, which we will examine later, specifically, the unacceptability of the government undertaking, "even on the solicitation of the parties concerned, to provide beforehand the means of practicing certain indulgences with safety" (CDA 354).

Mill's strong and well-known convictions about women's suffrage led him to say that the CDAs have "genuine characteristics of tyranny." One supporter of the CDAs argued that a law that applies only to one sex is not problematic because, after all, the enlistment law for military service applies only to men. However, Mill retorted in a letter, "the laws that regulate enlistment are not made by women only, themselves not liable to it, and then applied to men only, who have no voice in making them." Furthermore, women are not accepted as soldiers even when they volunteer for that role; hence, "being a soldier must be taken as a privilege, and not a penalty, of sex." Finally, no woman can be a prostitute "without a man for her accomplice: yet when it comes to the punishment, or, if you prefer to consider it, the discipline, we hear no more of him. Thus, the man only is a soldier, and he subjects himself voluntarily to the discipline: a man and a woman must be associated in prostitution, the woman only is subjected to discipline, and that without her own consent" (Letter 1625/1790).

There is a danger of misinterpreting Mill's overall argument if we focus only on respect for liberty and the equality precept of justice. In response to questions before the Royal Commission, Mill observed that the CDAs would be less objectionable if they applied to men and women and if women voluntarily chose the examinations (CDA 353). In doing so, Mill focused on degrees of ethical justifiability of different possible versions of the CDAs. Despite distinguishing degrees of ethical justifiability in response to specific questions at the inquiry, he nevertheless had one final and unyielding argument that targeted the CDAs' fundamental rationale. Even if the CDAs were equal between men and women—or limited to men—and more voluntary, Mill indicated he would still be implacably opposed to them because they express what we might call, in contemporary terms, the Harm-Reduction Principle.

Opposition to the CDA's (Preventive) Harm-Reduction Laws and Policies

For Mill, the CDAs should be evaluated not merely according to their object—for him the strongest reason, a violation of the harm-to-others principle (CDA 356), was the protection of innocent spouses and children who did not voluntarily consent to the risks—or on their unequal impact on the liberties of men and women. They should also be evaluated in light of their symbolic and communicative significance and, connectedly, their overall probable effects on citizens' sentiments and actions. These stem from the legislation's incorporation of the Harm-Reduction Principle, now common in public health.

The Harm-Reduction Principle holds that it is legitimate and perhaps even imperative to establish policies and practices that may (1) involve the government—or others—in the harmful and perhaps immoral activity it opposes, and (2) may even increase the incidence and prevalence of that activity, all in an effort to reduce the activity's overall harmfulness.[27] The goal is to make the harmful and immoral activity less harmful to those continuing to engage in it, rather than to stop the activity itself. (Of course, several goals may be combined in a comprehensive public health program). In modern public health, major examples of harm-reduction policies include

government-sponsored needle-exchange programs to reduce HIV exposure, and the provision of condoms in public schools. For Mill, the primary
example—and the only one he could identify—was the CDAs. These acts
sought to provide "safeguards" for actions—voluntary sexual relations between military personnel and prostitutes—deemed immoral and highly
risky under normal circumstances.

It might be supposed that Mill as a committed utilitarian and a vigorous
proponent of the harm-to-others principle could endorse harm-reduction
policies. Such policies could perhaps even be viewed as an outgrowth or
extension of the harm-to-others principle, but, even if not, they are clearly
congruent with and, depending on the circumstances and calculation of
consequences, could even be required by a utilitarian framework. However,
Mill's concern about immoral and generally injurious conduct (which
is still immoral even when rendered noninjurious or less injurious) and
about the symbolic and communicative significance of governmental laws
and policies led him to oppose the CDAs on principle. He also thought, as
we will see, that they would have bad overall consequences. His principled
and consequentialist objections to the CDAs would hold even if his initial principled objection (the unequal distribution of restrictions on liberty
between men and women) could be addressed—that is, even if the acts
were more voluntary, eliminated the "gross inequality between men and
women," or perhaps applied only to men. These principled and consequentialist objections constitute a thoroughgoing rejection of harm-reduction
policies.

Harm-reduction policies create "moral hazards." Mill did not use this
precise language even though it was available at the time.[28] In this context, concerns about moral hazards focus on individuals' reduced motivation to take personal precautions against risks by avoiding ordinarily risky
conduct, because of available protections against the harmful effects of that
conduct. From Mill's standpoint, individuals need to face the consequences
of their actions, rather than have those consequences eliminated or miti-
gated through "safeguards," either to prevent harm to themselves or to prevent harm to others. In effect, the CDAs "provide beforehand the means of
practicing certain indulgences with safety" (CDA 354).

Mill's concerns about harm-reduction policies and about moral hazards
affect his prioritization of remedial and penal policies over preventive policies. He was generally suspicious of the preventive function of government,
"which is far more liable to be abused, to the prejudice of liberty, than the

punitory function; for there is hardly any part of the legitimate freedom of action of a human being which would not admit of being represented, and fairly too, as increasing the facilities for some form or other of delinquency" (OL 89).

In addition, Mill had strong suspicions about these particular preventive laws, the CDAs, because they sought to reduce harm by providing "safeguards" to immoral and generally injurious conduct. While these safeguards could reduce the conduct's risk of harm, both to soldiers and sailors and to their spouses and children, they could not reduce the conduct's immorality.[29] For Mill, the state may seek to avert evil if and only if it "endeavours to avert [the evil] by any means which are not objectionable in a greater degree than the evil itself" (CDA 360).

Mill combines attention to the law's symbolic and communicative significance with concerns about its consequences. This law creates the general impression that the actions for which it provides "safeguards" are not so bad after all. "The interpretation certain to be put upon regulations of this description, even if entirely false, is so mischievous that a very great balance of well-ascertained practical good effects would not, perhaps, be sufficient to compensate for it"[30] (Letter 1513/1683). This interpretation—or misinterpretation—constitutes one of the "indirect evils" of the CDAs (Letter 1513/1682).

Mill can find "no parallel case of an indulgence or pursuit avowedly disgraceful and immoral for which the government provides safeguards" (Letter 1625/1781). Imagine, he says, the government providing "stomach pumps for drunkards." Through the CDAs, the legislature indicates that it views this specific conduct with "less disfavour than any other practice generally considered immoral and injurious to society" (Letter 1625/1781). Hence, the "public evidence" expressed in law "must of necessity tend to remove feelings of shame or disapprobation connected with it" (Letter 1625/ 1781). Against those who dismiss this objection as merely "sentimental," Mill contended that "men's sentiments have a good deal to do with regulating their conduct; and no law can be a good one which gives a bad direction to men's sentiments" (Letter 1513/1682).

Mill's consequentialist objections flow from what the legislation symbolizes and communicates. He notes that the CDAs encourage vice: "even if there were the strongest reasons of other kinds for the Act, it would also have this for one of its drawbacks. To soldiers and ignorant persons it cannot but seem that legal precautions taken expressly to make that kind of indulgence safe, are a license to it" (Letter 1625/1781). In effect, the government is providing "safeguards" for immoral and generally injurious conduct.

Given the CDA's communicative significance and encouragement of vice, through establishing these "safeguards," Mill was convinced that, even under a harm-reduction approach, the CDAs could not be justified. Noting the division among medical experts about the CDAs' efficacy, he concluded that their "medical efficacy" is "doubtful" (Letter 1513/1681). If, however, these acts were efficacious for their intended purposes, Mill conceded, this would provide "an additional argument for the Acts" (CDA 364). Nevertheless, this additional argument would not "overbear the very strong arguments of other kinds against the operation of such Acts" (CDA 364).

One questioner at the hearing of the Royal Commission asked Mill to view the public health problem of sexually transmitted diseases as a "plague," albeit with a "moral element," and then to consider whether the legislature would be not be "justified in the interests of the innocent in endeavouring, so far as it can, to stamp it [the plague of venereal diseases] out, even if there is no hope of complete success" (CDA 356). In response, Mill indicated that "the degree of hope . . . of complete success" would very much affect his answer to this question. He even suggested that if, contrary to expert medical opinion, there were a high probability that the CDAs would totally eradicate sexually transmitted diseases, at least in the context he discussed, then they could conceivably be justified (CDA 356). However, in his judgment, there was no reasonable prospect of such an outcome.

> It seems to me there ought to be a very good prospect of complete extirpation to justify anything of that kind [i.e., the CDA], and I do not understand that such hope is entertained by those who are now most in favour of the Acts. (CDA 356)

Furthermore, any realistic scenario must also include the CDAs' probable negative effects. These negative effects include not only the probable increase in the incidence and prevalence of risky and immoral behavior and possible increase in sexually transmitted diseases—but also the violations of liberties and equality, along with the concomitant oppression and abuses of power. The oppression of women and the abuse of power are not "mere accidents" but rather are the "necessary consequences" of any serious attempt to implement the program completely, in order to "stamp out" as much as possible this "plague" (Letter 1513/1681; see CDA 355). This is especially true because the law, as previously noted, did not define "common prostitute," thus leaving enforcement up to the judgment the officers engaged in surveillance.

Assessment of Remedial and Punitive Interventions

Remedial Interventions

Earlier I indicated that Mill, in general, had more reservations about *preventive* governmental interventions, in public health and elsewhere, than about *punitive* and *remedial* interventions. He accepted the legitimacy of individual, social, and governmental efforts to provide remedial measures by treating individuals who suffer the consequences of their sexual and other conduct. For Mill, the key distinction is between providing security through "safeguards" beforehand and treating the consequences of actions later, and he contended that we may and should do the latter (CDA 358). Despite this distinction, he admitted that efforts to rescue individuals after their diseases have occurred could still be subject to the same charges he leveled against efforts to prevent harms by making risky actions safer (CDA 359). Nevertheless, individual benevolence and communal benevolence remain important. According to Mill,

> Apart from any metaphysical considerations respecting the foundation of morals or of the social union, it will be admitted to be right that human beings should help one another; and the more so, in proportion to the urgency of the need.[31]

This applies even when those urgent needs have resulted from an individual's risky conduct: indeed, "we should help one another very little" if we were "never to interfere with the evil consequences people have brought upon themselves, or are likely to have brought upon themselves" (CDA 358). Even though a remedial approach after the exposure and the harms have occurred can also lessen individuals' motivation to avoid risky and immoral conduct, still, Mill insisted, "a marked line can be drawn there":

> You may draw a line between *attacking evils when they occur*, in order to remedy them as far as we are able, and *making arrangements beforehand which will enable the objectionable practices to be carried on without incurring the danger of the evil*. (CDA 358, italics added)

Mill believed these can be distinguished conceptually and kept distinct in practice (CDA 359).

Even in the context of remedial actions, it is important not to single out certain diseases when there is no defensible reason for doing so and when doing so appears to give these diseases "special favor."

> the grand objection I have to it [providing Lock Hospitals for treatment of sexually transmitted diseases] is to any measure taken specially with reference to this class of diseases. The general impression it would make, however contrary to the intention of those who support it, would be that the State patronises the class of practices by which the diseases are engendered, since it considers those who contract "these" [transcriber error] diseases as worthy of more attention and takes more pains to remedy the consequences, than those who have other diseases equally serious. (CDA 370)

Mill's concerns about the symbolic, communicative significance of laws and policies are evident throughout. Sometimes he insisted that sexually transmitted diseases should not be singled out from other *serious diseases*, sometimes he maintained that they should not be singled out from other *contagious diseases*, including consumption (tuberculosis). Mill was not opposed to the state's efforts to reduce the overall amount of disease by establishing hospitals: "providing always it is not done with special favour to the class of diseases, but forms part of a general system, such a system as it may be thought advisable by the State to adopt, with a view of getting rid of serious and especially contagious diseases, as far as possible, throughout the community" (CDA 370). Whatever is done for sexually transmitted diseases should, at the very least, be done for all contagious diseases (CDA 358).

As I noted earlier, Mill recognized and emphasized both individual benevolence and social benevolence (CDA 366), including that expressed through the state, in addressing diseases in the community. One questioner at the hearing before the Royal Commission tried to paint Mill into a corner by asking whether he would "leave these women to rot and die under the hedges, rather than pass Acts such as these [the CDAs] to save them" (CDA 366). Mill indicated that he would do more for these women, but not more than he would for people with other serious, particularly contagious, diseases. What is provided for relief from some diseases should be provided "in common to all others who have an equal claim to it" (CDA 367). However, in doing more for these women and others with equal claims, Mill would not do what is done through the CDAs, because they "do a great deal of mischief in other ways" (CDA 367).

Not only individuals acting benevolently but also state policies could legitimately, that is, within their "proper function," undertake to enable "common prostitutes" and others to "understand that they are not considered as totally unworthy of any kind of regard or consideration by the rest of their fellow-creatures." In effect, there should be a concerted effort to reclaim them, to "do them as much good as their condition makes them susceptible of." What Mill objects to is "having special legislation for those women, which would have the effect of singling them out to a special cure, to which persons with other equally bad diseases are not subject." Laws should not "take special care" of either the soldiers and sailors or the prostitutes who provide their services. It is sufficient to offer them "the means of care provided they accept it" (CDA 366). The goal should be to protect the "innocent," that is, the spouses and children who do not consent to the risky conduct.

Questions arose about who should pay for the costs of either preventive or remedial efforts. In some European countries, similar laws—but often involving explicit licensing—were self-supporting because the prostitutes paid for the licenses (and, of course, passed the costs on to their customers). Such policies raise questions not only about justice and fairness in covering their costs but also about their symbolic significance. In a *preventive* context, Mill worried that having the prostitute pay for the services would be construed as even more of a "license" than the CDAs. Much of this is a matter of degree—all of the objections against the CDAs apply with greater force to a formal system of licensing prostitutes (CDA 356). And, he noted, "the expense could not be charged on the prostitutes themselves without in a manner licensing their profession" (CDA 357). Mill conceded that there was only a fine line between the CDAs and the formal licensing of prostitutes, and that in England, under the CDAs, some prostitutes presented their orders and certificates to customers. However, requiring the prostitutes to pay would move the policy even closer to formal licensing with all that it would symbolize.

In addition, there is a question of fairness and justice in the distribution of the costs. If the CDAs are "sanitary measures" for the whole community and have as their object the protection of the community, including innocent persons within the community, then, according to Mill, it is only fair and just for the taxpayers to pay (CDA 356). After all, the "health of the community . . . is within the province of Government," and if these measures are justifiable at all, it would not be "unjust to make a charge on the whole community" (CDA 357).

Punitive Interventions

Mill's very simple principle and maxims from *On Liberty* set certain constraints on punitive governmental interventions, including the criminalization of sexual activities. He was opposed to criminalization of voluntary sexual activities by persons in the "maturity of their faculties," whether fornication for pleasure or fornication for money. (As noted, prostitution was not illegal at the time in England.) However, Mill called for stronger laws, with more severe penalties, to protect girls and young women (at least up to seventeen or eighteen years of age) who might be lured into prostitution[32] (CDA 369). And in both *On Liberty* and in his testimony to the Royal Commission, Mill recognized the legitimacy of governmental regulations for public order—for example, by stopping solicitation in the streets (CDA 369).

For Mill, some other issues were on the border between respect for personal liberty and the harm-to-others principle. While *On Liberty* emphasized that fornication "must be tolerated," Mill held that the question whether a person should "be free to be a pimp," and solicit prostitutes, fell "on the exact boundary between two principles," thus supporting arguments for both toleration and prohibition (OL 91–92). In his testimony to the Royal Commission, Mill similarly indicated that, in light of all the pros and cons, he found it "very difficult to make up [his] mind" about whether brothels should be banned but, in any event, did not think it was "material" to the question of the justifiability of the CDAs (CDA 369; 359–360).

Mill supported disciplinary and penal policies that targeted soldiers and sailors. He called for the exercise of military discipline, which could help deter undesirable conduct and prevent the spread of venereal diseases. In response to a question by a commissioner about whether Mill thought that "the State had better rather continue to suffer from the evil than to pass such Acts as these for its prevention," Mill stressed: "I think the State had better continue to suffer as much of that evil as it cannot prevent in other ways, by the application of military discipline and the correction of these practices among the soldiers," including through the imposition of penalties following the detection of venereal diseases through their own medical examinations, which some commissioners emphasized were more regular and valuable than Mill had supposed (CDA 360).

Other possible laws could also be effective deterrents, including making the communication of a sexually transmitted disease a penal offense, at least where the victim did not knowingly and voluntarily consent to the risk, in contrast, for example, to seeking the services of a prostitute. These laws could include "very severe damages in case a man is proved to have communicated this disease to a modest woman" (CDA 354).

> If it was proved that a man had been the means of communicating to his wife, she being a modest woman, or to his children, any of these diseases, the law should grant the woman a divorce, and compel the man in proportion to his means to pay very heavy damages to them for their support apart from himself. (CDA 355)

Mill conceded that it would be difficult to enforce such a law and that it would probably not be enforced in the majority of cases. Nevertheless, he believed that the possibility of its enforcement "would operate as a considerable check on the evil." Here again he appealed to the symbolic, communicative significance of the law, in this case a law that declares the transmission of sexually transmitted diseases "a very great crime," which subjects the transmitter to "heavy penalties" and which is deemed "so serious" as to warrant the dissolution of the marriage as "a matter of right." Legally branding the immoral and risky conduct in this way "would have very great influence," by marking this crime, "as in truth it is, one of the gravest a man could possibly commit" (CDA 355).

Conclusions

Insofar as scholars and policy-makers have focused only on Mill's principle of liberty, antipaternalism, and the harm-to-others principle, drawn mainly from *On Liberty*, they have not adequately unpacked his thought, and potential legacy, for public health ethics, that is, for the ethical analysis and assessment of public policies directed at the public's health. These key themes, so prominent in *On Liberty*, remain important, and yet their application to contemporary public health issues remains somewhat uncertain in part because of serious challenges to the sharp lines Mill drew between voluntary and nonvoluntary and between self-regarding and other-regarding conduct. Furthermore, through a close examination of Mill's but extensive and impassioned, but relatively neglected, critique of the CDAs of his day, we see that he actually invoked a much wider range of additional ethical considerations that are relevant to public health ethics. In his vigorous and uncompromising opposition to the CDAs, Mill's arguments deployed the full array of other ethical considerations identified above, moving well beyond—but not necessarily contradicting—the framework of *On Liberty*. From the standpoint of public health ethics, perhaps most surprising and troubling is how Mill's moralism shaped and limited his responses, particularly in the context of a potentially effective harm-reduction strategy that sought to limit the harm involved in certain activities without supposing that those activities could be completely stopped.

Notes

1. Some references will appear in parentheses in the text. OL = John Stuart Mill, *On Liberty*, ed. David Spitz (New York: W.W. Norton & Company, Inc., 1975).

    CDA = *The Evidence of John Stuart Mill, Taken before the Royal Commission of 1870 on the Administration and Operation of the Contagious Diseases Acts of 1866 and 1869*, in *The Collected Works of John Stuart Mill*, Vol. 21: *Essays on Equality, Law, and Education*, ed. John M. Robson (Toronto: University of Toronto Press; London: Routledge and Kegan Paul, 1984), pp. 349–371. Also available online at http://oll.libertyfund.org/titles/mill-the-collected-works-of-john-stuart-mill-volume-xxi-essays-on-equality-law-and-education.

    Letters = references to Mill's letters will appear by letter #, followed by the page number *The Collected Works of John Stuart Mill*, Vol. 17: *The Later Letters of John Stuart Mill 1849–1873, Part IV*, ed. Francis E. Minkea and Dwight N. Lindley (Toronto: University of Toronto Press; London: Routledge and Kegan Paul, 1972). Also available online at http://oll.libertyfund.org/titles/mill-the-collected-works-of-john-stuart-mill-volume-xvii-the-later-letters-1849-1873-part-iv.

2. Mill, *The Principles of Political Economy*, Bk 5, Chap. 11, #2; in *The Collected Works of John Stuart Mill*, Vol. 3: *The Principles of Political Economy with Some of Their Applications to Social Philosophy* (Books 3–5 and Appendices), ed. John M. Robson (Toronto: University of Toronto Press; London: Routledge and Kegan Paul, 1965). Also available on line at http://oll.libertyfund.org/titles/mill-the-collected-works-of-john-stuart-mill-volume-iii-principles-of-political-economy-part-ii

3. Joel Feinberg used the terms "harm principle" and "harm-to-others principle" in his classic essay, "Legal Paternalism," *Canadian Journal of Philosophy* I, No. 1 (September 1971): 117. I will often use the latter to emphasize the other-directedness of Mill's principle; it did not include self-harm.

4. Mill, *The Principles of Political Economy*, Bk 5, Chap. 11, #1.

5. Ibid., #2.

6. Ibid, #7.
7. Ibid.
8. Ibid, #2.
9. Feinberg, "Legal Paternalism," p. 124.
10. See Ronald Dworkin, *Taking Rights Seriously* (Cambridge, MA: Harvard University Press, 1978), pp. 262–263.
11. Mill, *The Principles of Political Economy*, Bk 5, Chap. 11.
12. See Cass R. Sunstein and Richard H. Thaler, "Libertarian Paternalism Is Not an Oxymoron," *University of Chicago Law Review* 70 (Fall 2003): 1159–1202, and Richard H. Thaler and Cass R. Sunstein, "Libertarian Paternalism," *American Economics Review* 93 (2003): 175–179.
13. Feinberg, "Legal Paternalism," pp. 111–112.
14. See Mill, "Whewell on Moral Philosophy" (1852), in *The Collected Works of John Stuart Mill*, Vol. 10: *Essays on Ethics, Religion and Society*, ed. J. M. Robson (Toronto: University of Toronto Press, 1969; Indianapolis, IN: Liberty Fund, Inc., Paperback reprint, 2006), pp. 197–198. Also available at http://oll.libertyfund.org/titles/mill-the-collected-works-of-john-stuart-mill-volume-x-essays-on-ethics-religion-and-society.
15. Ibid.
16. See Mill, *Utilitarianism* (1861), *The Collected Works of John Stuart Mill*, Vol. 10: *Essays on Ethics, Religion and Society*, p. 257. Also available at http://oll.libertyfund.org/titles/mill-the-collected-works-of-john-stuart-mill-volume-x-essays-on-ethics-religion-and-society
17. John Stuart Mill, *Collected Works of John Stuart Mill*, Vol. 28: *Public and Parliamentary Speeches, November 1850–November 1869*, ed. John M. Robson and Bruce Kinzer (Toronto: University of Toronto Press, London: Routledge, 1988), pp. 501, 504.
18. Judith R. Walkowitz, *Prostitution and Victorian Society: Women, Class, and the State* (Cambridge, UK: Cambridge University Press, 1980), p. 49.
19. Ibid.
20. Ibid., p. 50.
21. See Paul McHugh, *Prostitution and Victorian Social Reform* (London: Croom Helm, 1980), pp. 16, 18. Military regulations at the time permitted only 6% of enlisted men to be married.
22. See Walkowitz, *Prostitution and Victorian Society*, p. 2.
23. See Jeremy Waldron, "Mill on Liberty and on the Contagious Diseases Acts," in *J.S. Mill's Political Thought: A Bicentennial Reassessment*, ed. Nadia Urbinati and Alex Zaharas (Cambridge, UK: Cambridge University Press, 2007), pp. 11–42. This is a very important article, particularly in regard to Mill's views on general principles of legislation in the context of the CDAs. My approach, by contrast, attends primarily to the ethical principles and values that Mill invokes, beyond those emphasized in *On Liberty*, to address a complex public health policy.
24. Mill's lack of accurate and complete information on all of the specifics of the legislation's implementation did not affect his overall argument.

25. The Royal Commission's report drew a sharp distinction between soldiers and sailors on the one hand and common prostitutes on the other: "With the one sex the offence is committed as a matter of gain; with the other it is an irregular indulgence of a natural impulse." (Quoted in Waldron, "Mill on Liberty and on the Contagious Diseases Acts," p. 14 fn 23.) This differentiation according to motivation would have made no difference for Mill in this context.

26. Mill stated, "that which is compulsory seems to me always more degrading in its effects on the character than what is done voluntarily." See CDA 368.

27. This does not indicate the full range of harm reduction policies. For reviews of such policies, see *Harm Reduction: Evidence, Impacts and Challenges* (Lisbon: European Monitoring Centre for Drugs and Drug Addiction, April 2010); Susan E. Collins, Seema L. Clifasefi, Diane E. Logan, et al., "Current Status, Historical Highlights, and Basic Principles of Harm Reduction," as well as other chapters, in *Harm Reduction: Pragmatic Strategies for Managing High-Risk Behaviors*, 2nd ed., ed. G. Alan Mariatt, Mary E. Larimer, and Katie Witkiewitz (New York: Guilford Press, 2012); Diane Riley, Richard Pates, Geoffrey Monaghan, and Patrick O'Hare, "A Brief History of Harm Reduction," as well as other chapters, in *Harm Reduction in Substance Use and High-Risk Behaviour: International Policy and Practice*, ed. Richard Pates and Diane Riley (Chichester, Eng.: Blackwell Publishing Ltd, 2012); Barbara Krasner, ed., *Harm Reduction: Public Health Strategies*, Opposing Viewpoints Series (New York: Greenhaven Publishing, 2019).

28. See Allard E. Dembe and Leslie I. Boden, "Moral Hazard: A Question of Morality?" *New Solutions: A Journal of Environmental and Occupational Health Policy* 10, No. 3 (2000): 257–279. According to Dembe and Boden, several early mathematical discussions, as far back as the early eighteenth century, viewed "moral" as equivalent to "subjective" or psychological, rather than a matter of morality.

29. Mill's praise for "experiments in living" in *On Liberty* should not obscure the fact that he accepted much of conventional morality, whether or not he always provided a utilitarian defense for it. He comfortably used the language of "vice" in the hearing before the Royal Commission.

30. At times, Mill states this for the general population; at times, he focuses on the ignorant, etc.

31. Mill, *The Principles of Political Economy*, Book 5, Chapter 11, #13.

32. Mill was willing to consider raising this age. See CDA.

Index

For the benefit of digital users, indexed terms that span two pages (e.g., 52–53) may, on occasion, appear on only one of those pages.

in formulating criteria for triage in
public health crisis, 283–86
See also engagement
paternalism
active versus passive, 40
definition of, 39
in Donald/Dax Cowart case, 61–66
justificatory conditions for
pure, active, strong
paternalism, 42–43, 50
libertarian paternalism (Thaler and
Sunstein), 47, 296
neopaternalism/new paternalism,
6, 38, 46
pure versus mixed (third-party
effects), 44–46
soft versus hard, 46–50
weak versus strong, 40–44, 51n10
See also antipaternalism; John Stuart
Mill; *On Liberty*
Perry, Michael, 112, 114
Peters, Thomas, 190
*Playing God? Human Genetic Engineering
and the Rationalization of Public
Bioethical Debate* (John H. Evans), 7,
87–98, 103
pluralistic society. *See* liberal pluralistic
democracy
Poe, Edgar Allan, 155–57
Presidential Commission for the Study of
Bioethical Issues, 121
President's Commission for the Study
of Ethical Issues in Medicine and
Biomedical and Behavioral
Research, 164. See also *Splicing Life*
President's Council on Bioethics (PCB),
15n13, 97, 119–120, 161
Human Cloning and Human Dignity,
report of, 119
principles, prima facie, 21, 29, 40, 42,
55–56, 58–59, 63, 91, 108, 204,
236, 237, 240, 243, 275
See also moral norms
Principles of Biomedical Ethics (Tom
L. Beauchamp and James
F. Childress), vii, 5, 29, 86–97, 89, 91,
95, 184
principlism, 58–59, 85, 87–88, 90

viewed as professional bioethics' mode
of argumentation, 90–92
Prottas, Jeffrey, 189, 214
public, meanings of, 234–35
public bioethics
activity of, 1–2
contribution of academic bioethicists to, 4
definition of, 1–2
structures of, 2–5
public engagement. *See* engagement
public health
definition of, 232–34
expressing versus imposing community
for immunization programs, 267
general moral considerations in, 235–39
goals of, 255–57
human rights in, 247–49
meanings of public in public health, 234–35
public accountability in, 243–45
public health interventions
distinguished from paternalistic
interventions, 245–47
reasoning about means (absolutist,
contextualist, and presumptivist
approaches), 253–55
resolving conflicts among general moral
considerations in, 239–41
scope of (J. S. Mill's view), 297–300
screening in, 241–43
social justice in, 247–49
specifying and weighting general moral
considerations in, 238–39
public policy
conscientious exemptions from, 141–46
emotion and imagination in
forming, 104–07
meaning of, 1
religious voices in, chaps. 4 and 5
symbolic significance of (Mill's
interpretation), 301, 306–08, 311–14
thick and thin debates regarding, 86–87,
91, 93, 95–97, 108
See also public reason/reasoning
public reason/reasoning, 104
emotion in, 104–07
imagination in, 104–07
presumptivist, contextualist, absolutist
approaches to, 253–55